Sharing
Innovation

Edited by Neil G. Kotler

Sharing Innovation

Global Perspectives

on Food, Agriculture,

and Rural Development

Papers and Proceedings

of a Colloquium

Organized by the

Smithsonian Institution

Smithsonian Institution Press
Washington and London

Volumes in this series are based on annual colloquia organized at the Smithsonian Institution, in cooperation with the Kraft General Foods Foundation and the Winrock International Institute for Agricultural Research.

Previously published:

Science, Ethics, and Food, edited by Brian W. J. LeMay (Washington, D.C.: Smithsonian Institution Press, 1988).

Completing the Food Chain, edited by Paula M. Hirschoff and Neil G. Kotler (Washington, D.C.: Smithsonian Institution Press, 1989).

Library of Congress Cataloging-in-Publication Data

Sharing innovation : global perspectives on food, agriculture, and rural development / Neil G. Kotler, editor.
p. cm.
"Papers and proceedings of a colloquium organized by the Smithsonian Institution."
ISBN 0-87474-874-7 (Smithsonian)
ISBN 971-104-221-5 (IRRI)
1. Nutrition policy — Congresses.
2. Agricultural productivity — Congresses.
3. Rural development — Congresses.
I. Kotler, Neil G., 1941- .
II. Smithsonian Institution.
TX359.S48 1990
363.8 — dc20   90-53151

Contents

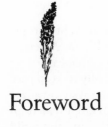

Foreword

Robert McC. Adams
Secretary, Smithsonian Institution

The challenge of world agriculture, in meeting a surging demand for food, is, according to the World Commission on Environment and Development, "colossal both in...magnitude and complexity."

Our Common Future, the Commission's report to the United Nations, stated: "Thus to achieve global food security, the resource base for food production must be sustained, enhanced, and where it has been diminished or destroyed, restored.... [New] realities require agricultural systems that focus as much attention on people as they do on technology, as much on resources as on production, as much on the long term as on the short term."

An additional one billion human beings will inhabit the earth by the end of this century. In 2025, according to UN projections, the world population could reach more than 8 billion people. Population growth, coupled with rising income in developing countries, will generate an enormous demand for food, most notably in the nations of Asia, Africa, and Latin America. Yet, despite the remarkable growth in food production in the past three decades, an estimated 750 million people today lack the food and healthful diets necessary to lead fully productive lives.

The breakthrough in agricultural productivity generated by "Green Revolution" technologies, particularly in Asia, will be extended in future years to other regions of the world. Yet production systems that fail to preserve the ecological integrity of land, forests, and water resources and ensure the sustainability of agricultural systems over generations no longer constitute viable solutions.

Virtually every region of the world is experiencing the processes of depletion and loss of arable land, the reversal of which is a paramount consideration: soil erosion in North America, soil acidification in Europe, and deforestation and desertification in Asia, Africa, and Latin America. The task of world agriculture, then, is complex, though measurable: to increase global food production by 3 to 4 percent annually to keep pace with rising demand; safeguard the resource base of farming systems; adapt technologies to resource-poor regions; raise income and employment in rural communities, in which much of the growth will occur; and build effective and equitable food distribution systems, which presupposes a further shift of productive capacity to food-deficit nations.

Policies and programs underway in the nations of Asia, Africa, and Latin America to a large extent will determine the quantity, quality, and availability of the global food supply. Vital to the outcome is the need to strengthen agricultural science and research, rural education, and extension services and to advance the cooperative enterprise of farmers, researchers, and policy makers.

The colloquium, "Sharing Innovation: Global Perspectives on Food, Agriculture, and Rural Development," will examine agricultural strategies and food policies in Asia, Africa, and Latin America; the central role of knowledge and technology transfer within and among nations; and successful innovations and national solutions that hold the promise of advancing food development throughout the world. The Smithsonian Institution is honored to sponsor this international exchange among distinguished leaders as part of a series of forums on food and agricultural development held in conjunction with the awarding of the World Food Prize.

Acknowledgments

This volume represents the papers and proceedings of an international colloquium on food and agriculture convened at the Smithsonian Institution in Washington, D.C., on October 17-18, 1989.

The colloquium and published volume form the third in a series examining developments in food and agriculture and the responses of the nations of the world in alleviating hunger and malnutrition. The first colloquium, convened on October 6-7, 1987, produced a volume entitled *Science, Ethics, and Food* (Smithsonian Institution Press, 1988). The second colloquium, held on October 4-5, 1988, resulted in a volume entitled *Completing the Food Chain: Strategies for Combating Hunger and Malnutrition* (Smithsonian Institution Press, 1989).

Each colloquium was organized in conjunction with the awarding of the World Food Prize, sponsored by the Kraft General Foods Foundation. The prize is the most significant international award given to an individual anywhere in the world whose work in the judgment of the selection committee has substantially improved and expanded the quantity, quality, or availability of food in the world. The prize laureate in 1987 was M. S. Swaminathan, the architect of India's "Green Revolution," and then director of the International Rice Research Institute (IRRI) in the Philippines. The 1988 prize laureate was Robert F. Chandler, Jr., founding director of IRRI and a former director of the Asian Vegetable Research and Development Center in Taiwan, whose leadership led to Asia's "Green Revolution."

The prize laureate in 1989 was Verghese Kurien, chairman of the National Dairy Development Board in Anand, India, who spearheaded India's unique dairy development program known as "Operation Flood," a cooperative-based organization of more than 60,000 milk producers marketing dairy products to an estimated 170 million consumers. Dr. Kurien was honored at the Smithsonian Institution in evening ceremonies on October 17 following the colloquium program.

The awarding of the World Food Prize, the convening of the colloquium series, and publication of the colloquium volumes share a common purpose: to expand knowledge of the applications of agricultural science, research, and technology in feeding the world's population; to bring scientists, scholars, and policy leaders together from the nations of the world to exchange ideas and perspectives and to advance solutions to the world's food problems; and to honor leaders in agriculture, food policy, and nutrition, in the universities, in industry, and in government, who have devoted their careers to the goal of generating an ample supply of wholesome food in the world.

The 1989 colloquium, "Sharing Innovation: Global Perspectives on Food, Agriculture, and Rural Development," examined agricultural development strategies, food policies, research management, and technological innovations in the nations of Asia, Africa, and Latin America. The morning session highlighted broad-gauged issues and developments: rural institutional development and technology transfer in Nigeria; the emergence of agricultural markets and technological growth in the People's Republic of China; and the role of water resource management, specifically rainfed agriculture, in India's agricultural development. The afternoon session examined national innovations and solutions: rice research and production in Indonesia; the growth of fruit and vegetable production and exports in Chile; and the development of a successful community-based food, nutrition, and infant feeding and public health program in the Republic of Tanzania.

On the morning following the colloquium, the participants, together with the 1988 and 1989 World Food Prize laureates, and other scholars and policy specialists, gathered at the International Food Policy Research Institute (IFPRI) in Washington, D.C., to probe the implications and opportunities for future research presented in the colloquium papers and discussion the previous day. An edited version of the transcript of that two-hour discussion, which was chaired by John W. Mellor, IFPRI director, is included in this volume.

The publication is enriched by Dr. Kurien's World Food Prize address, delivered on the evening of October 17 before an audience of more than 700 people who gathered to honor him in Baird Auditorium of the Smithsonian's National Museum of Natural History. The volume also is enriched by Robert F. Chandler, Jr.'s, lecture on world agriculture, population growth, and the environment, first delivered at Cornell University on September 20, 1989, which provides a comprehensive overview of future directions in food and agriculture development.

The colloquium and the publication owe a considerable debt to the sixteen distinguished individuals who agreed to participate in the program, many of whom traveled considerable distances and experienced the difficulty of long hours of travel compressed in an all-too-brief visit in Washington, D.C. Their expert knowledge and willingness to share and exchange their experiences and insights with one another and with the public contributed enormously to the success of the events. One of the speakers invited to the colloquium, Dr. Justin Yifu Lin, Deputy Director of the Development Institute in Beijing, China, was unable at the last moment to travel to the United States. The paper he prepared for the colloquium was presented, at his request, by his colleague, Zhigang Chen, an agricultural economist at the Université Laval in Quebec, Canada.

The colloquium program was organized at the Smithsonian Institution by Neil G. Kotler of the Office of Interdisciplinary Studies and by Cheryl B. LaBerge and Karen Harmon of the Office of Conference Services. The colloquium benefited from the supportive oversight of Robert S. Hoffmann, assistant secretary for research, and Wilton S. Dillon, chairman of the Office of Interdisciplinary Studies, the Smithsonian Institution.

The colloquium conveners and the editor of this volume wish to acknowledge several individuals who helped to shape and implement a remarkable set of events: John W. Mellor, IFPRI director, who generously contributed his time and resources; Edward S. Williams, administrator of the World Food Prize at the Winrock International Institute for Agricultural Development in Morrilton, Arkansas, who assisted so ably in coordinating the colloquium and World Food Prize ceremonies; A. S. Clausi, chairman of the Council of Advisors of the World Food Prize, who painstakingly organized support for the events and committed generous support to the colloquium program; and Norman E. Borlaug, who conceived of the World Food Prize as a fitting honor to agriculture, himself a recipient of the Nobel Peace Prize in 1970 for his achievements in plant genetics research that resulted in "Green Revolution" technologies.

Invaluable assistance also was provided by: Robert Bordonaro, Laurie Goldberg, and Edith Yalong of IFPRI who helped to organize the IFPRI roundtable; Anita Timrot for the fine transcription of portions of the colloquium proceedings; Elaine Sullivan and Robin Cormier of Editorial Experts, Inc., in Alexandria, Virginia, who supervised the production of the manuscript for publication; and Carla M. Borden of the Office of Interdisciplinary Studies who offered helpful assistance as a copyeditor of the manuscript.

The publication of this volume, as well as the publication of the 1987 and 1988 colloquium volumes, benefited enormously from collaboration with the International Rice Research Institute (IRRI) in Los Baños, Philippines, that serves as copublisher of the volume. Thomas R. Hargrove, IRRI's head of communications and publications, worked ably with the Smithsonian

Institution Press in making this volume available to readers throughout the world.

Acknowledgments would not be complete without expressing appreciation to the Kraft General Foods Foundation for sponsoring the colloquium program, and to the Elanco Products Company and Eli Lilly and Company for their generous support of the editorial and publication work entailed in the production of this volume.

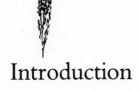

Introduction

Robert W. Herdt
Director, Agricultural Sciences
The Rockefeller Foundation, New York, New York

All developing countries face the challenge of providing adequate employ-ment and food entitlements to the present populations, slowing the rate of population growth to a steady-state level, and producing an annual increase in food output of about 4 percent using farming systems that can be sustained over the long run. While it is not necessary, and indeed would be extremely costly, for all nations to be self-sufficient in all foods, most governments desire that a large fraction of their food be produced domes-tically to assure a certain level of food security. In addition, the economic base of most developing countries is agriculture—it employs 60 to 80 percent of the work force and generates 25 to 50 percent of national income—and in most countries agriculture is an important national concern.

Thus, agricultural growth is a natural focus for participants in the Smithsonian Institution colloquium, organized in association with the awarding of the World Food Prize. The address of the 1989 laureate, Dr. Verghese Kurien, as well as many of the other papers in this collection, highlight the interdependence of technology, policy, and institutions in achieving adequate rates of food production growth. It is the interaction of these three factors that determines the pace of food production growth, along with, of course, its consumption and the rate of growth of food demand, which responds to all three.

The papers of Ojetunji Aboyade, Justin Yifu Lin, and Anthony Wylie emphasize institutions, the procedures by which they operate, and the methods they use to link producers and consumers. Lin traces the extraor-dinary rate of development of China's agriculture since 1947. In his view, the commune-collective system imposed a drag on agricultural output that was overcome with the shift in 1978 to the household responsibility system. Lin argues that the absence of growth in foodgrain production since 1985 is not an indication of lack of success, but rather that one ought to look at the growth of total agricultural output, which substantially exceeded that of foodgrain. Judged on the basis of that performance, the institutions in place between 1985 and 1989 would be considered part of a successful system.

Anthony Wylie discusses another success case that can be traced in part to a new set of institutions and to changes in economic policy that opened the Chilean economy to international trade. The Fundación Chile, established to transfer proven technologies to Chile, with initial focus on agribusiness, forestry, and marine resources, is one such important institution. The contributions of fruit production technology transferred directly from corresponding latitudes in the United States are part of the story, but the ability of a key organization to borrow and operate that technology is equally important.

Aboyade stresses the role of organization in the case study of Awe, Nigeria, whose success he attributes to a "bottom-up" approach and to the ability to provide credit for small producers. He contrasts this with the failure of many "top-down" organizations typified by the World Bank's agricultural development projects. Aboyade prescribes a policy of "selective closure" of African economies to protect farmers from international competition. Michael Lipton, a colloquium discussant, argues with this policy prescription, emphasizing the need to exploit the comparative agricultural advantages of different regions and to invest in new technology, fertilizer production, and expanded irrigation in Africa.

S. W. Sadikin, Bruce Stone, and R. P. Singh all stress the role of technology. The remarkable success of Indonesia in raising its rice production from a level of 10 million tons in 1965 to 15 million tons in 1975, and to nearly 30 million tons by 1988, moving that country from a position of being the world's largest importer of rice to a self-sufficient position, is recounted by Sadikin. Technology acquired from the International Rice Research Institute (IRRI) was important, but institutions to adapt that technology and deliver it to farmers, as well as policies to stabilize prices to farmers, also were important.

Stone's account of the contribution of agricultural technology in China gives insight into how rice varietal development, fertilizer production, and irrigation worked together to increase grain output in that country. In contrast to Lin, Stone believes that progress will continue even if China returns to more of a command economy, but both agree that it will be relatively challenging for China to increase its food output at the necessary rate over the next several decades.

Singh explores the potentials of rainfed agricultural systems in India. Arguing that over half the land and farmers will continue to produce without irrigation well into the twenty-first century, Singh is optimistic that improved rainfed agricultural and water response management technologies already available or still to be discovered can raise production and income to meet the needs of these farmers and of the population.

A counterpart to the emphasis on food production was provided by Calister N. Mtalo's exploration of the origin and evolution of a unique nutrition, child feeding, and public health program in the Republic of Tanzania, the Iringa Integrated Nutrition Program. A leading program of its kind in Africa, affecting behavioral changes in a population that until recently suffered greatly from hunger, malnutrition, and infant mortality, the paper describes yet another critical factor in the equation of agricultural development in the world — namely, the search for new ways to make food, healthful diets, and the knowledge of sound public health practices accessible to all peoples.

Dr. Kurien's inspirational remarks, delivered on the occasion of his acceptance of the 1989 World Food Prize, are wide ranging, touching on food aid, international trade, milk production, marketing, farmer psychology, and his encounters with prime ministers. His views on some of these topics are bound to raise eyebrows and perhaps even the ire of some readers, but it is difficult to argue with the success of the institutions he has helped create.

Each of the papers includes examples of sharing agricultural innovations. Some are more explicit than others; some are innovations in technology, others in organizations, and still others in policy, for there is truly "nothing new under the sun." A notable sharing occurred from the very beginning of the discussion, in the interpersonal exchange and innovation that took place when the authors, discussants, and audience met for the colloquium.

CHAPTER 1

Perspectives on African Food Policy and Agricultural Development in the 1990s: A Nigerian Perspective

Ojetunji Aboyade
Chairman, Presidential Advisory Committee, Lagos, Nigeria

The Micro Viewpoint

Awe, in the Oyo State of Nigeria, is a fairly representative African local community based substantially on a food and agricultural economy. In all, it occupies about 422 square kilometers of a typical tropical subhumid climatic region with marked wet and dry seasons and lies in the derived savannah belt at an average 300 meters above sea level. The pivotal settlement is a small town with a population of about 25,000, which serves as a center for an additional 5,000 or so people residing in some 200 adjoining villages, hamlets, and farmsteads. Farmers are engaged in the production of annual crops such as maize, cowpeas, yam, cassava, and vegetables. There are also some tree crops and citrus.

The importance of the Awe community to our subject matter lies in the sustained experiment of autonomous integrated rural development that it embarked upon in 1983. Differing from the World Bank's sponsored agricultural development programs (ADPs), the Awe experiment is basically an organizational model of indigenous development with interesting physical, economic, social, and managerial linkages. Lessons from the community's experiment can provide a small window from which to view the larger problems and prospects of African food policy and agricultural development over the next decade.

First, the ultimate testing ground of the efficacy of any policy or development program in food and agriculture is what happens at the community level. Costs can be incurred anywhere, but direct benefits are more location specific in terms of their impact on village-level production

1

and productivity. Microeconomic considerations and household behavior in the rural economy provide both the starting and finishing points of any policy analysis of African food and agriculture, the latter strongly characterized by smallholder family proprietorships. The Awe experiment has clearly brought out the necessity for sharply concentrating on local communities in order to gain an understanding of the precise constraints which African farming families face and for monitoring the policy measures for addressing those constraints.

Second, if any additional evidence were needed on the integrated nature of African farming systems and their delicate ecological balance, the Awe experiment is providing strong empirical support. Integration does not simply consist of the known mixed field cropping practices, but more importantly of the interactions between tree crops, food crops, fibers, animal products, off-farm activities, agro-processing, and income-producing activities including handicrafts. Moreover, there have been noteworthy demographic shifts taking place in the rural economy, a noticeable reverse flow back from the major cities into smaller towns since the mid-1980s, as the internal terms of trade have become favorable, rural transportation has improved, and peri-urban farming has expanded as a secondary occupation or as a supplement to nonfarming incomes. The character of internal food trade has changed as well, as more value is added within the local community through postharvest processing.

Third is the dynamics of traditional social interactions and institutional arrangements. Whatever organizational structures are designed and introduced by outside modernizing agents, African local communities have a way of adjusting to their own rhythm and style of achieving the same broad objectives. Organizationally, the Awe experiment was conceived as a four-stage hierarchical structure beginning with settlement units at the bottom, and then grouping these into primary production units, development areas, and a growth center at the apex. As it turned out, however, the farmers largely ignored the first two stages, participated actively at the level of the nine development areas, and added at the top their own farmers' union with the capability of securing farming inputs, tractor hire, and rural credit. As for the growth center at the top of the structure, this has been evolving via a different route under the impetus of a new state government-sponsored Rural Community Development Centre that is being established in the localities, as well as from diverse activities of the federal Directorate of Food, Roads, and Rural Infrastructures.

Fourth, the mobilization of rural credit has provided the strongest engine that drives the Awe experiment, far out of proportion to the designers' initial recognition of its importance. A branch of a major commercial bank was established in the town soon after the experiment started. The nine development areas which were set up, as well as the farmers' own union, have provided the actual viable organizational vehicles for both the

2

bank and the community's Development Corporation, mobilizing and supervising the community's rural credit program. Perhaps more than anything else, successful operation of the credit system furnishes not only the institutional anchor, but also serves as the entry point for on-farm trials of new technological packages, more orderly marketing, linkage with the nearby feedmeal processing industry, and as a veritable lobby for the resurgence of local democratic governance.

Fifth, the apparent controversy over the relative advantages of a price-incentive versus a technological-leverage approach to smallholder agricultural development would appear to be a futile one, at least in the African context. The mainstream of food policy researchers seems to hold to the view that policy makers do not really need rising food prices in order to provide farming incentives; rather, the true way forward lies in technological changes which can reduce costs, as embodied, for example, in new high-yielding crop varieties. The Awe experiment demonstrates, however, under prevailing traditional farming systems—which incidentally have been confirmed to be economically efficient—new technological packages often are not, in fact, available. Furthermore, the time lags involved in their diffusion and adoption are often so long that the supply shortages in the food equation would remain unbridged and create further distortions in the national economy under the prevailing conditions of diminished import capacity.

As the internal terms of trade have turned more favorable for domestic food and agricultural production, the Awe farmers suitably responded over the past four years by bringing both more labor and more land into the production process. Some of the additional labor is provided by the reverse urban migration flow, some by intensified incorporation of women and children in both on-farm and off-farm activities, and some by the farmers themselves through a greater number of on-farm work days. All these have been evident in the expanded local production of maize and cassava, for example.

Finally, while waiting for more research-intensive technological packages, the Awe farming households have been improving their household incomes through product diversification within their existing range of technological knowledge. As organizational units, farming families (not just the main farmers) in the Awe community have extended their activities to producing soybeans, citrus, aquaculture, snails, and vegetables, in addition to the normal staples of coarse grains and tubers. Interest also has been revived in palm produce, fibers, and marginally in cocoa.

When asked to look forward over the next decade and indicate their probable greatest needs for still greater output, the farmers have been almost unanimous in pinpointing tractor hire service and irrigation water from small earth dams, in addition to their continued access to rural credit. Perhaps because they are already being fairly well served with improved

3

rural roads, on-farm storage, and rural markets, these did not rank as high in their identification of production constraints. This should, therefore, remind us of the analytical danger of generalizing from particular case studies in spite of the inevitably sharper focus that they provide and their imperative as an ultimate policy starting point.

Sectoral Issues

The question might then be asked: why has the Nigerian food and agricultural economy performed so poorly in recent decades if the Awe experiment offers so much promise? Lack of representativeness and the invalidity of generalizing from particular cases are tempting explanations. In fact, however, in terms of the Nigerian context there is no gap or asymmetry in development. The critical explanatory factor is timing. The gradual turn-around in the Awe experiment has occurred only since 1985, largely mirroring the changing fortunes of the Nigerian food and agricultural economy in the second half of the 1980s. Actually, our interest in community-level case studies may be providing a useful signpost in resolving the apparent dilemma in cross-country African comparative studies about the sources of growth in the food and agricultural sector.

The seminal work, *Managing Agricultural Development in Africa*, recently completed under sponsorship of the World Bank, covered six African countries (Cameroon, Kenya, Malawi, Tanzania, Nigeria, and Senegal) from about the early 1960s to the mid-1980s. Although it was able to identify and compare the better-performance countries (Kenya, Malawi, and Cameroon) with the poor-performance countries (Tanzania, Nigeria, and Senegal), the study concluded by affirming the imperfect understanding of the real sources and causes of growth in African agriculture. For this reason, micro-focused, community level case studies of the Awe variety can, indeed, provide greater understanding of the various sources and causes of recent growth, as well as indicate the policy way forward for the 1990s.

The importance of the macroeconomic policy environment has to be emphasized, nevertheless. Inappropriate foreign trade and exchange-rate regimes, lopsided internal terms of trade, undisciplined monetary-fiscal measures, and unproductive national investment patterns only lead to a distorted food and agricultural economy and compromise its future performance.

Exploiting comparative cost advantages and initial conditions and moving only gradually to product diversification and new production processes are other important considerations. As the World Bank studies suggest, a large share of the production increases in the near future is likely to come from the expansion of cultivated land and from shifts to higher-value crops rather than from greater crop yields per se, given the present prevailing mixed-cropping farming systems. Furthermore, dramatic increases in land intensity in response to greater population density are likely to be constrained by environmental considerations (e.g., soil fragility), by factors proportion (e.g., favorable land-labor ratio), and by low-level water management (e.g., involving rainfed farming).

Given the long lead time necessary for technical progress (including institutional, political, and human capital considerations) to permeate African agriculture, imaginative programs are called for in production organization and policy management. Compared to the underdeveloped regions of Asia and Latin America, African agriculture is characterized by a combination of a gentle-sloping production function, high equitability in land distribution, a low income-employment multiplier effect of next-available technologies, an inherent tendency for the marginal productivity of labor in the nonagricultural sectors to rise above the average rural income, and a historically high incidence of labor loss to nonagricultural activities. There is, in addition, a serious lack of congruency between the food items produced and the food items consumed. Finally, there is also a growing gap between international food aid and national food import capacities.

A major conclusion of the World Bank studies is that it is difficult, indeed, to find much connection between the effects of external donor assistance, on the one hand, and the growth that has occurred in African agriculture, on the other. This leads to an important point: namely, the search for models of production organization and structures of household food consumption that are not tuned to the preferences and predilections of external institutions. On the domestic front in Nigeria, this would argue for a preference toward the DIFRRI (Directorate of Food, Roads, and Rural Infrastructures) approach over the ADP approach, with regard to social mobilization, diffusion effects, technological perspective, and internal sustainability.

On the external front, this translates to a trade regime of "selective closure" for the African food economy, especially in the West African subregion where the lack of congruency is greatest between production and consumption. Structurally, that subregion already suffers the multiple disadvantages of an inefficient and costly urban-industrial sector, severe agroclimatic uncertainties, great variabilities in output, natural resources fragility, out-migration of farm labor without a compensatory increase in rural labor productivity, and profound inadequacies of rural infrastructures. In such a setting, it is a counterproductive policy to close the widening food demand gap either through normal competitive international food trade or through regular international food aid.

Whatever ingenious policy measures or social experiments are introduced as stopgaps, the long-term imperative of raising factor productivity in African agriculture must be addressed. This is, indeed, more compelling than policy analysts in Africa tend to realize, given the magnitude of the food deficits being projected for the region in the 1990s by various international research institutes, the probability that traditional farming systems are reaching their agroclimatic limits in several production zones, and the mounting urban population pressures combined with low farm labor supply elasticities. The choice is thus not whether there must be a higher rate of agricultural intensification, but rather it is one of speed, content, and cost. Agricultural scientists and agricultural economists tend to argue generally for a quick switch to modern science and technology in farming practices. It can be argued, however, that from a community-level perspective, the fears and uncertainties surrounding nontechnological solutions may have been overstated, at least in the short-to-medium run of the 1990s.

Various policy experiments in structural adjustment in several African countries since the mid-1980s are demonstrating that the aggregate agricultural supply may not be as inelastic as the technologist-minded critics had feared. Both the observed labor shortages and the declining food production of the past fifteen years may have been caused by the long accumulated neglect of producer price incentives and of market infrastructures, and for the moment at least, there are in fact few relevant scientific and technological solutions readily available to the vast majority of African smallholder peasant farmers.

In some other cases, the impact of the external trade regime is a complicating factor, as, for example, in the internal marketing, storage, and food security of white maize in Kenya in relation to comparable available imports. There have also been situations in several African countries (in both bimodal and unimodal production systems) in which the prices of agricultural export commodities rose more than the prices of domestic food products, and farmers consequently switched their land and labor away from the domestic marketable food surplus. The result: the high food prices signaled by the domestic market could not bridge unsatisfied demand by translating this into an appropriate supply response. From a policy standpoint, the objective lesson is not so much the weakness of a pricing solution relative to a technology solution to the African food crisis. Rather, it is the more fundamental issue of what should properly constitute food security in African nations.

Food security, at least in the African context, must be conceived in terms of both the level *and* composition of a basket of food commodities the consumption *and* production of which can be *sustained* at succeeding stages of per capita real incomes for the majority of households. These would consist at present of home-produced staples of coarse grains, tubers, citrus, nuts, vegetables, ruminant small animals, and aquacultural products, all of

6

which substantially reflect culturally determined tastes, rather than externally induced by the demonstrated effects of acquired elite behavior.

The production challenge facing African agriculture, therefore, involves meeting a supply that the slowly moving resource capacity of the national economies can deliver to a large segment of the population over any given period. For the majority of African countries, as we approach the 1990s and as indicated by farmers from the Awe community, this means: (a) in the short to immediate term, emphasize producer price incentives, expanded rural credit, liberalized marketing, sustenance of poststructural adjustment macroeconomic reforms, and lateral expansion of land and labor; and (b) in the long run, improve the technological packages appropriate to smallholder farming systems; establish small-scale earth dam-based water management that can extend production cycles and reduce interseasonal output variabilities; and expand postharvest agroindustrial processing linkages.

Macroeconomic Framework

As we have defined it, food security is clearly only one element in the complex web of food and agricultural policies. The literature on the subject has shown unambiguously that food policy itself encompasses the collective efforts of public authorities to influence the decision-making environment of food producers, food marketers, food processors, food distributors, and food consumers, in order to foster desirable and achievable social welfare goals. Therefore, food policy analysis and thus food security considerations must be concerned with all food-related issues in a macroeconomic setting.

This position is further highlighted by the lessons of empirical experience, that apart from its dominance in household consumption and expenditure patterns at the early stages of economic growth, food and access to food constitute the analytical core and political economy of a nation's development process. As that process picks up momentum, shifts in the food and agricultural sector shape and are, in turn, shaped by the speed and character of industrialization. We can thus see the policy entry points to considerations of exchange rate, trade tariff, money supply, public finance, investment expenditures, employment generation, and income distribution. Above all and ultimately, there is the bottom line of a nation's management capacity. This is because the real essence of development consists of a people's capacity to understand, predict, respond flexibly to, and manage change, whether such changes are exogenously determined or internally induced.

In the social milieu of Africa and, in particular, considering the trauma and pains that have accompanied the current policy reform measures of structural adjustment, the rising pressure of unemployment has assumed great and urgent concern of political economy management. What John W. Mellor initially had argued for South Asia has now become an immediate challenge to African policy makers: namely, the critical role of agriculture in the propagation and amelioration of unemployment.

A country with a large agricultural sector and a large underemployed labor force, which tries to move employment at a pace greater than the domestic production of food and agricultural commodities (i.e., wage goods) and which tries to bridge the gaps substantially with imports, would soon discover that: (a) large-scale imports begin quickly to impact adversely on the real exchange rate; (b) real food prices will rise quickly and drag along with them the real wage rates; and (c) the narrow employment base gets even more squeezed.

In order to break this pressure and create more employment-enhancing breathing space: (a) savings and investment rates must be expanded; (b) capital spreading must be encouraged beyond supply tinkering with choice of techniques; and (c) a trade regime has to be put in place that imports capital-intensive goods and services while exporting labor-intensive goods and services.

How far Mellor's analytical and policy prescriptions can be applied operationally in the contemporary African context is conditioned by the import capacity that structural adjustment programs in Africa succeed in fostering. Past failures of the region's efforts at food and agricultural development are not just a reflection of unproductive resource allocations and weaknesses in macroeconomic policies. Rather, the succession of cycles of economic stagnation, bouts of hunger, sociopolitical crises, and short-lived episodes of export-based prosperity are as much a reflection of technical and economic structures that are vulnerable to both international and ecological uncertainties.

All that we can say for the present is that a great deal of the post-structural adjustment prospects of the African food and agricultural economy in the 1990s will depend on understanding the underlying macroeconomic issues, and on the acceptance by African policy makers of the strategies that we have tried to outline above. Sector-specific measures will clearly be compromised unless the macroeconomic policy environment is conducive, holistic, mutually consistent, and regularly kept under review.

The main macroeconomic issues are well known and embrace foreign exchange rates, tariff regimes, savings, investments, money supply, credit and interest rates, wage rates and income distribution, relative prices, taxation, and subsidies. Long-term issues such as demographic pressure and environmental protection also have to be factored in. But from our perspective, African policy analysts have to give greater emphasis, in addition, to issues of human capacity building, public administration, and political governance, in order to achieve a more democratic and responsive polity.

As an integral part of the ongoing structural adjustment policy reforms, the one central macroeconomic issue that needs to be kept constantly in view is the relationship of import capacity to African food security. This would mean that the existing revealed demand preferences, for example, cannot be taken as a given in a proper conceptualization of what constitutes food security. The region's food security problem is not simply a challenge from the supply side. Indeed, as the Nigerian experience over the past three years has shown, the supply deficiencies cannot be effectively addressed without at least simultaneously also correcting the built-in distortions on the demand side. A cardinal objective and starting point of social policy has to be a commitment to national self-sufficiency in *staple* foods, closely and culturally defined.

The International Environment

This reconceptualization of African food security differs in a significant way from what appears to be the mainstream approach of food policy analysis. For example, in a research volume edited by Alberto Valdés, *Food Security for Developing Countries*, food insecurity is viewed essentially in terms of weather-induced variability of supplies, a combination of production as well as price fluctuations from both food and nonfood sectors, and fluctuations in a country's real incomes. Once such fluctuations in real incomes can be smoothed, it is assumed, food security is attainable. The analytical and policy backdrops to all this lie in the scaffold of open competitive international trade, based on comparable cost advantages in food production, and supplemented by international stock adjustments and hunger alleviation programs.

In spite of the promising (though still limited) achievements of many African structural adjustment programs over the past four years, there is still great doubt about the extent of the benefits to African food and agricultural economies that derive from bold efforts at the liberalization of external trade and payments. Indeed, it was precisely the excessive exposure of African economies to the vicissitudes of world trade and payments that drove African policy makers in the 1960s and 1970s to seek alternative internal prime movers of growth. Because of the unpleasant experiences of colonial and neocolonial resource exploitation, policy makers became wary of foreign capital and management. Because of the continuing unfavorable factoral terms of international trade and despite efforts to increase the production of internationally traded commodities, faith in the existing international economic order weakened considerably.

Irrespective of their structural adjustments and policy reforms, African countries remain wary of full liberalization in the security-sensitive area of staple foods, as they plan for the 1990s. They can point to the example of the European Community's agricultural policy as well as the probable fallouts from Europe's 1992 economic integration on Africa's lagging exports of food and agriculture that exist under the African-Caribbean-Pacific Lomé Convention. They can point to the many flaws in the record of external assistance to African agriculture over the past two decades: the mismatching of international resource flows and national sources of growth, the negative impact on both environmental quality and social institutions, the overestimation of the utility of physical plants and expatriate technical assistance, and the failure to develop enduring human capabilities for sustainable growth with equity.

They can document the tariff and nontariff protectionist blocs and the cultural pressures that African food and agricultural commodities run up against in several industrialized countries. The well-known example of Japanese policy insistence on domestic agricultural production in spite of all economic logic for trade liberalization and its impact on the rice export markets of Southeast Asia is a lesson which cannot be ignored by African policy makers. To be factored into the projections for the 1990s must be the fact of continued dumping of food products in the African countries, bolstered by artificially high subsidies offered by industrialized countries to their own domestic producers.

It is, of course, true that some key studies have demonstrated a historical correlation between agricultural growth and increased food imports in several developing countries; and that, by inference, African nonfood agricultural prosperity may not be inconsistent with rising food imports in the region. The empirical basis for such an assertion is the increased demand for livestock products, animal feed, dairy goods, and non-coarse grains, as real incomes increase, urbanization quickens, and urban elite life styles begin to show a preference for convenience foods. The reality of African structural adjustment experience over the past four years, however, has unmistakably established the severe limitation of foreign exchange availability, net-of-servicing the huge external debt burden. It has also shown that a food-deficit country already hooked on imported tastes that run counter to its domestic resource endowments is unlikely to be able to import sufficiently to prevent a dangerous escalation in food price inflation.

The question might then be asked, why African countries cannot mitigate their import incapacity (net of external debt servicing) through enhanced export performance. Why, in other words, is Africa not able to expand its exports commensurate with its objective demand for food imports? The last four years have shown clearly that African countries require substantial foreign exchange. In the absence of significant exchange reserves and given the diminished inflow of foreign investment (whether private, governmental, direct, multilateral, or bilateral) outside the purely extractive industries, the needed foreign exchange has to be earned through intensified export activities. Substantial devaluations of national currencies have contributed to some degree to increased export activity under the structural adjustment programs of the past four years. Nor can African nations be accused of pursuing policies of autarky or economic isolation.

But what are the realistic prospects of sustaining this new momentum of expanded agricultural export earnings? For the 1990s, the prospects do not appear cheerful for Africa. First, those agricultural exports that compete directly with temperate-zone products (e.g., non-coarse grains, sugar, oilseeds, and cotton) face rather severe competition (tariff and nontariff barriers) in the large markets of the industrialized countries. With respect to tropical products such as cocoa, coffee, tea, and tubers, the prospects are greatly diminished by the near-saturation of demand levels and low-income elasticities of demand.

Second, experience has shown that a policy movement toward cash-crop production for exports often can dissipate the potential benefits by way of negative effects on domestic food production and nutritional status. In such a setting, the low-income groups and the children in particular are the most vulnerable groups that bear the brunt. It is true that in some exceptional cases, cash crop export production and sustained domestic food expansion have been complementary rather than competitive (e.g., Malaysia in Asia, Botswana and Rwanda in Africa). But in the vast majority of African countries, experience has shown that the foreign exchange generated through export cropping has neither been sustainable over a long period of time nor actually expended for imports of goods and services that can positively affect the food consumption and nutritional status of the majority of poor households.

Yet African countries have little choice but to press ahead with exploiting and reinforcing available export market opportunities. Experience of the past few years has shown that some scope does exist in the imaginative promotion of non-traditional agricultural exports, especially in the realm of vegetables, nuts, fruits, flowers, exotic forest products, and herbs for both medicinal and cosmetic purposes. But given Africa's long historical experience with both the instability and the secular decline in its commodity export earnings (agricultural as well as mineral), it would seem that the safest strategy for African decision makers is to pursue a careful and deliberate policy of selective closure in food and agricultural trade relations, using both tariff and nontariff measures. This would combine vigorous export promotion with appropriate fiscal disincentives for imported fine exotic grains, animal products, dairy, fish, beverages, and wines.

Policy Considerations and Future Prospects in Africa

Much of the performance outlook for Africa's food and agricultural economies in the 1990s already has been determined by today's established capital stock and production relations. There is evidence that, in several countries, the past declines in output and aggregate consumption have been arrested; and, in some, the trend has indeed turned positive over the past two years. But several significant pockets of poor performance still remain and are likely to persist until at least the early part of the 1990s. There are cases of continued civil strife, drought, crop failure, and incipient famine in the Sudan, parts of the Sahel, Ethiopia, Angola, and Mozambique. The West African subregion exerts a disproportionate pressure on the continent's food equation; and, there, the food deficits are still large in magnitude. Even if the gaps there have stopped widening in the aggregate, the per capita food gaps are still worsening as compared to the East and Central African subregions.

West Africa has a faster rate of population growth relative to comparable levels of food availability; it experiences a higher rate of rural-urban migration; it exhibits a wider income disparity socially as well as geopolitically; it is experiencing a disproportionate rise in food prices relative to the increases in wages; and it suffers from an increasing shift in dietary habits and consumption behavior toward unsustainable food imports. For Africa as a whole, it is therefore unlikely that the food deficit problem will have been fully resolved by the end of the 1990s, at least in terms of adequate per capita nutritional standards. Domestic output expansion is unlikely to be spectacular enough to change the current status of the continent as the most marginal of all major regions of the world economy in terms of food self-sufficiency and self-reliance ratios.

If West Africa looms large in the African food profile, Nigeria in turn occupies a premier statistical position in West Africa. Here, the prospects are slightly better, but not spectacularly different. The momentum of the past two years, driven by Nigeria's traumatic program of structural adjustments and improved internal terms of trade, is likely to be maintained into the 1990s, barring any unusually adverse climatic conditions. An average growth rate of about 4 percent per annum is being projected as achievable for the Nigerian food and agricultural economy over the next five years. Much of the growth is likely to come from increased land use and rural labor supplies, from privately managed, low-cost, small-scale irrigation systems, and from improved seeds and fertilizer applications, in spite of the expected reduction in fertilizer subsidies. Nigeria seems to have come a long way in its development of food products, especially with respect to post-harvest processing of grains and tubers. Peri-urban farming has also become a significant phenomenon in the towns.

But even then, Nigeria is not likely to have realized its full potential or completely eliminated its food deficits so as to achieve acceptable per capita nutritional levels by the end of the next decade. Some of the obstacles likely to be evident in the 1990s include the enormous area of arable land (some 95 percent) that would still not be served by any form of irrigation; the probable drop in the application of fertilizers (a consequence of expected subsidies reduction), which is unlikely to be fully compensated for by the expected greater labor supply deriving from reverse urban migration; the long lead time normally required for viable new technological packages to move from agricultural research systems to farm-level applications; the enormous funds required for widespread construction and maintenance of rural infrastructures; the continued gaps and deficiencies in statistical and non-statistical data that preclude better policy design and program monitoring; and the inadequacies in capacity building for both public and private operators in the agricultural sector.

At whatever level African food and agricultural issues are discussed (household, community, zonal, national, subregional, continental, and international), a constant factor for the policy analyst is the interrelationship with nonfood and non-agricultural considerations. There are primary, secondary, and tertiary impacts resulting from shifts in agricultural output, income, and expenditure. Not only do initial increases in farm incomes lead to other increases in income and employment (via related activities in farm inputs, processing, transport services, and marketing); but increases in consumption expenditures also provide ripple effects well beyond the food and agricultural sector. Again, dynamic interactions have been documented by researchers in the region between farm and nonfarm activities, between tradeables and nontradeables, and between size distribution of farms and patterns of human settlement. Running through all these are concerns about environmental quality and the integrity of the ecosystem.

Given the high locational specificity of agriculture, the complexity of all those interactions, and the compelling need for new forms of social mobilization for expanded production, there is hardly a better perspective for viewing and addressing African agricultural problems than analyzing and mobilizing the local communities themselves. At least, in the social setting of Africa with the constraints of communications and transportation, local communities represent the pivotal point for the agricultural researcher, the policy analyst, and the decision maker. It is in that context that the Awe experiment in Nigeria is providing a small but useful window for viewing the continent's present challenges and future possibilities.

Readings

Aboyade, Ojetunji. 1987. "Growth Strategy and the Agricultural Sector." In *Accelerating Food Production in Sub-Saharan Africa*, eds. John W. Mellor, Christopher Delgado, and Malcolm J. Blackie. Baltimore: Johns Hopkins University Press.

Lele, Uma. 1990. *Managing Agricultural Development in Africa*. Washington, D.C.: The World Bank.

Mellor, John W. 1976. *The New Economics of Growth: A Strategy for India and the Developing World*. Ithaca: Cornell University Press.

Valdés, Alberto, ed. 1981. *Food Security for Developing Countries*. Boulder: Westview Press.

CHAPTER 2

Farming Institutions, Food Policy, and Agricultural Development in China

Justin Yifu Lin

Deputy Director, The Development Institute, Research Center for Rural Development, Beijing, People's Republic of China

Introduction

China is highly acclaimed for its ability to feed over one-fifth of the world's population with only one-fifteenth of the world's arable land.[1] When the People's Republic of China was founded in 1949, cultivated land per capita was only 0.18 hectare. Due to rapid population growth, per capita cultivated land dropped to 0.1 hectare in 1978.[2] The government, nevertheless, was able to keep grain production ahead of population growth. Meanwhile, per capita national income increased from 66 yuan (U.S. $18.3) in 1949 to 312 yuan (U.S. $182) in 1978.[3] The economy also experienced a dramatic transformation. The share of industrial sector income in total national income expanded from 12.6 percent in 1949 to 46.8 percent in 1978.[4] The strategy that the Chinese government adopted to obtain the necessary accumulation for industrial development and to cope with the increasing food demand from rapid population growth was a collective farming system in agriculture and a restricted food-rationing system in urban areas. This Chinese strategy was often considered as a development model for densely populated Third World countries.[5]

Really remarkable achievements in Chinese agriculture, nevertheless, did not occur until the recent farm sector reforms launched in 1979. Between 1952 — when the Chinese economy recovered from twelve years of war and destruction — and 1978, the growth rate in grain production was 2.4 percent per year, which was only 0.4 percent above the population growth rate in the same period. Per capita availability of grain, therefore, increased only 10 percent over a quarter of a century (see Table 2-1). Frustrated by the

15

inability to raise living standards substantially after thirty years of socialist revolution, the moderate veteran leaders, who were purged during the "Cultural Revolution" and came into power again after the death of Chairman Mao Zedong in 1976, initiated in 1979 a series of sweeping reforms in agriculture. The new policies included diversification of the rural economy, production specialization, crop selection in accordance with regional comparative advantage, expansion of free markets, and a marked rise in state procurement prices. The most important change, however, was the emergence and eventual predominance of the household responsibility system, which restored the primacy of the individual household in place of the collective team system as the basic unit of production and management in rural China. While the population grew at 1.3 percent per year, as an average, between 1979 and 1984, the value of agricultural output and grain output grew annually at 11.8 percent and 4.1 percent, respectively, in the same period (see Table 2–1).

The success of agricultural reform, especially the remarkable growth of grain output, greatly encouraged the moderate political leaders. As a result, a series of more market-oriented reforms were undertaken at the end of 1984 in both the urban and rural sectors. The urban economy in China is much more complicated than the agricultural sector. Any policy change, good or bad, is not likely to manifest itself in a short period. A policy essential for the long run may even cause great difficulties in the short run. A continuous flow of successful experiences, however, is essential for maintaining the momentum of any reform. Therefore, the question of whether the market-oriented reforms in the Chinese economy will be carried forward may depend, again, on the performance of agricultural reforms.

Although agriculture as a whole grew at a respectable average annual rate of 3.5 percent after 1984, grain production, nevertheless, stagnated after reaching a peak of 407 million tons in 1984 (see Table 2–1). Over the many dynastic transitions in the several thousand years of Chinese history, political leaders in China have come to recognize the crucial importance of food production to political and social stability.[6] Therefore, the optimism that robust agricultural development generated during the first five years of rural reforms was swiftly replaced in the subsequent downturn by a pessimistic mood.[7] There even has emerged a call for recollectivization of the individual household-based farming system under the banner of pursuing economies of scale in agricultural production.

Chinese reform is at a crossroad. In this paper I will argue that the poor performance of grain production in the past four years did not arise from the small size of the household farm. Rather, the main reason is the failure of the government to change the urban food-rationing policy and to implement a market-oriented price system reform for grain. In this view, a

Table 2–1

Population, Agricultural Output, and Grain Output in China

Year	Population (million) (1)	Agri. Output (1952 baseline = 100) (2)	Grain Output (million tons) (3)
1952	574.8	100.0	164
1953	588.0	103.1	167
1954	602.7	106.6	170
1955	614.7	114.7	184
1956	628.3	120.5	193
1957	646.5	124.8	195
1958	659.9	127.8	200
1959	672.1	110.4	170
1960	662.1	96.4	143.5
1961	658.6	94.1	147.5
1962	673.0	99.9	160
1963	691.7	111.5	170
1964	705.0	126.7	187.5
1965	725.4	137.1	194.5
1966	745.2	149.0	214
1967	763.7	151.3	218
1968	785.3	147.6	209
1969	806.7	149.2	211
1970	829.9	166.4	240
1971	852.3	171.4	250
1972	871.8	169.6	240
1973	892.1	183.8	265
1974	908.6	190.1	275
1975	924.2	196.0	284.5
1976	937.2	195.3	286
1977	949.7	194.3	283
1978	962.6	210.2	305
1979	975.4	226.0	332
1980	987.1	229.2	320.6
1981	1,000.7	244.0	325
1982	1,015.9	271.5	355
1983	1,027.6	292.6	387
1984	1,038.7	328.5	407
1985	1,050.4	339.7	379
1986	1,065.3	351.2	391
1987	1,080.7	371.5	405

Source: State Statistical Bureau, *Zhongguo Tongji Nianjian, 1988* (China Statistical Yearbook, 1988) Beijing: China Statistics Press, 38, 97, and 248

market-oriented food policy reform should be the focus of further economic reforms in China.

The paper will be organized as follows. The relationship between China's development strategy and the choices of food policy and farming institutions are investigated in section II. Section III discusses the motivation and achievements of the 1979 farming institution reform. Section IV describes the current status of food policy in China. A proposal for food policy reform is outlined in section V. Concluding observations are presented in section VI.

Development Strategy, Food Policy, and Farming Institutions

Food and farming institution policies prior to the 1979 reform were shaped by the development strategy that the Chinese government adopted in the early 1950s.

At the founding of the People's Republic of China in 1949, the Chinese government inherited a war-torn economy in which 89.4 percent of the population resided in rural areas, and industry was limited to only a 12.6 percent share of national income.[8] Heavy industry is a major characteristic of a developed country's economic structure. In order to strengthen national power, China adopted in 1952 a Stalin-type heavy-industry-oriented development strategy, as the economy was recovering from wartime destruction. The goal was to build as rapidly as possible the country's capacity to produce capital goods and military materials.

Capital was extremely scarce at that time and the voluntary saving rate was far too low to finance the high rate of investment in heavy industry sought by the development strategy. To facilitate rapid capital expansion, a policy of low wages for industrial workers evolved alongside the heavy-industry-oriented development strategy. The assumption was that through low wages, the state-owned enterprises would be able to create large profits and to reinvest the profits for infrastructure and capital construction. The practice of establishing low prices for energy, transportation, and other raw materials, such as cotton, was instituted for the same reason.

To implement low wages, the government was required to provide urban dwellers with inexpensive food and other necessities, including housing, medical care, and clothing. A strict food-rationing system was instituted in 1953, and has been kept in effect ever since.[9] Food rationing for urban residents consists of two elements: 1) a basic ration which varies according to sex and age, and 2) a professional ration which is related to the intensity of labor in the workplace. The ration varies from year to year according to the supply situation. On the average, the food ration per capita is about 15 kilograms (kg) a month. Meanwhile, in order to secure the food supply for rationing, a compulsory grain procurement policy was imposed in rural areas in 1953. The grain trade in China has been virtually monopolized by the state since then.

The industrial development strategy also resulted in a great demand for agricultural products. First, the urban population increased dramatically from 57.65 million in 1949, to 71.63 million in 1952, and to 99.49 million in 1957.[10] Since the industrial strategy would not permit the use of large amounts of scarce foreign reserves to import food for urban consumption, satisfying the increasing food demand in urban areas hinged on the growth of domestic grain production. Second, since the bulk of China's exports consisted of agricultural products, the country's capacity to import capital goods for industrialization depended on agriculture's growth.[11] Third, agriculture was the main source of raw materials for many industries, such as textiles and food processing. Agriculture, therefore, was clearly viewed as the bottleneck and major point of intervention in pursuing the overall economic development strategy in China in the early 1950s.

Under these conditions, agricultural stagnation and poor harvests would not only affect food supply but also have an almost immediate and direct adverse impact on industrial expansion.[12] Since the government was reluctant to divert resources from industry to agriculture, a new agricultural development strategy was adopted that would permit and foster the simultaneous development of agriculture alongside the development of industry. The core of this strategy involved mass mobilization of rural labor to work on labor-intensive projects, such as irrigation, flood control, and land reclamation, and to raise unit yields in agriculture through traditional methods and inputs, such as closer planting, more careful weeding, and the use of more organic fertilizer. Collectivization of agriculture was the institution that the government believed would perform these functions.

Collectivization also was viewed as a convenient vehicle for effecting the procurement of grain and other agricultural products to carry out the industrial development strategy. As noted by an economist:

A still more fundamental reason for the collectivization of agriculture, however, was the fact that China had embarked on the construction of a planned socialist economy in 1953. For large-scale development of the national economy, it was imperative that changes be effected in the small peasant economy to enable it to provide the large quantities of grain, cotton, oil-bearing crops, sugar crops and other industrial raw materials needed by developing industry . . . the solution of which could only be found in the collectivization of agriculture.[13]

The independent family farm was the traditional farming institution in rural China for thousands of years prior to the founding of the People's

Republic. The typical farm not only was small, but also fragmented. In the wake of the socialist revolution, nearly half of the cultivated land in rural China was owned by landlords who rented land out to peasant families. Rent was often as high as 50 percent of the value of the main crops. A land reform program was implemented in areas under the Communist Party's control beginning in the 1940s. Under this program, land was confiscated without compensation from the landlord and distributed to the tenants. The land reform program continued after the success of the revolution and was completed in 1952.

Experiments with various forms of cooperatives began even before the completion of land reform. The first type of cooperative was the "mutual aid team," in which four or five neighboring households pooled together their farm tools and draft animals and exchanged their labor on a temporary or permanent basis, with land and harvest belonging to each household. The mutual aid team was the predominant form of cooperative up to 1955. The second type was the "elementary cooperative," in which about twenty to thirty neighboring households pooled together farm tools, draft animals, as well as land under unified management. The net income of a cooperative was distributed in two categories: payment for land, draft animals, and farm tools; and remuneration for work performed. Land, draft animals, and farm tools were still owned by member households. The third type was the collective farm, or the "advanced cooperative," in which all means of production, including land, draft animals, and farm tools, were collectively owned. Remuneration in an advanced cooperative was based solely on the amount of work each member contributed and took the form of work points. The income of a family in an advanced cooperative depended on the amount of work points earned by the family members and on the average value of a work point. The latter, in turn, depended on the net production of the collective farm. The size of an advanced cooperative initially consisted of about thirty households, and later evolved to include all households in a village, or approximately 150–200 households.

The official approach to collectivization, initially, was cautious and gradualist. Peasants were encouraged and induced to join the various cooperatives on a voluntary basis. However, proponents for accelerating the pace of collectivization in the summer of 1955 won the debate within the Party. There were only 500 advanced cooperatives in 1955. By the winter of 1957, 753,000 advanced cooperative farms, with 119 million member households, were established on a nationwide basis.[14]

Collectivization was surprisingly successful in the initial stage. It encountered no active resistance from the peasantry and was carried out relatively smoothly. The gross value of agriculture (measured at constant prices in 1952) increased 27.8 percent and grain output increased 21.9 percent between 1952 and 1958 (see columns 2 and 3, Table 2–1). This experience greatly encouraged the leadership within the Party and led them to take a bolder approach. The main rationale of collectivization was rooted in the notion that mobilizing rural surplus labor would increase rural capital formation and, hence, increase production. However, while a collective farm of 150 households provided a basis for mobilizing labor for work projects within the collective, the collective farm did not solve the problem of mobilizing labor for large-scale projects, such as digging irrigation canals, building dams, or the like. These kinds of projects would in general require the simultaneous participation of labor from several dozen collective farms.

The obvious solution for the large-scale labor mobilization was to pool twenty or thirty collective farms of 150 households each into a larger collective unit. In this way, the "People's Commune" came into existence in 1958. From the end of August to the beginning of November, within only three months, 753,000 collective farms were transformed into 24,000 communes, which consisted of 120 million households, or 99 percent of total rural households in China in 1958. The average size of a commune was about 5,000 households with 10,000 laborers and 10,000 acres of cultivated land. Payment in the commune was made according to subsistence needs and partly according to the work performed. Work on private plots, which existed in the other forms of cooperatives, was prohibited.

Billions of person-days of labor were mobilized as expected. However, the communal movement ended up in a profound agricultural crisis between 1959 and 1961. The gross value of agriculture, measured at the constant prices of 1952, dropped 14 percent in 1959, 12 percent in 1960, and another 2.5 percent in 1961. Most importantly, grain output was reduced 15 percent in 1959, another 16 percent in 1960, remained at the same low level for another year, and did not recover to the level of 1952 until 1962. As compared to 1952, the population by 1959 had increased 17 percent, and the dramatic reduction in grain output had resulted in a widespread and severe famine. Thirty million people were estimated to have died of starvation and malnutrition during this crisis (see Table 2–1).[15]

Communes were not abolished after the great crisis. However, starting in 1962, agricultural operation was divided and management was delegated to a much smaller unit, the "production team," which consisted of about twenty to thirty neighboring households. In this new system, land was jointly owned by the commune, brigade, and production team. However, the production team was treated as the basic operating and accounting unit. Income distribution, based on work points earned by each member, was undertaken within the production team. A similar remuneration system occurred in the advanced cooperative. After 1962, some experiments to improve the grading of work points were made. The production team nevertheless remained the basic farming institution until the household responsibility system reform began in 1979.

A more realistic approach toward agricultural development was adopted after the 1959–61 crisis. The mobilization of rural labor for public irrigation projects continued. Greater emphasis was given to modern inputs. Irrigated acreage increased gradually after 1962. Additional acreage resulted from increasing powered irrigation rather than from the construction of labor-intensive canals and dams. The utilization of chemical fertilizers was accelerated after 1962, accompanied by the promotion of high-yield fertilizer-responsive modern varieties. Dwarf varieties of rice and wheat were introduced in the early 1960s. By the end of the 1970s, about 80 percent of the traditional varieties of rice and wheat had been replaced by the modern dwarf varieties. After 1976, dwarf varieties of rice were replaced by higher-yielding hybrid rice. Modern varieties of corn, cotton, and other crops were also introduced and promoted in the 1960s and 1970s. The pace of mechanization also accelerated after 1965, especially during the 1970s.

Despite dramatic increases in modern inputs in the 1960s and 1970s, the poor performance of agriculture and grain production continued. Although great emphasis was given to self-sufficiency, China changed from a net grain exporter in the 1950s to a sizable grain importer after 1961, and per capita consumption of food grain in 1978 was no higher than it was in 1957. Poor agricultural performance had its origin in the collective farming system and defective food policy.

Household Responsibility System Reform

The main defect of the production team as an institution for agricultural development is its incentive structure. Team members, working under the supervision of a team leader, were accredited with work points for the jobs they performed. At the end of a year, net team income was distributed according to the work points that each member accumulated during the year. Work points were supposed to reflect the quality and quantity of effort that each member contributed to the team's work. The work-point system is not inherently an inefficient incentive scheme: if the monitoring of each peasant's work is perfect and complete, the incentives to work will be strong rather than weak. The return on a peasant's additional increment of effort has two components: a share of the increase in team output, and a larger share of the total net team income, as now he contributes a larger share of total effort and thus obtains a larger share of work points. The sum of these two components is likely to lead a worker to exert himself or herself beyond the point at which what he or she adds to the value of output equals his or her valuation of the foregone leisure. On the other hand, if the monitoring of work effort is deficient or nonexistent, a peasant is not likely to obtain additional work points for his additional contribution of effort. In this case, the return on his increase in effort has only a single component, namely, a share of the increase in team output. The incentives to work then would be insufficient. The extent to which a work-point share is increased for an additional unit of effort depends on the degree of monitoring. Incentives to work in a production team are positively correlated with the degree of monitoring in the production process. The higher the degree of monitoring, the higher the incentives to work, and thus the more effort contributed.

However, monitoring is costly. The management of the production team has to balance the gain in productivity due to an increase in incentives against the rise in the cost of monitoring. The monitoring of agricultural operations is particularly difficult because of agricultural production's sequential nature and spatial dimension. In agricultural production, the process typically spans several months over several acres of land. Farming also requires peasants to shift from one job to another throughout the production season. In general, the quality of work provided by a peasant does not become apparent until harvest time. Furthermore, it is impossible to determine each individual's contribution by simply observing the outputs, because of the random effects of nature on production. It is thus very costly to provide close monitoring of a peasant's effort in agricultural production. Consequently, the optimum degree of monitoring, even under the best circumstances, has to be very low. The incremental income for each additional unit of effort will be only a small fraction of the marginal product of effort. Therefore, the incentives to work for peasants in a production team are also likely to be low.[16]

The commune, brigade, and production team system of agricultural production management, with its work-point system of compensation, has been challenged ever since its establishment. After the disaster of the Great Leap Forward, land was reallocated to individual families, and households were restored as the units of production in many parts of China, especially in Anhui Province. Production soon recovered in these areas. Nevertheless, this practice was prohibited and criticized as capitalistic, and those people responsible were punished. Although the reallocation of land to individual households, secretly or sometimes openly, was never totally extinguished in some areas, real change was not possible until 1978, when moderate leaders came into power again after the chaos of the "Cultural Revolution" and the death of Chairman Mao.[17]

At the end of 1978, the government proposed a sweeping change in rural policies.[18] In place of a lopsided stress on grain production, the new policy encouraged the development of a diversified economy. Better prices were set for the state purchase of farm produce. Production teams were granted more freedom in making decisions about their own affairs. Private plots and the country fairs in which farm people sold their surplus products were revived and expanded. It had been recognized at that time that solving the managerial problems of agriculture within the production team system was the key to improving work incentives. Yet the household-based farming system reform was considered the reverse of the socialist principle of collective farming and, therefore, was prohibited. The official position at that time maintained that the production team was to remain the basic unit of production, income distribution, and accounting.

Nevertheless, a small number of production teams, first secretly and later with the blessing of local authorities, began to experiment with a system of contracting land, other resources, and output quotas to individual households. Toward the end of 1978 this was done in Feixi County and also in Chuxian Prefecture in Anhui Province, two areas that had been frequently damaged by flood and drought. A year later, these teams brought in yields far larger than those of other teams. The central authorities later conceded the existence of these practices and named them "the household responsibility system." However, the authorities required that this system be restricted to poor agricultural regions, such as hilly, mountainous areas, and to poorly functioning teams in which people had lost confidence in the collective. In practice, this restriction could not be put into effect at all. Rich regions welcomed the household responsibility system as enthusiastically as poor regions. Full official recognition of the household responsibility system as universally acceptable eventually was given in late 1981. By the end of 1983, almost all the households in China's rural areas had adopted this new system. Under the arrangement of the household responsibility system, land is contracted to individual households for a period of fifteen years. After fulfilling the procurement quota obligations, farmers are then entitled to sell their surplus on the markets or else retain it for their own uses.

In the household-based farming system, the difficulty of monitoring work performance does not exist. By definition, a peasant becomes the residual claimant. He does not need to measure his own effort. The marginal return on his effort is the marginal product of his own effort. Although economies of scale are sacrificed in the household-based system, it can be demonstrated that the incentive structure in the household-based system exceeds that of the team system.[19] Therefore, the incentives to work are improved by shifting from the production team system to the household responsibility system. Peasants feel happier and contribute more effort to production under the household responsibility system.

The change from a production team system to a household farming system is found empirically to have improved the incentive for adopting new technology, a key ingredient for agricultural growth over a long period of time.[20] The most conspicuous effect has been the one-time discrete impact on productivity arising from the increase in working incentives. It is estimated, for example, that total factor productivity — i.e., the total output produced by given amounts of inputs — increased 15 percent as a result of improvements in the incentive structure resulting from the shift from the production team system to the household responsibility system.[21] The household responsibility system reform that was begun in 1979 was fully established in 1984. During this period, agricultural output increased by 45 percent (see Table 2-1). About one-third of the output growth between 1979 and 1984, therefore, can be attributed to the improvements in incentives that resulted from the household responsibility system reform.[22]

The Status of Food Policy

As discussed in section II, the basic framework of existing food policy was set up in 1953. It was instituted to secure the government's control of grain supply, on the one hand, and to meet the demand of urban residents for low-priced grain, on the other hand. As in many other countries, grain is more than just a commodity. Once the government is involved in the distribution of grain, the shift in the sale price of grain becomes a political event. To avoid possible political unrest such as occurred in Poland and in other countries, ration prices have changed little since the ration system was first instituted in 1953.[23]

The compulsory grain procurement program can be divided into two categories: the "basic quota" and the "above quota," the latter having been introduced in 1960. Both categories together specify the amount of obligatory grain delivery required of a farm unit. The only difference between these two categories is that the government pays a price premium for the above-quota delivery. The total amount of the basic quota was generally fixed although it has actually declined slightly since 1953.[24] Most increases in grain procurement over the years have fallen in the category of the above quota. When the quota system was introduced in 1953, procurement prices were set at a level at which the state grain procurement and marketing agency could make a small profit.[25] However, after the great agricultural crisis in 1959–61, grain procurement prices were raised on an average of 25.3 percent in 1961 to improve the incentives for grain production. After that, four other major price adjustments were made, in 1966, 1979, 1985, and 1988. Because the ration prices were kept nearly constant, each raise in the procurement price resulted in an increase in the amount of the government subsidy.[26]

At the beginning of the 1979 reforms, political leaders in China reached an agreement that farm income was too low and grain output was barely sufficient to meet subsistence needs. As a measure to increase farm income and boost grain production, procurement prices for grain and other major crops were increased by a big margin in 1979. The basic-quota price of grain was raised 20 percent, and the above-quota price was raised

25

from 130 percent to 150 percent of the basic-quota price (the weighted-average increase was 33 percent). Furthermore, the state monopoly on grain marketing was gradually lifted. Private as well as collective traders were allowed to handle grain marketing alongside the state marketing agency.

The household responsibility system reform along with the marked price increase brought in an upsurge of grain output. The annual growth rate, for example, increased from an average of 2.4 percent annually in the period 1953–78 to 4.1 percent in the period 1979–84. Since the output growth rate was about twice as large as the growth rate of consumption in 1979–84, China became a net grain exporter in 1985, after having been a net importer for a quarter century. The sudden success, nevertheless, also brought with it new issues which the Chinese government had never handled before. According to the regulation at that time, the government was obliged to buy all grain at the above-quota price after a farmer fulfilled his quota obligation. Consequently, the greater the output growth, the larger the government's financial burden. Food subsidies (including edible oils) increased from 5.6 billion yuan in 1978 to 32.1 billion yuan in 1984, representing 21 percent of the government's budget in that year.[27] Further-more, there existed a serious shortage of storage facilities. Because the government was unable to buy all the grain that farmers wanted to sell, the market price for grain dropped substantially throughout the country. In some grain surplus areas, the market price at harvest time even approached the basic-quota price set by the government.

As a measure to reduce the government's financial burden and to increase the role of the market in the production and distribution of grain, the mandatory quota procurement system was changed to a contract procurement system at the beginning of 1985. According to the new system, procurement quantity was to be determined by contracts based on mutual agreements between the government and individual farmers. The contract price was calculated as a weighted average of the original basic-quota price (30 percent) and the above-quota price (70 percent). This price was 135 percent of the original basic-quota price and about equivalent to the market price in major grain production areas at the harvest time in 1984. However, it was 10 percent lower than the above-quota price. As a supple-ment to contract procurement, the government agreed, in addition, to purchase certain amounts of grain on the market at the market price.[28]

The contract procurement system, however, met with a host of prob-lems in its first year. Management costs incurred in signing contracts with millions of agricultural households were tremendous, and the means to enforce contracts were limited. The contract price did not provide enough incentives to farmers, especially in areas where the contract price was lower than, or even roughly equalled, the market price in 1984. Enforcement of contracts was made difficult because of a 6.9 percent drop in grain output in 1984. The drop in output led the market price of grain to register a 10 percent increase in 1985. As a result, the gap between the contract price and the market price had widened, and farmers were reluctant to fulfill the contracts.

As a reaction to this experience, contract procurement reverted to the original compulsory quota procurement system by the end of 1985, even though the term "contract" was not abolished. The quantity of procurement was reduced and the quantity of market purchase was increased. To minimize administrative costs, procurement quotas in each region were allocated to households in proportion to the cultivated land that each household operated under the household responsibility system. To compensate for losses, the government promised to provide farmers with fertilizer, diesel gas, and credit at subsidized prices. Farmers, nevertheless, frequently complained that these promises had not been realized.

The enforcement of procurement contracts is carried out by local governments. The central government established a policy that a local government is obliged to use its budget to purchase grain in the market in order to offset deficits in cases where farmers failed to fulfill their contracts. Since the market price of grain is higher than the contract price, the enforcement of contracts is a very demanding job. As a measure to overcome the difficulty, local governments often blockade the grain market under their jurisdiction until the compulsory procurement quotas are completed. During the period of blockade, all sales of grain by farmers and purchases of grain by traders other than at the local state grain station are prohibited. In areas that have two harvests per year, the blockade can last as long as four or more months each year. As a result of local government blockades, the market price of grain varies greatly from region to region.[29]

A Proposal for Food Policy Reform

The main problem with food policy in China arises from the combination of procurement practices and consumer prices. Because the sale price to consumers has changed little since the institution of a food-rationing system in 1953, the procurement price is thus strongly constrained by the sale price. Under this situation, an increase in procurement price means an increase in the government's subsidy. Because of the existence of a gap between the government-set procurement price and the market price, the government is confronted with a dilemma. If the government tries to make the procurement price as competitive as the market price, its financial burden becomes unbearable. If the government, on the other hand, attempts to limit the procurement price so that the amount of food subsidies can be controlled, a peasant's incentive to produce grain and to fulfill his or her quota obligations is impaired. Since individual households have been

27

given more autonomy in the production decision and the government's enforcement measures have been weakened as a result of the household responsibility system reform, the latter issue becomes particularly severe.

Low procurement prices also greatly limit the potential of exploiting regional comparative advantage in agricultural production. The gap between the market price and government-set price is an implicit tax. The more quota grain a region sells to the state, the more tax that region pays. As a consequence, no area is willing to increase the quota obligation. When the demand for food rations increases in an area due to economic development or to an increase in urban population, the area has to produce the grain itself. Local self-sufficiency has become a policy. All thirty provinces and thousands of counties in China are involved in the production of grain. Moreover, to make this tax contribution equitable, the procurement quota in an area is evenly assigned to each household.

Procurement price has to be low because the sale price of rationed grain to consumers is low. Unless the urban food-rationing policy is removed and the sale price of grain is liberated, the above-mentioned dilemma cannot be solved. The attempt to keep the grain price at a low level was justifiable in the 1950s because expenditure on grain alone represented in 1957 22.8 percent of total household expenditure for an average urban household. The share of grain expenditure in an urban household's total budget, however, declined to 7.6 percent in 1987.[30] Even though the sale price of grain has doubled, the expenditure on grain in an urban household's total budget should still not exceed 15 percent.

From the above discussion, we find that the obstacle to reforming the food-rationing policy does not arise from the urban dweller's inability to pay the market price of grain. The low-price food ration is, in fact, a vested interest of urban residents. It is a rule that a reform will not be supported by a group of people whose vested interests are weakened by the reform, even though the reform is beneficial to the economy as a whole and indirectly to this particular group of people. All workers in state enterprises and the majority of workers in the collective enterprises are entitled to food rations. Since over 90 percent of government income is obtained from the state and collective enterprises, the government is thus particularly conscious and protective of the support of workers. In addition, all cadres in the government system enjoy the same privilege. The government's reluctance to change the low-price food ration policy is, therefore, understandable.

A food policy reform, to be successful, should meet the following conditions: it should improve the welfare of the vested interest group directly; reduce the government's financial burden of food subsidies; and at the same time increase the farmer's incentive for producing grain. Such reform is possible.[31]

The low-price ration is not completely appreciated by the vested interest consumers. Since farmers treat the fulfillment of the obligatory quota as an obligation and the quota is prescribed in terms of quantity, to meet the obligation farmers tend to produce the kind of grain which has high yield but is of low quality. Consumer complaints over the quality of rationed grain are pervasive.

It is a well-known fact that the income elasticity of grain is very low.[32] Nevertheless, the income elasticity of high-quality grain differs greatly from the income elasticity of low-quality grain. According to a 1988 household survey in a city in southern China, the income elasticity of rice as a whole is −.02. Since the quality of rationed rice was poor, most households bought some high-quality grain in free markets. The income elasticity for the low-quality rationed grain is estimated to be −.99, while the income elasticity for the high-quality grain is estimated to be 1.36. Moreover, 22 percent of the surveyed households voluntarily gave up their grain ration privilege and bought only the market-priced, high-quality rice. The average income of this group of households was 13.5 percent higher than the income of the group of households which bought both the low-quality rationed rice and high-quality market rice. From the above survey, we find that it is possible to utilize the differences in the income elasticity between high-quality grain and low-quality grain as a way to reform the food-rationing policy.

The reform proposal is the following. The government guarantees the supply of a low-quality grain ration at a subsidized price as usual, but simultaneously provides high-quality grain at market prices. Urban dwellers are entitled to purchase as much of the low-quality grain at the subsidized ration price as before; however, they shall pay the full market price for the high-quality grain. The more they purchase the high-quality grain, the less the low-quality grain will be purchased. Since the government only subsidizes the low-quality grain, the greater the sale of high-quality grain, the less becomes the subsidy.

The income of urban dwellers will increase along with the development of the economy. As a consequence, there will be more demand for the high-quality grain and less for the low-quality grain. The government's grain subsidies will disappear when the demand for the low-quality grain is completely replaced by demand for the high-quality grain. On the procurement side, farmers still have to fulfill the quota obligation of low-quality grain at the previously set price as usual. This quantity, however, will be reduced gradually according to the changes in demand for low-quality grain from urban residents. As for high-quality grain, the price is determined by market demand and supply. Once urban demand for the subsidized low-quality grain disappears, the food policy reform is achieved. By that time, the price of grain for both producers and consumers will be completely determined by the demand and supply of the market. The role of government will be reduced to crisis relief and market stabilization by way of international trade and adjustments in domestic grain storage.

The above-outlined reform represents a Pareto-superior (i.e., optimizing) change for all parties concerned.[33] For urban residents, their original privilege in obtaining the food ration at a subsidized price is still protected. They are, nevertheless, under my proposal given one additional choice, namely to purchase high-quality grain. This choice increases their degree of freedom in making adjustments to their diets in accordance with changes in their income. For the government, the fiscal burden of the grain subsidy will be reduced, while food reforms are strengthened. The subsidy eventually will disappear when the development of the economy leads to the replacement of the demand for low-quality rationed grain by a demand for high-quality grain. For the farmers, the obligatory low-price quota will gradually disappear along with the grain ration. Grain production then will be increasingly determined by the market as the demand for high-quality grain increases.

This food policy reform is market-oriented. It is consistent with the overall direction of economic reform in China. The only drawback to this proposal is the time horizon. It may take quite a long time to complete this reform. However, if growth in the economy can be sustained at an annual rate of 7 percent, as is planned, the reform might be carried out in the space of a decade.

Concluding Remarks

China's experiences with agricultural development, both the successes and the failures, provide many valuable lessons for other developing countries. It is remarkable that China has been able to use only one-fifteenth of the world's arable land to feed over one-fifth of the world's population. China, however, paid a very high price for this achievement prior to the 1979 reform. The collective farming system was detrimental to work incentives. Regional comparative advantages, an important element in agricultural development, were also lost, because the low-price compulsory procurement system required that each region become self-sufficient in grain. Therefore, despite sharp increases in modern inputs to farming in the 1960s and 1970s, grain production in China was barely able to keep up with population growth.

The individual household-based farming system reform in 1979 greatly improved a peasant's incentives. Agriculture as well as grain production registered unprecedented growth between 1979 and 1984. However, the increase in work incentives derived from the household-based reform was a one-time, discrete jump and had become depleted by 1984. Compared to the agricultural growth rates in other developed as well as developing countries, the average growth rate of 3.5 percent per year in 1984–88 is, indeed, quite remarkable. Grain production in China, however, has stagnated after reaching a peak in 1984. This stagnation is mainly due to the fact that reform in food policy lagged behind the reform in farming institutions. Individual households were given more autonomy to produce after the household responsibility system was instituted. Peasants began to allocate greater resources to the crops which command higher profits. After the household responsibility system reform took effect, the markets of most crops had been decontrolled. Grain is among the exceptions. Farmers are still required to meet the grain quota obligations at government-set prices. In addition, local governments still can impose blockades on grain markets. The result is to reduce grain prices in areas with comparative advantage in producing grain. The stagnation of grain production in the postreform period, contrasted with a sizable growth of agriculture as a whole, therefore, can be attributed to the decline in the profitability of grain as compared to the profitability of other crops.

Most people in China, including political leaders and economists, assign grain the top priority. With the stagnation in grain production, optimism about Chinese agriculture quickly shifted to pessimism. The small size of farms and the fragmentation of cultivated land under the household-based farming system are often wrongly blamed for the poor performance of grain production after 1984. In the name of pursuing economies of scale in agricultural production, some areas have begun to recollectivize and replace the household-based farming system. This practice is especially appealing to some government officials because it makes easy the fulfillment of the obligatory grain procurement requirement. Market-oriented reform in China is, therefore, at a crossroad.

The ultimate way to break out of the stagnation in grain production is to allow agricultural prices to communicate the right signal to farmers. As long as the grain price yields farmers the same competitive profits as the prices of other crops, household-based farmers in China will be able to produce enough grain to feed China's population. This requires, however, a market-oriented food policy reform.

In this paper I have proposed utilizing the differences in the income elasticity between high-quality and low-quality grain as a way to introduce this reform. This approach will not only increase the welfare of urban consumers and rural producers but also reduce the government's burden of costly food subsidies. The success of a market-oriented reform in a socialist economy, however, depends more on the determination of political leaders than on the wisdom of economists.

Notes

1. World population and China's population in 1986 were 4.916 billion and 1.051 billion, respectively, while the arable lands were respectively 13.76 billion hectares and 0.96 billion hectares. See State Statistical Bureau, *Zhongguo Tongji Nianjian, 1988* (China Statistical Yearbook, 1988) (Beijing: China Statistics Press, 1988), 993–94.

2. Cultivated land and population were 97.9 million hectares and 541.7 million, respectively, in 1949, and 99.4 million hectares and 962.2 million in 1978.

3. The official exchange rate was 3.58 yuan/dollar in 1950 and 1.72 yuan/dollar in 1978. See James T. H. Tsao, *China's Development Strategies and Foreign Trade* (Lexington, Massachusetts: Lexington Books, 1987), 156–57.

4. See State Statistical Bureau, *Guominshouru Tongji Ziliao Huibian* (A Compilation of National Income Statistical Data) (Beijing: China Statistics Press, 1987), 11.

5. See Joan Robinson, "Chinese Agricultural Communes," *Co-Existence* (May 1964), 1–7. Reprinted in Charles K. Wilber, ed., *The Political Economy of Development and Underdevelopment* (New York: Random House, 1973), 209–15.

6. This political wisdom is captured in an often-cited motto, "Wu nong bu wen" (Without a strong agriculture, the society will not be stable).

7. In China both the general public and most economists often regard grain as constituting the entire sector of agriculture. Despite a respectable growth rate for agriculture as a whole in the past four years, agriculture is widely regarded as stagnant and declining as a result of the grain situation.

8. *Zhongguo Tongji Nianjian, 1987*, 89; and *Guominshouru Tongji Ziliao Huibian*, 11.

9. In addition to grain, edible oils, pork, and sugar are included under rationing.

10. See *Zhongguo Tongji Nianjian, 1988*, 97.

11. Agricultural products alone in 1953 represented 55.7 percent of the total value of China's exports with another 25.9 percent consisting of processed agricultural products. Up to the mid-1970s, agricultural and processed agricultural products represented over 70 percent of the total value of exports. See Editorial Board of the Almanac of China's Foreign Economic Relations and Trade, *Almanac of China's Foreign Economic Relations and Trade, 1986* (Beijing: Zhongguo Zhanwang Press, 1986), 954.

12. This argument is clearly supported by the fact that the heavy-industry-oriented development strategy had to temporarily give way to the "agricultural-first-strategy" after the harvest failures caused by the collectivization in the late 1950s.

13. Luo Hanxian, *Economic Changes in Rural China* (Beijing: New World Press, 1985), 53.

14. Ibid., 59.

15. The commonly accepted explanations for this crisis were bad weather, poor management, and the disincentives of working in the commune. If these explanations were the main causes of this crisis, agricultural productivity should have returned to the pre-crisis level by 1962 or shortly thereafter because the size of the production unit was reduced to the pre-crisis level after 1962. However, the total factor productivity in Chinese agriculture in 1962 was less than three-quarters of the 1957 level and remained at that low level until the early 1980s. These explanations can thus be rejected. An explanation consistent with empirical evidence was the

switch in 1958 from voluntary to compulsory collectivization. Because of the difficulty in supervising agricultural work, the success of an agricultural collective depends on a self-enforcing contract of self-discipline, which can only be sustained as a repeated game. The nature of the collective farm was changed from a repeated game to a one-time game when the principle of the collective movement was changed from volunteerism to compulsion. As a result, the self-enforcing contract could not be sustained and agricultural productivity collapsed. See Justin Yifu Lin, "Collectivization and China's Agricultural Crisis in 1959–1961," Working Paper 89-01 (Beijing: The Development Institute, RCRD, 1989).

16. For a formal theoretical model and empirical testing of the above argument, see Justin Yifu Lin, "The Household Responsibility System in China's Agricultural Reform: A Theoretical and Empirical Study," *Economic Development and Cultural Change* 36 (April 1988): 199–224.

17. It was found recently that a village in Guizhou Province had adopted this practice secretly more than ten years prior to the recent reform. The villagers did not dare to admit it until the new policy was announced. See Du Runsheng, *China's Rural Economic Reform* (Beijing: Social Science Press, 1985), 15.

18. The policy changes were proposed in the Third Plenary session of the 11th Central Committee of the Communist Party of China, held in December 1978. The session adopted the "Decisions of the Central Committee of the Communist Party of China on Some Questions Concerning the Acceleration of Agricultural Development (Draft)." The draft was promulgated nine months later in September 1979 by the Fourth Plenary Session of the CPC Central Committee. For the text of the decision, see the Editorial Committee on the Agricultural Yearbook of China, *Zhongguo Nongye Nianjian, 1980* (China Agriculture Yearbook, 1980) (Beijing: Agriculture Press), 56–62.

19. See Justin Yifu Lin, "The Household Responsibility System in China's Agricultural Reform: A Theoretical and Empirical Study."

20. See Justin Yifu Lin, "The Household Responsibility System Reform and the Adoption of Hybrid Rice in China," Working Paper 89-02 (Beijing: The Development Institute, RCRD, 1989).

21. See Justin Yifu Lin, "The Household Responsibility System in China's Rural Reform," forthcoming in *Proceedings of the XX International Conference of Agricultural Economists*.

22. The other two-thirds of the output growth is attributable mainly to increases in inputs.

23. For example, the procurement price of rice in 1986, compared to 1953, increased 128.7 percent. The ration price of grain, however, only increased 9.4 percent in the same period.

24. The total amount of the basic quota was 36 million tons in 1965–67. It dropped to 35 million tons in 1979 and to 30.3 million tons in 1982–84.

25. The procurement price is a weighted average price of the basic quota price and the above-quota price, the weight being the share of above-quota grain in the total grain sold to the government.

26. The subsidy per 50 kg of grain sold at the government-set ration price was 2.65 yuan in 1965, 3.22 yuan in 1970, 3.56 yuan in 1978, 7.83 yuan in 1979, 15.11 yuan in 1984, and 18.67 yuan in 1987.

27. *Zhongguo Tongji Nianjian, 1988*, 763.

28. The amounts purchased on the market were 19.64 million tons in 1985, 32.32 million tons in 1986, and 42.28 million tons in 1987, which were respectively 17.0 percent of the total procurement in 1985, 24.0 percent in 1986, and 30.0 percent in 1987.

29. For example, in December 1988, the market price of rice in the five rice-surplus provinces, Jiangsu, Jiangxi, Anhui, Hunan, and Hubei, was 1,161 yuan per ton, while in the three rice-deficit provinces, Guangdong, Guangxi, and Fujian, the price was 1,839 yuan per ton.

30. *Zhongguo Tongji Nianjian, 1986*, 668; and *1988*, 807.

31. The following discussion draws on a policy proposal made to the government in the spring of 1988, and on a paper by Justin Yifu Lin and Cai Fang, "The Good Quality Grain: A Proposal for Food Policy Reform," *Jingji Yanjiu* (Economic Research Monthly), no. 6 (1988): 12–16.

32. The income elasticity of a commodity is the percentage change of a commodity purchased by a consumer with respect to the consumer's percentage change in income. It measures how a consumer's demand for a commodity varies with respect to the change in his income. For example, if a commodity's income elasticity is $-.1$, a 10 percent increase in income will result in a 1 percent decline in the demand for that commodity.

33. Pareto-superior change means that the proposed change will at least increase the welfare of certain members but bring no harm to the rest.

Readings

Du Runsheng. 1985. *China's Rural Economic Reform*. Beijing: Social Science Press.

Editorial Board of the Almanac of China's Foreign Economic Relations and Trade. 1986. *Almanac of China's Foreign Economic Relations and Trade, 1986*. Beijing: Zhongguo Zhanwang Press.

Editorial Committee on the Agricultural Yearbook of China. 1980. *Zhongguo Nongye Nianjian, 1980*. Beijing: Agriculture Press.

Lin, Justin Yifu. 1988. "The Household Responsibility System in China's Agricultural Reform: A Theoretical and Empirical Study." *Economic Development and Cultural Change* 36 (April supplement): 199–224.

———. 1989. "The Household Responsibility System Reform and the Adoption of Hybrid Rice in China." Working Paper 89-02. Beijing: The Development Institute, RCRD.

———. Forthcoming. "Collectivization and China's Agricultural Crisis in 1959–1961." *Journal of Political Economy*.

———. Forthcoming. "The Household Responsibility System in China's Rural Reform," in *Proceedings of the XX International Conference of Agricultural Economists*.

Lin, Justin Yifu, and Cai Fang. 1988. "The Good Quality Grain: A Proposal for Food Policy Reform." *Jingji Yanjiu* (Economic Research Monthly), no. 6: 12–16.

Luo Hanxian. 1985. *Economic Changes in Rural China*. Beijing: New World Press.

Robinson, Joan. 1964. "Chinese Agricultural Communes." *Co-Existence* (May): 1-7. Reprinted in Charles K. Wilber, ed. 1973. *The Political Economy of Development and Underdevelopment*. New York: Random House.

State Statistical Bureau. *Guominshouru Tongji Ziliao Huibian* (A Compilation of National Income Statistical Data). Beijing: China Statistics Press, 1981 to 1988.

———. *Zhongguo Tongji Nianjian* (China Statistical Yearbook). Beijing: China Statistics Press, 1981 to 1988.

Tsao, James T. H. 1987. *China's Development Strategies and Foreign Trade*. Lexington, Massachusetts: Lexington Books.

CHAPTER 3

Evolution and Diffusion of Agricultural Technology in China

Bruce Stone
Project Director for Chinese Research, International Food Policy Research Institute, Washington, D.C.

The diffusion of technological innovation in agriculture involves transfers across national boundaries, among regions within countries, and among subgroups and population strata. For the process to reach all farmers and potential beneficiaries of farming technology, diffusion along each of these paths is necessary. Focusing on the People's Republic of China, this paper examines progress in diffusing the most critical elements of staple foodcrop technology.

Innovation affecting agriculture is not limited to agricultural techniques but also includes improvements in organization to facilitate their use, extending the range of beneficiaries, and ensuring the sustainability and stability of the entire process. The paper reviews fundamental changes during the 1980s in China's economic organization and the interactive effects on technological change in the staple foodcrop sector. New agricultural technology involves an array of innovations, and discussion, therefore, has to focus on critical subcategories. The definition of what is critical depends upon national objectives, factor proportions, and the stage of development within a particular country. For China, identification is rendered more complex by its size and geographic diversity.

The first section of the paper places the elements of innovation in a theoretical framework. The second section focuses on China's progress

Financial support for the research on which the article is based comes primarily from the International Food Policy Research Institute and the Rockefeller Foundation. Wang Sangui, of the Agricultural Economics Institute, Chinese Academy of Agricultural Sciences, assisted with data collection.

overall in diffusing the most fundamental technical components for the first stage of agricultural transformation and food consumption development. The third section tracks during the last decade the diffusion process for these components within China's 29 provinces and major municipal areas, and then within China's poorest and most remote counties.

The fourth section reviews economic system reform in China and its implications for the diffusion process. The fifth section identifies several areas of applied scientific research related to agriculture, state-of-the-art farmer practices for which China is a principal source of innovation, and discusses the primary mechanisms of diffusion. The final section summarizes the main arguments.

Two Stages of Food Consumption Development and Technological Transformation of Agriculture

The key elements of an agriculturally based strategy of economic development were identified between the mid-1950s and the mid-1970s.[1] Among the elements associated with agricultural development in developing countries in Asia, only three have been indispensable to rapid and prolonged growth in yields at the initial stage: improved water control; abundant supplies of fertilizer; and high-yielding seed varieties responsive to these inputs.[2] The introduction of one or more of these normally provides some growth in average yields, yet much greater returns accrue when all three are applied appropriately. These are the fundamental ingredients of the "Green Revolution," which have provided rapid growth in cereal yields throughout most of Asia and elsewhere in the developing world.

The principal criteria for judging technical change at the initial stage of modern agricultural development in a large but land-scarce peasant economy include yield growth of principal staple foodcrops, and various indicators relating to the three fundamental inputs. The latter includes growth in irrigated area, multiple cropping, capacity of irrigation and drainage machinery in use, fertilizer use, and area sown with high-yielding and early-maturing staple crop varieties.

Should yield growth greatly exceed the growth in these input indicators, it might be concluded that factors other than technical change were at work. Should yield growth fall short of what might be expected from the pace of technical progress, the quality of the inputs, the efficiency or allocative coordination of their use, the strength of the back-up systems, and other factors may be examined to explain the deficiency. Finally, the adequacy of the pace of technical progress and yields in terms of China's development strategy may be evaluated by examining the growth of production per capita nationally, and for greater detail, the growth in rural-to-urban marketing per urban resident, and in production per agricultural laborer.

It may be argued that China during the last decade or so has entered a second stage of agricultural development, which may be defined in a number of ways. One may focus, for example, on the levels of per capita supply of basic staple crops. In Asian agricultural economies, when aggregate staple crop production per capita reaches around 300 kilograms per capita per year, emphasis on improvements in quality and diversity of diet increasingly displaces concentration on elevating calorie intake by the most readily available means.[3]

Agricultural requirements of the second stage of food consumption development in a poor land-scarce economy include: rapidly rising yields of a wide variety of nonstaple crops and a rapid increase in the production of livestock products. Although direct consumption of staple foodcrops will not increase as fast as income in the second stage, and will eventually decline, the need for continued rapid growth in staple crop yields is greater than ever. Several conditions characterize this stage: 1) supplying calories via livestock products requires much greater quantities of feedgrains than the foodgrains displaced; 2) adequate supplies are required to cover population growth and increases in consumption levels among the poor, which depends on continued rapid growth in aggregate production; 3) a larger proportion of farmland will have to be allocated to nonstaple crops; and 4) acceleration in nonfarm employment associated with the second stage normally will be accompanied by a reduction in cultivated area and/or multiple cropping, particularly on lands near cities and towns; in a peasant economy, this involves high-quality land. As Figure 3–1 indicates, Asian countries, in particular socialist countries, tend to increase direct staple crop consumption even after high-average levels have been reached.

Figure 3–2 summarizes the two stages of food consumption and technical transformation. It indicates there has to be increasing emphasis on other criteria, particularly when the second stage of food consumption development coincides with a second stage of technical transformation. Entry into the latter may be defined as the point at which increases in efficiency and quality of the three critical inputs become more important, more feasible, or more cost effective than continued growth in their gross supply.[4]

This is the context in which technological progress for Chinese agriculture in the 1980s and 1990s must be viewed. This paper, however, concentrates on the first-stage indicators that are so important in the effort to increase the consumption of basic staple crops to adequate levels: namely, water control; high-yielding seed varieties; and chemical fertilizer. Despite high-average per capita grain consumption levels, and the entry of the more advanced areas of the country into the second stage of food

Figure 3–1.

International Cross-Section Relationship between per Capita Grain Consumption per Year, and per Capita Calorie Intake per Day of All Food

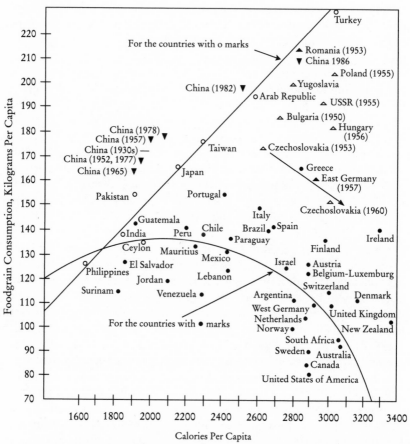

Calories Per Capita

Notes: The figures for per capita foodgrain consumption are calculated as the sum of the weights of processed foodgrains consumed directly by humans, and one-fourth the weight of root and tuber crops. To conform with other international data, the entries for China omit soybean consumption and have reevaluated root and tuber crops from one-fifth to one-fourth natural weight. Consumption per capita of foodgrains in Chinese data includes rice and millet at "trade grain" weight (partially processed paddy and millet weight). Rice has been converted to processed weights according to FAO convention at the time the international data were published (67.5 percent paddy weight). The 1982 calorie figure is calculated from the most authoritative data base yet generated in China, by the country's premier nutrition research organization, although estimation procedures have not been reviewed in detail for possible biases. The international data are for 1965 unless otherwise specified.

Sources: Bruce Stone, "China's 1985 Foodgrain Production Target: Issues and Prospects," in *Food Production in the People's Republic of China*, Anthony M. Tang and Bruce Stone, Research Report no.15 (Washington, D.C.: IFPRI, 1980), 93. For China, the 1982 and 1986 figures have been added and the 1952–78 figures have been recalculated on the basis of population and consumption per capita figures in ZGTJNJ 1987, 89 and 711, adjusted population data in ZGTJZY 1988, 14, and crop production data in ZGTJNJ 1987, 170. It was assumed that 50 percent of soybean production (average of cited and previous year) were included in SSB foodgrain consumption per capita figure, on the basis of Alan Piazza, *Trends in Foodgrain and Nutrient Availability in China 1950–81*, World Bank Staff Working Paper no. 607 (Washington, D.C.: The World Bank, 1983). Seventy percent of root and tuber crops in 1978 are assumed included in the SSB direct foodgrain consumption figure and 80 percent for previous years, for the purpose of recalculating foodgrain equivalents; these were adjusted to 50 percent for sweet potatoes and 60 percent for white potatoes in 1982 and 1986 on the basis of Charles Gitomer and Bruce Stone, "Sweet Potato and White Potato Development in China," a paper prepared for the International Potato Center, IFPRI, Washington, D.C., November 1, 1988. The 1982 average calorie consumption figure (2485 kcal) is based on nutritional material collected with the 1982 census and calculated by the Chinese Academy of Preventive Medicine; provided to author by Dr. Chen Chunming, President, May 1986 and confirmed June 9, 1988, Beijing. Calories not accounted for among the SSB data categories are assumed to derive from liquor, dairy products, fruits, vegetables, and other miscellaneous categories. Estimates for other years for these categories are indexed against the 1982 residual figure.

consumption development, the first-stage indicators remain relevant to less advantaged Chinese localities. This is due to the barriers in factor and product markets even more inhibiting in China than in most developing countries.[5] Thus the first question the paper addresses is the extent to which Chinese farmers throughout the country are participating in the fundamental processes of the "Green Revolution."

Progress in Water Control, Use of Fertilizer, and High-Yielding Varieties

China's performance with first-stage requirements for rapid agricultural transformation has been discussed in detail elsewhere[6] and requires no more than a brief summary here.

Water Control Development

Irrigated area increased rapidly during the 1950s and 1960s, partly based on recovery of operating systems built in the 1930s, and partly on new initiatives, both locally financed small-scale construction and nationally and

Figure 3 – 2.

Objectives, Critical Components, and Requirements for the First and Second Stages of Agricultural Technical Transformation and Food Consumption Development in Land-Scarce Peasant Economies

Stage	Principal Objectives	Critical Technical Components	Principal Success Indicators	Institutional Needs
First Stage of Technical and Food Consumption Development	↑Staple crop yields ↑Staple crop production per capita	– Water Control – Staple crop HYVs – Fertilizer use – Early maturing varieties[1] – Cultural practices	↑Staple crop yields ↑Staple production per capita ↑Irrigated area ↑Flood control area ↑Capacity of irrigation and drainage equipment ↑High- and stable-yield area ↑Multiple cropping index ↑Fertilizer application ↑Area under HYVs	– Water engineering contruction organization – Local water distribution authorities – Fertilizer distribution network – Seed production, distribution, and extension system – Agricultural research system – System for input purchase financing – Staple crop purchasing system – Some transport, power, educational, and statistical system infrastructure
Second Stage of Technical Transformation and Food Consumption Development	– Same as first state; and ↑Yields and production per capita of non-staples ↑Production per capita and efficiency in livestock sector	– Same as first state; and – Stress-tolerant staple crop varieties – Nonstaple crop HYVs – Higher quality varieties – Weed control	– Same as first state; and ↑Nonstaple crop yields ↓Feedgrain/meat, milk, egg output conversion ratios ↑Completion of ancillary facilities on irrigation projects ↑Within-project distribution of water ↑On-farm water management ↑Balance of fertilizer nutrients ↓Nitrogen losses	– Same as first stage; and – Farmer water management organization – Soil testing and fertilizer trial network – Meteorology network – Sophisticated statistical system – Agricultural education system – Animal breeding and weight station network – Machine parts supply and repair network

↓Labor per unit of staple crop production	– Pest and disease control for crops and livestock – Improved livestock breeds – Better livestock management – Animal nutrition – Mechanization	– Transport infrastructure – Communications infrastructure – Rural power – General education – Rural motor vehicle stocks – Fuel supply network – Rural credit – Fertilizer stock management and facilities – Farm product stock management and facilities – Others	↑Geographic distribution of fertilizers ↑On-farm analysis of nutrient needs ↑Farm chemical use ↑Biological control of pests and diseases ↑Seed breeding for local environments ↑Experimental yields of new HYVs ↑Mechanization ↑Fuel use for farm tasks ↓Labor application to farming	– Fuel supply network – Others
Market-Related Technical Change Associated with Second Stage	– Prevent local or temporary demand constraints from lowering supply growth and pace of technical change – Allocative efficiency for inputs to food production process			

Note: [1] China's considerable breeding concentration on early-maturing varieties is not duplicated elsewhere, but is a typical extension of land- and capital-scarce, labor-abundant factor proportions. (↑) denotes increase; (↓) denotes decrease.

Source: Bruce Stone, "Developments in Agricultural Technology," *The China Quarterly*, Special Issue on Food and Agriculture in China During the Post-Mao Period, no. 116 (December 1988): 768–770

Table 3-1.

Basic Indicators of Water Control Development, 1952–88, in Million Hectares (mill. ha), Kilowatts (kw), and Kilowatt Hours (kwh)

Years	Effectively Irrigated Area[a] Total	Power-Irrigated Area Share	High & Stable Yield Area[b]	Multiple Cropping Index[c]	Number of Tubewells Total	Number of Tubewells Outfitted	Small Hydropower Stations in Rural Areas Nos.	Small Hydropower Stations Generating Capacity	Electricity Consumed in Rural Areas[d]	Motors for Agricultural Drainage and Irrigation	
	(mill. ha)	(percent)	(mill. ha)		(1000 units)		(units)	(1000 kw)	(100 mill. kwh)	(1000 units)	(100 mill. watts)
1952	19.959	1.6	–	130.9[c]	–	–	98	8	0.5	–	0.9
1957	27.339	4.4	–	140.6	–	–	544	20	1.4	40	4.1
1962	30.545	19.9	–	136.3	–	–	7,436	252	16.1	367	45.2
1965	33.055	24.5	25-30	138.3	100	–	–	–	37.1	558	66.7
1970	36.000	41.6	–	141.9	–	–	29,202	709	95.7	1,471	134.2
1971	36.441	45.6	–	144.7	590	–	40,040	817	104.5	1,640	146.0
1972	38.005	46.9	–	147.0	800	–	47,227	902	132.8	2,078	181.3
1973	39.223	50.4	33	148.2	1200	–	52,765	1,060	139.9	2,880	254.6
1974	41.269	52.5	34	148.8	1600	–	61,378	1,277	156.1	3,422	300.6
1975	43.284	52.9	34	150.0	1700	–	68,164	1,445	183.1	3,891	357.9
1976	44.981	53.9	–	150.6	1800	–	74,125	1,610	204.8	4,262	398.4
1977	44.999	54.1	–	150.5	–	–	79,047	1,868	221.9	4,695	441.6
1978	44.965	55.4	22[f]	151.0	2300	–	82,387	2,284	253.1	5,026	482.3
1979	45.003	56.3	f	149.2	–	2100	83,224	2,763	282.7	5,384	523.8
1980	44.888	56.4	f	147.4	2599	2089	80,319	3,041	320.8	5,630	549.0
1981	44.574	56.6	–	146.6	–	2081	74,017	3,360	369.9	5,672	551.5
1982	44.177	56.9	–	146.8	2621	2095	66,256	3,530	396.9	5,803	564.1
1983	44.644	56.6	32.771	146.4	2621	2410	62,328	3,463	435.2	6,077	577.3
1984	44.453	56.4	33.038	147.4	2675	2400	60,062	3,615	464.0	6,150	577.7
1985	44.036	55.9	32.871	148.3	2628	2370	55,754	3,802	508.9	6,163	575.5
1986	44.226	56.6	33.155	149.9	2674	2364	54,136	3,879	586.7	6,507	604.4

| 1987 | 44.403 | 24.825 | 55.9 | — | 151.2 | 2623 | 2371 | 51,978 | 3,941 | 658.8 | 6,839 | 625.8 |
| 1988 | 44.376 | 26.083 | 58.8 | 33.571 | 151.3 | 2732 | — | 51,558 | 4,611 | 712.0 | 7,508 | 656.8 |

Notes: [a] *Youxiao guangai* defined as "level land which has water sources and complete sets of irrigation facilities to lift and move adequate water for irrigation purposes under normal conditions" (ZGTJNJ 1981, 521–22). Power-irrigated area includes area serviced by electric and fuel-injection facilities. Share of irrigated area with power facilities within total irrigated area are provided in the third column.

[b] "Fields with stable and high yields despite drought or excess surface water" (*han lao baoshou gaochan wenzhen tian*) are normally expected to have adequate facilities to withstand a once-in-ten-year drought or flood without crop damage. In some places, the requirements are more stringent. In Guangdong, 100-day drought resistance capability is required. Fields so designated are also supposed to surpass National Agricultural Development Program targets ranging from 3 to 6 tons/ha for major foodgrains, depending on the region.

[c] (Sown area / cultivated area) × 100. Cultivated area and the MCI have not appeared in major publicly distributed State Statistical Bureau compendia during most of the 1980s. During the early 1980s, the Bureau was reported to be considering upward revision of the 1986–87 cultivated area figure from less than 100 mha to "2 billion mu" (133.3 mha) or to "14 percent of total land area" (134.4 mha), based on revised analysis of satellite imagery which had provided an original estimate of around 150 million hectares. While methodological problems remain with satellite-based estimates, the idea that official cultivated area figures are substantial underestimates is widely shared in technical circles. Detailed aerial surveys of two counties in Jilin and Beijing, for example, showed cultivated area underestimated in official data by 7.6 percent and 25.8 percent, respectively. *Guangming ribao* has quoted Wang Xianjin, director of the State Land Administration Bureau, as giving 120 mha and 126.6 mha as cultivated area figures for 1987–88. The larger would be more or less consistent with the satellite-based estimate for 1980–81 and subsequent retirements. The official data, nevertheless, are occasionally published in Chinese books and articles, including the 1988 and 1989 Statistical Yearbooks. The MCIs are calculated from these questionable data and the somewhat more reliable sown area figures published by the SSB.

[d] Includes electricity provided by state power grid as well as by rural power stations, excluding electricity consumed by state-owned units located in rural areas.

[e] 133.5 as recalculated to correct for underreporting of cultivated area (Thomas B. Wiens, "Agricultural Statistics in the People's Republic of China," in *Quantitative Measures of China's Economic Output*, ed. Alexander Eckstein [Ann Arbor: University of Michigan Press, 1980]).

[f] The implied decline relative to the mid-1970s may reflect a tightening of standards or improved statistical precision rather than an actual deterioration in facilities. It is significant that there was severe drought on the North China Plain in 1977 and 1978, which may have revealed the inadequacy of facilities throughout the region. In 1979 HSYA was described as approximately that of 1978, and in 1980 as "half China's irrigated area of 700 million mu" (literally 23.3 million ha) and "less than one-fourth of the total cultivated land" (<24.8 mha).

Source: Bruce Stone, "Developments in Agricultural Technology," *The China Quarterly*, Special Issue on Food and Agriculture in China During the Post-Mao Period, no. 116 (December 1988): 772–73. Transcription errors appearing in the original publication have been corrected and data for 1988 and (for tubewells) for 1987 have been added on the basis of Zhongguo guojia tongjiu [State Statistical Bureau of China], *Zhongguo tongji nianjian 1989* [Statistical Yearbook of China 1989] (Beijing: Zhongguo guojia tongjiu, 1989), 174, 175, 184, and 192 (hereafter ZGTJNJ 1989) and ZGTJNJ 1988 (English edition), 188 and 206.

provincially financed larger-scale surface structures. Following setbacks in the early 1960s resulting from poor design and construction of a portion of the late 1950s' projects, irrigation development resumed with further reservoir construction and a major focus on tubewells.

These efforts facilitated the multiple cropping increases of the 1950s (see Table 3-1) centered in rice growing areas, and those of the 1970s, which provided for the rapid expansion of overwintering wheat on the North China Plain. Flood control and drainage efforts were similarly significant. These initiatives contributed to the establishment and expansion of high and stable yields guaranteed against drought and waterlogging.

During the 1980s, however, growth in effectively irrigated area stagnated, as did the proportion with pumping facilities. The multiple cropping index declined, recovering only between 1986 and 1989. High- and stable-yield area seems to have dropped sharply in the late 1970s, regaining but not surpassing the 1972–74 levels by the late 1980s.

A major part of the decline in high- and stable-yield area, and the lesser decline in irrigated area and multiple cropping, seems to involve corrections for exaggerated statistical claims of the 1970s. Another part represents rational adjustment correcting for economically irrational growth in the cropping index.[7] Yet there is no question that Chinese agriculture in the 1980s lost the important assistance of rapid growth in these indicators. An important question to be addressed in section III is that of the implications of this stagnation for technical change in poorer regions and localities.

Diffusion of HYV Seed
Characteristic of the 1950s were ambitious and well-oriented programs that imported desirable varieties from abroad and that selected attractive local cultivars for rapid dissemination on a provincial basis, while at the same time establishing a national network for breeding, testing, producing, and disseminating high-yielding varieties (HYVs). Some of the tasks were executed in a haphazard and overhasty fashion, and analytic and basic research had a weak theoretical base, which may have combined to produce or accelerate disasters. But the 1950s represented for China a large, if unsteady, first step in rapid varietal transformation.

During the 1960s and 1970s, excesses in management practices were considerably reduced, though not eliminated. The scientific community suffered from isolation and, to some extent, harassment, but China's own varietal breeding community became a formidable scientific force. The breeding of new varieties with superior traits was very strong, and the speed with which new varieties were tested and adapted to local environments was especially rapid. The system grew to be highly sophisticated for wheat and rice in China's major growing regions.

Table 3–2.

Area Sown with Hybrid Rice, Maize, Sorghum, and Semi-Dwarf Wheat and Rice, 1955–90

| | Area Under True Hybrids | | | Area Under All Dwarf and Semi-dwarf Varieties | |
	Maize	Sorghum	Rice	Rice (<100cm)	Wheat (<105cm)
	(percent of total area planted with crop)				
1955-59	a			a	a
1961	(20-40)			a	
1962	(0-20)[b]				
1964			c	c	
1965				14	d
1966	~40[b]				
1968				f	e
1971		20		f	
1973	40		f		g
1974				80	
1976			0.4		
1977		40	6.2	80	h
1978	60		12.6		
1979	65	55	14.9		
1980	69	57	13.9[i]		
1981	72	60	15.4	f	
1982	75	60	17.0		
1983			20.3		
1984			26.7	~56	(67-75)
1985			26.4	95	
1986		90	28.3		
1987			~34.0[j]		
1988	~90[k]				
1989	(86-91)[k]		(40-41)[j]		
1990	(89-94)[k] (plan)		(46-47)[j]		

~ = estimated value
cm = height in centimeters at maturity

Notes: [a] Experimental breeding work on semi-dwarf rice began in the early 1950s, but the first cross between dwarf and high-yielding varieties was accomplished in 1956. Semi-dwarf indica varieties were grown as an early crop in South China in the late 1950s; the first short stature japonica varieties (Nongken #58) were introduced in North China in 1957. The first semi-dwarfs were developed in China by cross breeding in 1959 (Guang Changai) and released in 1961. Experimental breeding work on semi-dwarf wheat varieties was initiated during the late 1950s. Chinese work on hybrid maize began in 1923 and double-cross hybrids were first released in Sichuan 1943-45. Work resumed throughout the

1950s in several institutions from which double-cross hybrids were released in 1958.

b Double-cross hybrids were decimated by corn blight in 1961 and 1966; total maize area declined by around 20 percent in 1962, presumably primarily in disease-affected hybrid areas; double-cross extension dropped after 1966; single-cross hybrids initially extended in 1966.

c Work on hybrid rice and broad-scale dissemination of semi-dwarf rice varieties initiated. Short stature (non-hybrid) indica varieties released in South China in 1963.

d First Chinese-bred (100 cm) variety of eventual commercial importance (Beijing #10).

e Dwarf wheats imported for the Chinese breeding program from Pakistan and elsewhere in 1968, 1969, and the early 1970s; the first Chinese-bred variety under 90 cm of eventual commercial importance (Fan #6) was bred.

f Cyctoplasmic male sterile, maintainer, and restorer lines necessary for producing hybrid seed developed 1970–73. IRRI's IR#8 was first planted in China 1968 and eventually used as restorer line for hybrid rice breeding; 3,335 varieties and advanced lines provided to China by International Rice Research Institute between 1971 and 1981.

g Large quantities of dwarf wheat seed imported from Mexico for direct planting 1972–74; maximum sown area reached 800,000 hectares, then declined sharply due to environmental stresses not problematic in Mexico; subsequent emphasis turned to Chinese-Chinese or Chinese-foreign crosses except in a few western regions.

h Chinese crosses with imported Mexican varieties and other Chinese-bred semi-dwarfs were sown throughout main winter wheat producing areas, and on 2 million hectares (~ 40 percent of national spring wheat area) in the northeast spring wheat region.

i Hybrid area was cut back in principal growing area (lower Yangzi Valley) due to susceptibility to yellow dwarf virus and discovery that in some localities increased hybrid yields did not compensate for losses on alternate crops as the maturation period for hybrid was normally longer than the crop it replaced. Rapid growth resumed in subsequent years with aggressive extension of new subtropical hybrids in South China (especially Guangdong and Sichuan). Some japonica hybrids were already extended in 1979-80: 43,000 hectares, with Liyou #57. These were not always successful and the total area under all japonica hybrids declined to 33,300 hectares in 1981. But more suitable varieties were developed and by 1986, 261,000 hectares were planted with japonica hybrids.

j Another large expansion of hybrid area in 1987; total reached "one-third" of China's rice area. Area increased 95 percent over the previous five years to almost 11 million hectares. Hybrid area grown as early rice grew substantially as new varieties proved superior to non-hybrids up to 30°N, compared with previous hybrids limited to 23°N. Better single-season hybrids for highland areas (especially Xianyou #63, up to 1,500 m) also extended, especially in the South, accounting for more large increases in hybrid area in Yunnan, Guizhou, and mountainous areas of other southern provinces. Planned hybrid area for 1990 is 15 million hectares, 1.9 million more than 1989.

k According to Chinese maize scientists attending the Colloquium on Agricultural Reform and Development, October 18–19, 1989, around 80 percent of maize area is covered with HYVs bred via the single-cross hybridization process popularized in the late 1960s; 5 percent with HYVs bred via the double-cross process used primarily in the late 1950s and most of the 1960s; and 5 percent with HYVs bred via a newer triple-cross hybridization process. Eighteen million hectares of hybrids are planned for 1990, reportedly 600,000 hectares more than 1989.

Sources: For complete references, see Bruce Stone, "Developments in Agricultural Technology," *The China Quarterly*, Special Issue on Food and Agriculture in China During the Post-Mao Period, no. 116 (December 1988): 792–94, as updated and amended with data appearing in Zhongguo nongxuyuyebu jihuaju [Chinese Ministry of Agriculture, Animal Husbandry and Fisheries, Planning Dept.], *Nongye jingji ziliao, 1949–1983* [Economic

Materials on Agriculture, 1949–1983] (Beijing: Ministry of Agriculture), 285 (hereafter NYJJZL); Li Meisen and Zhao Lijian, "National Conference on Hybrid Rice Development," *Agricultural Yearbook of China 1988*, 95–96; comments provided by Chinese maize scientists at the Colloquium on Agricultural Reform and Development in China, held in conjunction with the Annual Meetings of the American Society of Agronomists, Las Vegas, October 18–19, 1989; Wang Dongtai, "State Aims to Commit New Funds to Farming," *The China Daily*, December 26, 1989, 1; "Increased Harvests a Goal for This Year," *The China Daily*, January 22, 1990, 4. The 1989 and 1990 proportional ranges are based on 13.1 million hectares and 15 million hectares for rice and 17.4 million and 18 million hectares for corn cited in *The China Daily* articles, highest and lowest actual sown area figures recorded for these crops during the 1986–88 period based on ZGTJNJ 1989, 192.

Figure 3-3.

Rice, Wheat, Corn, Sorghum, and Root and Tuber Yields in China, 1952–88, Growth in Yields, Kilograms per Hectare (Kg/ha)

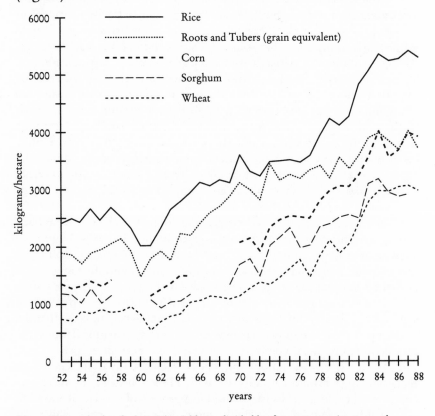

Notes: Root and tuber fresh weight yields are divided by four to approximate cereal equivalents for the dominant crop (sweet potato). Currently published Chinese yield and production data are recorded at one-fifth fresh weight and must be multiplied by 1.25 to approximate cereal equivalents. Although detailed data are not yet available, yields for most foodgrains increased in 1989, as total production surpassed the previous (1984) peak on substantially reduced area.

Sources: Root and tuber crop yields for 1984–88, all rice and wheat yields, and corn yields except those for 1961–62, are calculated from production and area data in ZGTJNJ 1984, 138, 141; and ZGTJNJ 1989, 192 and 198. Root and tuber crop yields are based on official series adjusted for statistical consistency and published in Bruce Stone, "An Analysis of Chinese Data on Root and Tuber Crop Production," *The China Quarterly* (September 1984): 596–97 (Series B). Sorghum yields except for those for 1961–62 are calculated from Zhongguo Tongjiju Nongye Tongjisi [State Statistical Bureau of China, Agricultural Statistics Department], eds., *Zhongguo nongye di guanghui chengjiu, 1949–84* [Glorious Achievements of Chinese Agriculture, 1949–84] (Beijing: Zhongguo tongji chubanshe, 1985) (hereafter ZGNYGHCJ), 42–47; He Kang, et al., eds., *Zhongguo nongye nianjin 1985*[Agricultural Yearbook of China, 1985] (Beijing: Nongye chubanshe [Agricultural Publishing House], 1986), 148 (hereafter ZGNYNJ 1985); ZGNYNJ 1986, 183; and ZGNYNJ 1987, 216–17. Corn and sorghum yields for 1961–62 are from NYJJZL, 147–48.

Chinese-bred varieties of rice, wheat, sweet potato, and to a considerable extent corn and sorghum, became comparable to the best varieties in the world in terms of yield, early maturity, and some stress factors, while lagging in resistance to other sources of stress and in taste characteristics. Average sweet potato yields surpassed those of all major world producers. Successful varieties of cassava and white potato were bred, selected, or imported prior to the late 1960s. Much of the rapid area expansion for white potatoes was based on these imported varieties or crosses among them, while area expansion for cassava was based on varieties selected for dissemination in the 1950s and early 1960s, but imported earlier. Unlike sweet potato, for which major varietal improvements continued into the 1970s, yields for cassava and white potato remain about average for Asia, although the very highest yields are comparable to the highest yields elsewhere.

Table 3–2 shows how rapid the dissemination of HYV cereals has been throughout the 1960s and 1970s and even including the 1980s. Figure 3–3 shows that yield progress for these crops has also been rapid. The contribution of yield-increasing technical change to foodgrain production growth is even greater than the impression provided by Figure 3–3, since area sown with staples has been increasingly allocated to these crops, for which especially productive varieties are available. Chinese data indicate that the crops represented in Figure 3–3 provided 79.2 percent of national foodgrain production in 1952, 94.0 percent in 1978, and 92.4 percent in 1988.[8]

But the Green Revolution cannot be characterized as a single period of replacement of traditional cultivars with HYVs. Instead, in successful countries like China, it is systematized in a process of sequential adoption of a steady stream of increasingly more desirable varieties. Table 3–3 illustrates this process for wheat. By 1984, varieties having a height at

Table 3-3.

Area Sown with Semi-Dwarf Wheat Varieties, 1980–84, in Hectares

	Fall-Sown	Spring-Sown	Total
	(million hectares)		
< 90 cm			
1980	2.863[a]	0.093[b]	2.956[ab]
1981	3.111[a]	0.141[c]	3.252[ac]
1982	4.739[b]	0.387[b]	5.126[b]
< 100 cm			
1983	8.364[b]	0.556[b]	8.920[b]
1984	9.362[b]	0.666[b]	10.028[b]
			(16.5) [d]
< 105 cm			
1977		~ 2.0[c]	
1984			(20–22)[d]

~ = estimated value
cm = height in centimeters at maturity

Note: Data upon which these compilations are based are incomplete, generally including only the more important semi-dwarf varieties sown over relatively large areas. The specific reference marks indicate figures that are based on compilations of data for semi-dwarf varieties including only those:

[a] With sown area exceeding 66.7 thousand hectares.

[b] With sown area exceeding 6.67 thousand hectares.

[c] With sown area exceeding 13.33 thousand hectares.

[d] With sown area exceeding 6.67 thousand hectares to which estimates have been added for remaining semi-dwarf plantings for 1984 or 1985, assuming 29 million hectares of coverage. Officially, wheat area was 29.577 million hectares in 1984 and 29.61 million hectares in 1985.

[e] Two million hectares of semi-dwarfs (< 105 cm) were sown in northeast spring wheat zones by 1977. Semi-dwarfs were commonly planted in main fall-sown wheat zones by that date.

Source: Bruce Stone, "Chinese Wheat Production and Technological Change," in International Center for Maize and Wheat Improvement (CIMMYT), *The Wheat Revolution Revisited: Recent Trends and Future Challenges*, a special issue of *World Wheat Facts and Trends* (Texcoco, Mexico: CIMMYT, 1989). For another presentation based on most of the same data, see also Dana G. Dalrymple, *Development and Spread of High-Yielding Wheat Varieties in Developing Countries* (Washington, D.C.: Bureau for Science and Technology, Agency for International Development, 1986).

maturity of under 105 cm had reached between two-thirds and three-quarters of China's wheat area. But varieties under 100 cm, with even greater yield potential, increased their area by 12.4 percent in 1984 to reach 57 percent of total plantings, while even shorter-stature varieties were increasing at a yet faster pace from a lower-base level. Another example of replacement of HYVs by even higher-yielding varieties is the increasing importance of hybrid rice.

Development of Fertilizer Use

Table 3-4 shows that fertilizer use has grown rapidly throughout the People's Republic period, and especially during the last decade (see Figure 3-4), when annual increments to use exceeded 1.2 million tons of nutrients.

China's relatively rapid growth in fertilizer use implies better handling of the four fundamental processes involved in sustained progress with fertilizer adoption: 1) influencing the agronomic potential for fertilizer use (primarily via development of water control and of agricultural research and extension systems); 2) converting the potential into farmers' effective demand for fertilizers (via market development or public-sector expedients to circumvent limitations imposed by poor market development); 3) determining the growth of aggregate supply (including planning for and execution of imports, capital construction investments to develop domestic production, and policy to fully utilize that capacity); and 4) developing the

Table 3-4.

Trend Growth in Manufactured Fertilizer Use, 1952–88

	Trend Growth Increments (1000 metric tons of nutrients/year)	Growth Rate Relative to Period Average (percent)
1952–57	59.7	29.0
1957–70	235.5	15.7
1970–78	555.8	10.4
1978–88	1,207.7	7.7

Sources:

1953–56: Zhongguo nongye kexueyuan turang feiliao yangjiusuo [Chinese Academy of Agricultural Science, Soil & Fertilizer Regionalization Plan] (Beijing: Zhongguo nongye keji chubanshe [Agricultural Science & Technology Publishing House of China], 1986), 6 and 7.

1978–88: ZGTJNJ 1989, 183.

All Others: Ibid. and/or NYJJZL 1949–83, 292.

Figure 3-4.

China's Production, Application, and Imports of Manufactured Fertilizers, 1970–88

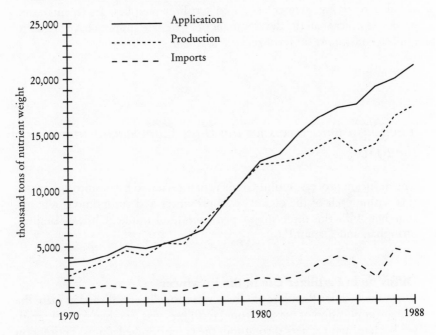

Sources:

Applications:
1970–78: NYJJZL 1949–83, 292.
1978–88: ZGTJNJ 1989, 183.

Imports:
1970–84: Converted from standard weight to nutrient weight estimated by multiplying by constant factor of 0.21. ZGTJNJ 1984, 410; ZGTJNJ 1985, 516.

1985–87: Converted from product weight found in ZGTJNJ 1987, 601; ZGTJZY 1988, 87; and ZGTJNJ 1989, 643, to nutrient weight estimates by multiplying by 0.43.

Production: ZGTJNJ 1989, 300.

fertilizer distribution system and determining the allocation of fertilizers among farmers.[9]

Yet even Chinese growth could have proceeded more rapidly. Of the four processes, aggregate supply of fertilizers seems to have been the most chronically constraining. Had more foreign exchange been allocated for fertilizer imports, had domestic capacity construction proceeded more quickly, and, particularly, had the decision to invest in large-scale efficient plants for producing high-quality fertilizers been undertaken earlier, the other three processes would have been sufficiently robust to have allowed for faster growth in fertilizer use and farm production.[10]

Aggregate fertilizer use has continued to grow rapidly during the last decade. Later we will examine whether this is primarily due to further intensification in advanced areas, or whether poorer regions and counties are also receiving greater access to fertilizer supplies. In recent years, processes other than the development of aggregate supplies have begun to impose constraints on fertilizer development.

The Diffusion Process for the Basic Components in the 1980s

The diffusion process within China is first reviewed by monitoring progress within each of the country's 26 provinces and autonomous regions, together with the three major province-level municipalities—Beijing, Shanghai, and Tianjin.[11]

Diffusion of Fertilizer Use in the Provinces

When the People's Republic of China was formally established in 1949, the average application of manufactured fertilizers was less than one kilogram per hectare, and farmers throughout the country relied almost entirely on green manure crops and the application of other organic manures to maintain soil health and supplement soil nutrients for better crop growth. Figure 3-5 shows that major differences had developed by 1980 in the intensity of fertilizer use among China's provinces: per hectare application within Beijing and Shanghai (on the left) and the populous coastal provinces (on the right) far exceeded average levels throughout the remainder of the country, with application especially lagging in Tibet and the far northern and northwestern provinces (two left panels).

Growth in fertilizer application during the 1980s, nevertheless, has been rapid and relatively steady within most jurisdictions. The five exceptions (left panel) include the three major municipalities where labor's rapidly rising opportunity cost has engendered a continuous state of frenzied economic growth, usually in directions away from agriculture; and Qinghai and Tibet—cold, mountainous, sparsely populated herding regions with relatively little agriculture and a variety of special problems. The decline in these minor agricultural regions since 1983 may relate closely to liberalization of pasture-based livestock development, other market liberalizations, and demographic movements.

Figure 3-5.

Provincial Fertilizer Application per Sown Hectare, 1980–88

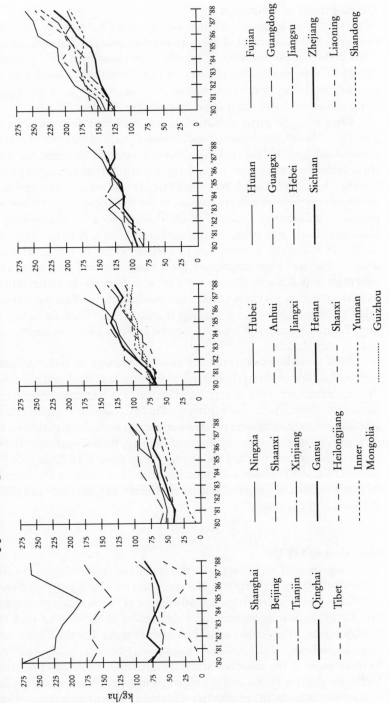

Sources: Bruce Stone, "Developments in Agricultural Technology," *The China Quarterly*, Special Issue on Food and Agriculture in China During the Post-Mao Period, no. 116 (December 1988): 806. Data for 1988 have been added, based on ZGTJNJ 1989, 182 and 192.

Development of Irrigation

While effectively irrigated area increased in most Chinese provinces during the 1970s, only one-third of them showed an unequivocal upward linear trend between 1980 and 1988, including three showing decline during the latter half of the period. Four others actually finished the period with more area irrigated than in 1980 (see Figure 3-6). In six provinces, the negative trend amounted to as much as one percent per annum.[12]

Over half the gross reduction in irrigated area took place in three provinces: Anhui, Guangdong, and Sichuan, totalling 152 percent of the net national decline. If Hubei, Henan, Shandong, and Guangxi are added, these values become 87 percent and 250 percent. So the aggregate problem is somewhat concentrated. Yet an analysis of these reductions suggests that an important portion reflects correction for statistical error. Of the seven provinces accounting for most of the decline, data for Guangdong and Guangxi clearly incorporate large statistical errors. A large share of the decline in Shandong, Henan, and, to a lesser extent, Anhui, reflects water sources that had been inadequate for a long time and the retirement of tubewells too densely placed, both of which point to corrections for overestimation in previous years. The same may be said for several of the other provinces and cities recording smaller net declines, including Beijing, Tianjin, Shanxi, and Inner Mongolia, and to a lesser extent, Zhejiang, Gansu, and Shaanxi.

Yet if the reductions are not as serious or widespread as they originally appeared, it is nevertheless irrefutable that Chinese agricultural growth lost the important assistance of very rapid increases in aggregate irrigated area during the 1980s. Those that experienced net increases in irrigated area at an average rate exceeding one percent per annum include relatively wealthy provinces (Jiangsu, Hebei, Fujian, and Hunan), those benefitting from an increase in national funding (Xinjiang, Ningxia, and Heilongjiang), and provinces that have been too poor historically to exhaust the supply of relatively attractive potential irrigation projects (the last three and Jiangxi, Yunnan, and Guizhou).

Diffusion of HYVs

The proportion of area sown with the major Green Revolution crops and covered with high-yielding varieties is so great (see Table 3-2) that there can be little question that the regional diffusion of HYVs is relatively complete. Of course, important interregional differences in the *level* of seed technology remain. This shows up in a number of ways. For the higher valued crops like wheat and rice, varietal turnover may occur as often as every two to three years in the most sophisticated growing regions of the Yangtze Valley, Pearl River Delta, and the Huang-Huai-Hai Plain of North China; four to five years in the productive Chengdu Plain of Sichuan; and six to

Figure 3–6.

Irrigated Area by Province, 1980–88

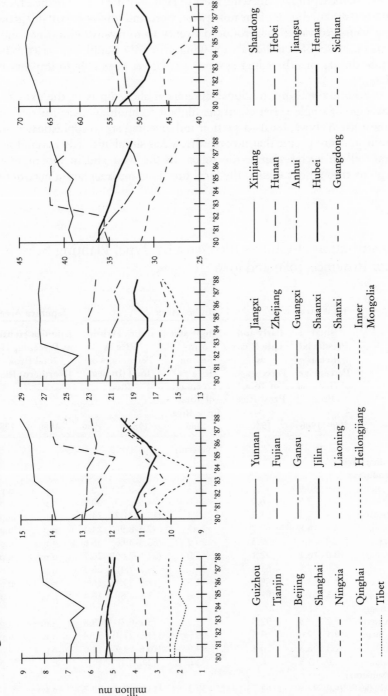

	Guizhou		Yunnan		Jiangxi		Xinjiang		Shandong
	Tianjin		Fujian		Zhejiang		Hunan		Hebei
	Beijing		Gansu		Guangxi		Anhui		Jiangsu
	Shanghai		Jilin		Shaanxi		Hubei		Henan
	Ningxia		Liaoning		Shanxi		Guangdong		Sichuan
	Qinghai		Heilongjiang		Inner Mongolia				
	Tibet								

Note: 15 mu = 1 hectare.

Sources: AGNYNJ 1981, 66–67; ZGNYNJ 1982; ZGTJNJ 1983, 198; ZGTJNJ 1984, 176; ZGTJNJ 1985, 282; ZGTJNJ 1986, 157; ZGTJNJ 1987, 147; ZGNYNJ 1988, 377; ZGTJNJ 1989 (English edition), 184

55

seven years in primary growing areas of Heilongjiang in the northeast. Less market-oriented areas of the northwest, west, and southwest are still growing improved varieties introduced twenty to thirty-five years ago, and a small number of counties are growing primarily traditional varieties because the regional breeding system has not yet been able to improve on them.[13]

Another way interregional differences show up is in the extent of coverage of single varieties. In the highest technology areas for rice and wheat listed above, local adaptation and breeding are so sophisticated and environment-specific that no one variety has simultaneously covered several million hectares since the 1960s. In the west and in mountainous regions throughout China, the local breeding and adaptation network is

Table 3 – 5.

Distribution of China's Rice Area by Type, Planting Season, and Province, 1980 and 1986

	Total Area		Indica Area				Japonica Area	
	Total Provincial Rice as Percentage of National Rice	Early and Late Rice as Percentage of Total Prov. Rice	Single and Mid- Season Rice as Percentage of Total Prov. Rice	Indica Hybrid Rice as Percentage of Total (Indica) Rice		Japonica Hybrid as Percentage of Total Prov. (Northern) Rice		
	1980 1986	1986	1986	1980ª	1986	1980	1986
	(percent)							
Indica Rice Producers								
Shanghai	0.9 0.9	47.7	50.3	(6.7-8.2)	0	n.p.	n.p.
Jiangsu	7.9 7.5	6.0	94.0	(24.5-29.9)	30.6	n.p.	n.p.
Zhejiang	7.4 7.3	91.7	8.3	(17.4-21.2)	24.1	n.p.	n.p.
Anhui	6.6 6.8	57.7	42.3	(7.3-8.9)	24.4	n.p.	n.p.
Fujian	5.0 4.6	79.3	20.7	(32.5-39.6)	38.6	n.p.	n.p.
Jiangxi	10.0 10.1	92.1	7.0	(22.6-27.6)	26.7	n.p.	n.p.
Hubei	8.0 7.9	61.3	38.7	(6.1-7.4)	26.2	n.p.	n.p.
Hunan	13.1 13.4	88.5	11.5	(18.9-23.1)	36.6	n.p.	n.p.
Guang- dong	12.3 11.2	98.4	1.6	(3.9-4.8)	19.4	n.p.	n.p.
Guangxi	8.2 7.8	92.8	7.2	(5.2-6.3)	19.8	n.p.	n.p.
Sichuan	9.1 9.6	3.5	96.5	(22.5-27.4)	57.8	n.p.	n.p.
Guizhou	2.3 2.3	0.1	99.9	(10.6-12.9)	14.6	n.p.	n.p.
Yunnan	3.0 3.3	6.4	93.6	(2.0-2.4)	10.3	n.p.	n.p.
Sub-total (Indica)	94.0 92.5	64.7	35.3	(14.8-18.0)	29.7	n.p.	n.p.

56

Japonica Rice Producers

Beijing	~0.2	~0.1	n.p.	n.p.	n.p.	n.p.	0	0
Tianjin	~0.2	~0.1	n.p.	n.p.	n.p.	n.p.	0	0
Hebei	0.4	0.4	n.p.	n.p.	n.p.	n.p.	(8.4-10.3)	0
Shanxi	<0.1	<0.1	n.p.	n.p.	n.p.	n.p.	0	0
Nei Menggu	<0.1	~0.1	n.p.	n.p.	n.p.	n.p.	0	0
Liaoning	1.1	1.2	n.p.	n.p.	n.p.	n.p.	(8.5-10.4)	6.6
Jilin	0.7	1.1	n.p.	n.p.	n.p.	n.p.	(4.8-5.9)	0
Heilong-jiang	0.6	1.2	n.p.	n.p.	n.p.	n.p.	(2.0-2.4)	0
Shandong	0.5	0.3	n.p.	n.p.	n.p.	n.p.	(7.1-8.7)	0
Henan	1.2	1.3	n.p.	n.p.	n.p.	n.p.	(5.3-6.5)	32.0
Xizang	<0.1	<0.1	n.p.	n.p.	n.p.	n.p.	0	
Shaanxi	0.5	0.5	n.p.	n.p.	n.p.	n.p.	(16.6-20.3)	55.5
Gansu	<0.1	<0.1	n.p.	n.p.	n.p.	n.p.	0	0
Qinghai	n.p.	n.p.	n.p.	n.p.	n.p.	n.p.	n.p.	n.p.
Ningxia	0.1	0.2	n.p.	n.p.	n.p.	n.p.	0	19.5
Xinjiang	0.3	0.2	n.p.	n.p.	n.p.	n.p.	0	0
Sub-total (Japonica)	6.0	7.5	n.p.	n.p.	n.p.	n.p.	(6.1-7.4)	10.0
China[b]	100.0	100.0	59.9	32.6	(13.9-16.9)	27.5	(0.4)	0.8

Notes: Northern rice areas plant primarily japonica varieties; others plant primarily indica varieties. The appearance of rigid boundaries differentiating these plantings coinciding with provincial boundaries reflects convenience in statistical presentation rather than an exact representation of reality. Japonica varieties are also grown in East Central China and in high altitude areas of the South for example.

"n.p." denotes that there is little or no cultivation of the type of rice or growing season in the indicated province according to available statistical data.

[a] Several figures have been published for national hybrid rice area in 1980 ranging from 72 million mu to 88 million mu (4.800-5.866 million ha.). Sources for the 72.1 million mu figure seem to be the most authoritative, but the only provincial data so far released add up to 88 million mu, although they appear with a figure for total paddy area of 542.43 million mu as opposed to 506.33 million mu (ZGNYNJ 1981, 23) or 508.18 million mu (ZGTJNJ 1984, 138 and elsewhere). The higher figures in the included ranges use the original hybrid rice area data divided by data for total area from ZGNYNJ 1981. The lower figures deflate those percentages by 0.82 (= 72.1/88.0).

[b] Data in this row provide percentages of indicated column categories in total rice area for the specified year.

Sources: 1980: Hybrid area in 1980 by province was provided to S. Virmani of the International Rice Research Institute (IRRI) and published in Robert E. Huke, *Rice Area by Type of Culture: South, Southeast, and East Asia* (Los Baños, Philippines: IRRI, 1982), 32. Other calculations are based on ZGNYNJ 1981, 23-24.

1986: Proportion of rice area under hybrids by province are unpublished data from Ministry of Agriculture, Animal Husbandry and Fishery. All other calculations are based on data published in ZGNYNJ 1987, 213-14.

For comparison of data from these sources with detailed data for Yunnan, see Table 3-7.

less dense and less capable; provincial academies of agricultural sciences are more dominant; and a single breakthrough, usually based on a variety developed elsewhere, will be extended successfully over vast areas. Furthermore, microclimatic variation in the west and in the mountainous areas is likely to be considerably greater than within China's principal growing regions.

The interregional pattern of adoption, as shown in Table 3–5 for hybrid rice, a high-technology Chinese innovation, is a complicated one. Interprovincial differences in the proportion of rice areas covered with hybrids in 1980 are largely explained by climate. Only indica hybrids for temperate climates had at that point been developed, which were superior to the non-hybrid dwarf HYVs in the region. Japonica hybrids provided less yield improvement over the Korean- and Japanese-based varieties with which they competed, and the poorer taste characteristics of early hybrids were more problematic for adoption in japonica areas, since a greater proportion of japonica production is for export or for higher-income urban consumption. For the same reasons, the adoption rate in Shanghai was relatively low, despite the city's sophisticated agricultural research program. As for the far south, successful semitropical and tropical indica hybrids had not yet been developed.

By 1986, successful semitropical indica varieties were being rapidly extended in Guangdong and Guangxi and in the warmer areas of Yunnan and Sichuan. Meanwhile, less cold-sensitive indica hybrids were being extended in medium-elevation areas of Hubei and Hunan, low-elevation areas of Anhui, Henan, and Shaanxi a little farther north, and higher-elevation areas of the southern provinces. Superior temperate hybrids were also beginning to replace the earlier successful varieties and expand their area. With continued rapid growth in cereal yields through the mid-1980s, the poorer-tasting hybrids were largely dropped in Shanghai and in the japonica areas. Ningxia, where rice is scarce and consumers are less discriminating, is a principal exception.

Diffusion of Fertilizer Use in Poor Areas

The data appearing in Table 3–6 have to be used with caution (see table notes), yet they provide some confirmation that growth in fertilizer use in the poorest one-third of China's counties and municipal areas, taken as a group, has progressed rapidly during the 1980s. Progress is still not as fast for the bottom one-third as for the national average, however, indicating that the gap in fertilizer use intensity between poor and wealthier counties is still widening. Moreover, a significant number of the very poorest counties, although awarded special quotas of subsidized supplies during the last decade, have not since that time received increased allocations at either subsidized or market prices, and consequently are suffering from severe fertilizer supply constraints on staple crop yields.

Table 3-6.

Comparison of Officially Designated Poor Counties (663) with All Counties in China: Various Categories of Agricultural Performance and Input Use, 1980–87, in Kilograms (kg), Hectares (ha), and Kilowatt Hours (kwh)

	1980	1985	1987
Fertilizer Use (kg of fertilizer nutrients per sown ha)			
NG	56.4	84.5	92.3
PPG	66.3	85.4	98.0
NAV	89.0	123.6	137.8
Rural Use of Electricity (kwh/sown ha)			
NG	105.2	158.0	187.8
PPG	108.8	162.9	214.1
NAV	220.3	354.3	454.5
Rural Use of Electricity (kwh/rural resident)			
NG	17.3	24.6	28.5
PPG	19.2	28.1	35.4
NAV	39.6	61.0	76.9
Cultivated Area with Effective Irrigation (percent)			
NG	16.9	11.8	16.1
PPG	25.0	16.0	21.8
NAV	45.3	45.5	46.3
Average Foodgrain Yields (kg/sown ha)			
NG	2,129	2,583	2,566
PPG	2,192	2,880	2,893
NAV	2,732	3,483	3,637
Foodgrain Production Per Capita (kg/rural resident)			
NG	296	315	310
PPG	321	376	373
NAV	392	454	472
Agricultural Output Value Per Rural Resident (in constant 1980 Yuan)			
NG		248	250
PPG		294	300
NAV		349	372

NG = 300 poor counties supported by the national government
PPG = 363 poor counties supported by the provincial and prefectural governments
NAV = National average of all 1,986 counties and 378 municipal areas (1987)

Notes: A number of strong reservations must be considered in drawing conclusions from this comparison. First, officially designated "poor" counties include large groups of counties that are not especially poor in the Chinese context, and exclude some groups which are quite poor. Second, the 663 poor counties constitute almost one-third of China's total poor population and one-fifth of China's total population—therefore comprising an appreciable portion of the national averages included; the comparison thus considerably underestimates the differences between "poor" and "other" counties.

Third, benchmark year comparisons are always problematic. An especially poor weather year was 1980, while 1987 weather was good. Weather was relatively poor in 1985, and there was considerable and costly confusion in markets for farm goods, fertilizer, and credit, coupled with public financial retrenchment. Thus the 1980–85–87 temporal comparison overstates positive trends for all groups.

In terms of intergroup comparisons, stronger-than-average performance by poor counties in several categories may reflect greater vulnerability during periods of poor weather, financial retrenchment, and input shortages (1980 and 1985) to a greater extent than constitutes evidence of any phenomenon of poor counties "catching up" with the average, which might be inferred from a superficial glance at the data. Finally, sown area and especially cultivated area are considerably underestimated in China. The proportional underestimation is certainly greater in poor areas.

"Foodgrains" consist of rice, wheat, corn, sorghum, millet, and other minor cereals, all evaluated at unmilled weight, sweet potatoes and white potatoes evaluated at one-fifth fresh weight, and soybeans and other bean crops.

"Effective irrigation" denotes level agricultural land which has water sources and complete sets of irrigation facilities to lift and move adequate water for irrigation purposes under normal conditions. The national increase in the proportion irrigated reflects retirement of cultivated area rather than net growth in irrigated area among official data. The degree of overestimation of official data in this category, however, has declined somewhat during the 1980s.

Sources: Guojia tongjiju nongcun shehui jingji tongjisi [State Statistical Bureau, Division of Rural Social and Economic Statistics], eds., *Zhongguo fenxian nongcun jingji tongji gaiyao* [Statistical Abstract of China's Rural Economy by County] (Beijing: Zhongguo tongji chubanshe [Statistical Publishing House of China], 1988), 639–42.

He Kang et al., eds., *Zhongguo nongye nianjian 1981* [Agricultural Yearbook of China, 1981] (Beijing: Nongye chubanshe [Agricultural Publishing House], 1982), 10, 21, 64, 65.

He Kang et al., eds., *China Agricultural Yearbook 1986* (Beijing: Agricultural Publishing House, 1987), 137, 156, 160, 267, 270.

He Kang et al., eds., *China Agricultural Yearbook 1988* (Beijing: Agricultural Publishing House, 1989), 200, 208, 214, 342, 345.

Bruce Stone, "Developments in Agricultural Technology," *The China Quarterly*, Special Issue on Food and Agriculture in the Post-Mao Period, no. 116 (December 1988): 767–822, especially 771–90.

State Statistical Bureau of the People's Republic of China, *China Statistical Yearbook 1988* (Hong Kong: International Center for Advancement of Science and Technology and China Statistical Information and Consultancy Service Center, 1988), 1.

Development of Irrigation in Poor Areas

While the irrigated area data listed in Table 3–6 are subject to the reservations discussed above, they suggest that poor counties bore the brunt of irrigated area losses during the 1980s. Reasons for this imbalance are discussed in Section IV.

Diffusion of HYVs in Poor Areas

There are a number of relevant dimensions to the diffusion process for improved staple crop technologies among poorer people: 1) the diffusion of improved and advanced technologies for the primary cereal crops into poorer prefectures and counties; 2) the access of the poorest farmers within poor counties to these technologies; and 3) technological progress and diffusion with other staple crops grown predominantly by poorer people.

Again, the HYV percentages within total area planted with these major staple crops are so high (see Table 3-2) that considerable diffusion into poorer prefectures and counties must have transpired. But what about the more advanced technologies such as hybrid rice? The two provinces with the largest numbers of very poor rice-dependent counties are Yunnan and Guizhou. These provinces displayed the lowest proportions of paddy area under hybrid rice among indica producers in 1986. This is not only because they are poor and their breeding systems are less developed. The geographic complexity of these provinces and their dependence upon developments for both semitropical and cold-tolerant indica rice (in their lowland and middle-elevation regions) as well as for japonica rice (for their highland regions) are major factors as well.

In Yunnan, the first hybrid variety developed was Nanyu #2, introduced from Guangzhou (Guangdong). In 1979, it was decimated by disease, accounting for reduction in hybrid area in 1980 and 1981 (see Table 3-7).[14] In Guizhou, the early hybrid varieties introduced were susceptible to cold fall winds which were especially severe in 1980, accounting for hybrid area declines in 1981 and 1982.[15]

In both cases, recovery was based largely on the introduction in 1982–83 of Xianyou #63, but the relatively late start with a suitable variety accounts for the low proportions of coverage in these provinces in 1986. Table 3-7 shows that hybrid rice area has expanded rapidly in both provinces since prior to the mid-1980s.

A logical question for those interested in diffusion is whether the increase is confined to relatively wealthy areas of these provinces, or whether diffusion is proceeding throughout Yunnan and Guizhou, including their poorest regions.

Table 3-8 indicates that hybrid diffusion has occurred and is increasing in all prefectures of Yunnan except Diqing, yet there are major differences in the proportions of paddy area covered and the speed of its increase in the 1980s. While the economic status of Yunnan's regions is not unrelated to these differences, the primary determinant is the agroclimatic environment, the most critical aspect of which is elevation. The administrative units with the highest average incomes, for example, as listed in Table 3-8, are Kunming and Dongquan Municipal Areas, and Yuxi and Dali Prefectures,[16] with low-to-average proportions of hybrids, each predominantly dependent on japonica varieties. Of the four, Yuxi, with the highest proportion of indicas, has the highest proportion of hybrids.

Table 3-7.

Area Sown with Hybrid Corn and Hybrid Rice Varieties, Selected Southern Provinces, 1976–95

	Hybrid Corn Area				Hybrid Rice Area				
	Yunnan	Guizhou	Hubei	Hunan	Yunnan	Guizhou	Hubei	Jiangxi	Jiangsu
				(thousand hectares)					
1976					...				
1977					0.2				
1978					2				
1979	98	53			24				
1980	116(10)	117(16)			16(2)	69(11)	165(6)	765(23)	656(25)
1981	89	87			12	decline			
1982	99	decline			14	decline			
1983	128	110			23	recovery			
1984	184	157			55	recovery			
1985	207	153			87	110			
1986	191(20)	169(27)			109(10)	113(15)	666(26)	868(27)	741(31)
1987	192(20)	178(29)	307(78)	53(47)	151(15)	160(22)			819(34)
1988	257(27)	233(39)	307(80)	70(63)	202(20)	302(41)	1200(47)		
1989	322	246	316	85	212	347	1400	1386	
1990 (plan)	333–366	300			233				
1995 (plan)	533								

Notes: Numbers in parentheses indicate the percentage of total provincial area sown with the specified crop that was sown with hybrid varieties.

Sources: Except for Yunnan and Guizhou, the 1980 (lower estimates) and 1986 data for hybrid rice are from Table 3-5. Sources for other data are:

Yunnan: Yunnansheng Zhongzi Guanlizhan [Yunnan Province Seed Management Station], *Yunnansheng zhuyao zuowu liangzhong tuiguang mianji (1979–1988)* [Yunnan Province Extension Area Statistics for Improved Varieties of Important Agricultural Crops (1979–1988)] (Kunming: Yunnan zhongzi guanlizhan, 1989), 1, 3, 7, 20, 28, 39, 55, 68, 87, 97, 119, 126, 145, 155, 174, 184, 206, 209 and Appendix tables (hereafter YZZLTM); Zhou Guorong and Cao Bingyi, Director and Deputy Director, Yunnan Province Seed Corporation, Kunming, January 9, 1990.

Guizhou: Wu Sikai, Production Dept., and Hong Ceyu, Agricultural Extension Station, Guizhou Province Bureau of Agriculture, Guiyang, January 2, 1990.

Hubei: Xiong Fengming, Hubei Seed Corporation, Wuhan, November 13, 1989.

Hunan: Liu Houau, Upland Grain Dept., Hunan Bureau of Agriculture, Changsha, November 24, 1989.

Jiangxi: Jiangxi Seed Corporation, Nanchang, December 2, 1989.

Jiangsu: "Hybrid Rice Harvested in Jiangsu," *The China Daily*, November 6, 1987.

Provincial data used to calculate hybrid area percentages: ZGNYNJ 1981, 23, 24, 27; ZGNYNJ 1987, 213, 216; ZGNYNJ 1988, 231, 234; ZGTJNJ 1989, 194.

The six prefectures with the greatest total area sown with hybrids are in the two southern rice zones, where most rice is grown at elevations below 1,500 meters (m) and where indica varieties predominate: Wenshan, Honghe, Xixuangbanna, Simao, Dehong, and Lincang. Some portions of Yuxi and Baoshan, with the seventh and eighth greatest areas under hybrids in 1988, are occasionally included with the northernmost of these two zones.[17]

Half of the hybrid area in Yunnan is sown with the indica hybrid Xianyou #63, originally introduced from Fujian Province in 1982 and now bred throughout much of the mountainous areas of the southern provinces. More than half of the remaining hybrid area in the province is sown with D-you #63, another indica variety.[18] These varieties increase yields by around 1,500 kilograms/hectare (kg/ha) over those of the improved varieties previously grown under similar conditions; and in the southern part of the province, by as much as three tons/ha.[19] An even newer hybrid, D-you #64, reportedly performs better than these two below 1,000 m and may become more dominant in the far south and lowland areas, but as of 1988, it was limited to 3,120 hectares.[20]

Guizhou's experience is roughly similar to Yunnan's with Xianyou #63 dominating the plantings (65 percent of total hybrid area in Guizhou) below 1,000 m, and Weiyou #64, another indica hybrid (accounting for 25 percent) predominant above 1,000 m. Availability of these two varieties over the past five years has substantially improved Guizhou's participation in the benefits from hybrid technology.

But not all of South China's mountainous areas are likely to grow even these shorter-season, cold-tolerant indica hybrids. There are no suitable hybrid varieties for northwest Guizhou, where (mostly japonica) rice is cultivated up to 2,000 m and which includes Guizhou's poorest counties.[21] Yunnan's North Central Japonica/Indica Paddy Zone includes most or all of Qujing, Chuxiong, Dali, Yuxi, Baoshan Prefectures, and Kunming Municipal Area. This region grew single-season indica rice almost exclusively until the 1970s, when japonica varieties partially replaced them owing to their superior taste and their greater ability to withstand cold, indispensable for the higher localities of the region. Most japonicas in this zone are grown between 1,700 m and 1,900 m (but 1,600-1,700 m in Baoshan),[22] which is beyond the most effective range of the leading indica hybrids. But the development of japonica hybrids has come later and more slowly. And the inferior taste characteristics of most hybrids relative to alternative japonica varieties may account for especially slow development in the wealthier areas of Kunming and Dali. The wealthier portion of the region grows japonicas even where indicas (and thus indica hybrids) could be grown.

This explains why the proportional coverage of hybrids is as great or

Table 3-8.

Area Sown with Hybrid Rice and All Improved Varieties in Yunnan Province, 1981–88, by Prefecture

	Area Sown with All Improved Varieties 1981	Area Sown with Hybrid Rice								Area Sown with All Improved Varieties 1988	Total Paddy Area Compiled 1988
		1981	1982	1983	1984	1985	1986	1987	1988		
		(thousand hectares)									
Kunming Munic. Area	33.23	–	–	–	–	–	0.02	–	0.05	63.03	64.91
Dongquan Munic. Area	–	–	–	–	–	0.01	0.08	0.11	0.23	1.47	1.87
Zhaotong Prefecture	18.19	1.42	1.23	1.45	2.03	2.43	3.07	4.94	8.61	25.94	31.72
Qujing Prefecture	55.33	–	–	–	–	0.43	1.88	1.89	4.65	66.56	73.38
Chuxiong Yi Minority Region	52.98	–	–	–	–	0.62	1.79	3.19	4.27	65.47	73.58
Yuxi Prefecture	42.13	1.60	2.63	4.79	6.80	5.94	6.36	7.99	8.75	41.64	48.70
Honghe Hani–Yi Minority Region	66.31	2.33	2.16	4.79	10.13	17.34	23.07	28.60	36.53	84.21	92.51
Wenshan Zhuang-Mao Minority Region	36.68	1.00	1.37	2.58	8.67	14.87	19.07	23.59	28.48	45.86	60.56
Simao Prefecture	17.92	0.65	0.93	3.25	7.16	11.80	12.21	20.33	28.00	62.86	87.06
Xixuangbanna Dai Minority Region	18.67	–	–	0.07	6.20	8.55	10.57	11.80	16.29	16.29	47.05
Dali Bai Minority Region	54.66	0.03	–	–	–	0.22	0.56	0.92	1.19	74.80	74.80
Baoshan Prefecture	43.26	0.65	0.59	0.73	1.35	2.51	3.95	6.87	11.08	68.65	68.65
Dehong Dai-Jingpo Minority Region	32.70	2.69	3.20	3.37	7.57	11.47	15.42	24.41	33.33	53.33	57.95
Lijiang Prefecture	11.57	–	0.17	0.24	1.19	2.07	1.64	1.80	2.33	15.37	22.69
Nujiang Lisu Minority Region	0.95	0.82	0.88	0.98	1.13	1.09	1.20	1.43	1.74	3.10	6.37
Diqing Zang Minority Region	2.13	–	–	–	–	–	–	–	–	2.67	2.90
Lincang Prefecture	13.86	1.00	0.73	0.66	3.07	7.72	8.07	13.47	16.00	16.00	69.10

Yunnan Province

Hybrids	500[a]	12.37	13.89	22.89	55.29	87.08	108.95	151.29	201.54	707.26[a]	—
Total Paddy (compiled)	1,078	1,078	938	927	951	922	912	890	884	883.79	883.79
Total Paddy (official)	1,104	1,104	1,078	1,107	1,130	1,075	1,049	1,020	1,009	1,008.80	1,008.80

Note: Improved varieties include, but are not limited to, hybrids. Area sown with improved varieties reached 500,000 hectares or almost half paddy-sown area in 1979 and 1981, and exceeded 600,000 hectares in 1980. These compiled data exclude minor varieties sown on less than 66.7 hectares in a given year. They therefore underestimate the prefectural and national totals for both hybrids and improved varieties. Both the compiled totals for paddy areas in each year (whether sown with traditional or improved varieties) as well as the total for all paddy areas, including minor varieties and adjustments for underestimates, as given in Ministry of Agriculture and State Statistical Bureau publications, are listed at the bottom of the table. [a] Refers to all improved varieties, including but not limited to hybrids.

Sources: YZZLMT, 1, 7, 28, 55, 87, 119, 145, 174, 206 and Appendix tables (hereafter YZZLTM). Official SSB totals are from ZGNYNJ 1981, 24; ZGNYNJ 1983, 56; ZGNYNJ 1984, 85; ZGNYNJ 1985, 146; ZGTJNJ 1986, 176; ZGTJNJ 1987, 166; ZGNYNJ 1988, 231; and ZGTJNJ 1989, 194.

greater in Zhaotong, Lijiang, and Nujiang, with generally higher elevation but poorer inhabitants than in the North Central Zone. The Northeastern Zone includes Zhaotong, Dongquan Municipal Area, northern Qujing, and northeastern Kunming, while Nujiang, Diqing, and most of Lijiang and northern Dali comprise the Northwestern Zone.[23] Most of the hybrids grown in the three northern zones are in areas low enough in elevation to grow cold-tolerant indicas. The main hybrid varieties, even in these three higher elevation regions, are Xianyou #63 and D-you #63,[24] grown predominantly in relatively lower-elevation localities. The (japonica) paddy areas of Diqing are generally above 2,000 m and are completely out of reach of indica hybrids.

But varieties for even the more demanding locations are being developed. A team from the Tropical Agricultural Research Institute in Japan has been cooperating with local breeders to produce a series of twenty-five japonica hybrids for extension between 1,700 m and 2,000 m in the Kunming area, of which four exhibit superior disease and cold resistance, as well as desirable taste characteristics. These may prove extendable to other North Central Zone locations,[25] but were still limited to less than 5,000 hectares in 1989.[26] Expansion is planned for approximately 30,000 hectares, although some features of these varieties have made extension more difficult.[27]

For more southerly locations Xunjiao #29 is an experimental japonica hybrid grown in Jianshui County of Honghe (Yunnan), which performs well up to 2,000 m and increases yields by 1.5-2.25 tons per hectare over varieties it replaces. And for more northern areas and especially high altitudes, He #16, developed in Dali, can grow well even above 2,000 m.[28] Although He #16 has been extended in 1988 to only 1,500 ha, entirely within the prefecture,[29] development of such varieties suggests that even Diqing may join the hybrid revolution before long.

It is one thing to move technology into poor regions, which is clearly occurring in Yunnan and Guizhou; it is another to extend it to the poorest people within those regions. Poorer inhabitants of a poor region are less likely to have paddy area, or as much paddy area; and even if they do, they are less likely to grow hybrids because they farm environmentally marginal fields (in Yunnan and Guizhou, usually at higher elevation) for which hybrids are only now being developed. They are also more likely to stand toward the end of the line of recipients as scarce hybrid seed is distributed. Seed distribution is governed more by local political considerations and the public interest in increased marketings than by poverty relief or equity.[30]

In Yunnan, the disadvantage of the poor in having access to technology is exacerbated by racial and language issues. Yunnan includes large populations of twenty-four officially recognized minority groups, concentrations of which are greatest in mountainous regions. If Han Chinese are farming as well as administrating and engaging in industry and commerce in a minority region, they are apt to be concentrated in the low-lying paddy fields near the rivers and towns rather than in highland areas. These areas get first crack at new technology because they supply the towns with food, the paddy cultivation conditions are relatively good, and they can more easily afford to finance the complete package of complementary inputs, combining with hybrid technology to greatly raise yields. But there are also barriers of race and language.

Chinese-run administrative, technical, and commercial organizations deal more readily with Chinese speakers, and especially with Han Chinese. While a portion of minority group populations attend Chinese schools, and some who become fully bilingual are then trained to be extension agents,[31] the technical extension coverage in minority regions is unquestionably poorer. During the 1980s, 1,005 new technical stations were established in Yunnan at the township level; but in roughly 500 townships, such stations have not yet been established, all in areas dominated by minorities primarily cultivating upland rather than paddy or other irrigated crops.[32] Of the hundreds of farmers contacted as part of Winrock International's technical development projects located in mountainous regions of Wenshan (SE), Simao (SW), Zhaotong (NE), and Nujiang (NW), heavily populated with minorities, none had ever met an extension agent.[33]

To some extent, extension shortcomings arise from and are reinforced by a research bias. The technical problems and local economies of such regions are very poorly understood because they have not been seriously researched. Even the seed breeding organizations have tended to concentrate on the major agricultural areas that supply Han Chinese-dominated urban areas. Early in the 1980s, however, the Chinese Academy of Agricultural Sciences officially reestablished priorities in favor of poorer environments and the crops that are more suited to them. Several of the provincial academies followed suit. It must be recognized, however, that this is generally a much more difficult scientific task than to develop varieties for areas where conditions are more favorable.

While there is still relatively little research leading toward productivity improvements for many locally specific highland crops, there is generally more research activity in China than in most developing countries. Among crops widely planted throughout the world in both highland and lowland areas and for which technical improvements are achieved with relative ease, corn and potatoes hold particular potential for China's highland areas.

Historically, the most important productivity limitations for potatoes in China have been the lack of high-yielding genetic stock, late blight, and various forms of potato virus. The varietal problem was addressed between the 1940s and the early 1960s, with imports from Japan, the United States, Poland, the Soviet Union, and East Germany. Several of the imported varieties exhibited resistance to late blight, and were widely propagated and distributed, and used extensively in the nascent Chinese breeding system. One such variety, Mira, introduced from East Germany in the mid-1950s, still covers 400,000 hectares in China,[34] including 80 percent of Yunnan's area planted with potatoes. However, it is susceptible to virus and after three decades its resistance to late blight has considerably diminished.[35]

The momentum in Chinese potato research dissipated in the late 1960s and did not revive until the development of virus-free stock in the late 1970s. The first virus-free seed farm in China was established in 1975 in Heilongjiang. By 1979, six others had been set up in Shanxi, Hebei, Shandong, Liaoning, Gansu, and Inner Mongolia, claiming yield increases of 150 percent for some forty virus-free cultivars. By 1982, one hundred such cultivars existed, and by 1987, ten farms provided seed to more than 114,000 hectares of fields.[36] Yet this accounted for less than 5 percent of the area planted with potatoes and, while these farms are continuing to serve new areas each year, the seed farm area is no longer expanding. This indicates that a greater portion of "virus-free" stock being used is of fourth, fifth, and sixth generation, no doubt losing its disease-resistance properties.[37]

In Yunnan, the only virus-free seed farm is located in Kunming and serves the relatively affluent surrounding areas. In northeastern and northwestern Yunnan, virus-free stock could improve yields with no additional inputs, by a factor of five or more, but none is available. Only very recently has this situation begun to improve. The International Potato Center (CIP) has provided forty varieties to a single potato scientist working at Yunnan Normal University. After two years of tests, he has identified three varieties that are promising for breeding and extension in east and central Yunnan. With limited funding from the Yunnan provincial government and the Qujing Prefectural Seed Corporation, and with assistance from a single staff member from the Kunming Municipal Bureau of Agriculture, along with farmers, county staff, and university students, Professor Wang Jun has set up a virus-free seed production base in a village at 2,500 m in Huize County (Qujing). Fifty thousand virus-free tubers were produced in 1989, primarily for local use. As the operation expands, the Qujing Seed Corporation will purchase the seed tubers for redistribution throughout the prefecture.[38]

This example shows the modest scale of research and dissemination of technology for even an important highland crop in poor areas of Yunnan and the role of serendipitous factors. It also demonstrates that human capital and institutions were already available to make rapid progress. In addition to the base at Huize, the selected virus-free CIP varieties have been sent on request to Xinping, Fuyuan, Guoshan, Menghai, Yuxi, Tengxiong, and Luquan Counties in Yunnan Province and to a few county leaders in Guizhou Province. Wang Jun has made contracts with Yunnan Agricultural University, Yunnan Genetic Engineering Laboratory, and Kunming Municipal Extension Station for rapid, including in-vitro, seed propagation.[39]

The long-term research picture for sweet potatoes has not been as spotty as for white potatoes. China's breeding system has continued to crank out improved varieties bred for, or adaptable to, more and more areas, gradually including some poorer ones still dependent on sweet potato as a major staple crop and for food security. Yet Xushu #18, a variety bred in northern Jiangsu in 1972, still covers 45 percent of the sweet potato area throughout the country, demonstrating the much slower rate of varietal turnover than for wheat, rice, and corn.[40] Critical problems of postharvest technology (as well as market imperfections) are not being addressed in many provinces; in some, losses can reach 60 percent under extreme conditions.[41] The ambivalence of the authorities in further developing potato and sweet potato production in advanced areas where surpluses have appeared has tended to inhibit research on these commodities, despite their importance for poorer localities and the difficulties in transferring those surpluses to poorer areas. The unresolved postharvest problem has led planning authorities to emphasize corn rather than sweet potatoes in low-cost feed development plans, even in areas more environmentally suited to sweet potato cultivation.[42]

The most energetic effort to develop and disseminate HYVs of staple crops, which could greatly benefit poor areas, has involved hybrid corn. In Hubei, hybrid corn yields average five to six tons per hectare as compared with three to four tons for the varieties it replaces, under similar conditions. In the poorer provinces of Guizhou and Yunnan, increments cited for hybrid corn are sometimes greater still.[43]

According to agricultural ministry and academy specialists in Beijing, hybrid corn now covers around 90 percent of China's corn area. Table 3–7 shows that dissemination is increasing in many southern provinces, including the poorest ones, and Table 3–9 shows that dissemination of hybrids is increasing in most prefectures of Yunnan. Yet the regions with the lowest proportions of hybrids are generally among the poorest.

In Yunnan, where most prefectures are poor, hybrid coverage for Kunming and Dongquan Municipal Areas, and for the Yuxi, Chuxiong, Dali, and Lijiang Prefectures all surpassed 44 percent in 1988, all but Lijiang among Yunnan's more prosperous jurisdictions (see Table 3–8). In Guizhou, significant inroads have been made during the 1980s, with hybrids covering around 40 percent of provincial corn area in 1988 and 1989 (see Table 3–7). But in Guizhou's poorest prefecture, Bijie, where most corn is grown at around 1,700 m, and with some fields above 2,000 m, there are no suitable varieties. Yet Bijie is one of Guizhou's principal corn-growing prefectures and is highly dependent on corn and potatoes. During the last two years, hybrids have been adopted at lower elevations in Bijie, with the use of plastic sheeting to protect early growth.[44]

In the somewhat wealthier provinces of Hunan and Hubei, corn is most heavily concentrated in the poorest, most mountainous prefectures with the lowest proportion of hybrids: Xiangxi, with 50-60 percent of Hunan corn area, and Woxi in Hubei. Yet the data presented in Table 3–7

Table 3–9.

Area Sown with Hybrid Corn and All Improved Corn Varieties in Yunnan Province, 1981–88, by Prefecture

	Area Sown with All Improved Varieties 1981	Area Sown with Hybrid Corn (thousand hectares)									Area Sown with All Improved Varieties 1988		Total Corn Area Compiled 1988
		1981	1982	1983	1984	1985	1986	1987	1988	(%)		(%)	
Kunming Munic. Area	3.07	1.20	1.33	1.47	18.05	17.73	17.95	19.11	24.87	(71)	31.42 (90)		35.01
Dongquan Munic. Area	—	—	0.20	0.03	0.79	2.67	2.60	1.13	2.47	(55)	3.20 (71)		4.50
Zhaotong Prefecture	112.84	11.93	10.67	15.67	21.33	21.33	20.49	18.49	29.93	(20)	100.65 (68)		147.61
Qujing Prefecture	94.00	27.63	42.61	62.04	63.33	73.13	43.58	39.23	50.47	(44)	50.47 (44)		115.91
Chuxiong Yi Minority Region	33.20	7.95	10.69	10.21	11.33	14.87	14.57	15.80	19.29	(52)	20.26 (54)		37.28
Yuxi Prefecture	11.40	4.28	3.11	3.80	8.20	7.67	9.98	8.94	12.01	(57)	20.13 (96)		20.89
Honghe Hani-Yi Minority Region	65.41	4.08	4.94	5.74	11.13	11.87	8.52	13.63	16.90	(21)	63.10 (80)		79.03
Wenshan Zhuang-Mao Minority Region	65.70	3.77	0.45	0.27	0.80	4.00	5.12	5.31	5.57	(5)	60.01 (50)		120.33
Simao Prefecture	1.40	2.47	0.73	0.80	3.87	3.67	5.88	6.93	12.08	(10)	26.30 (31)		84.60
Xixuangbanna Dai Minority Region	—	0.42	—	0.53	0.20	0.73	4.61	2.59	2.77	(17)	4.00 (24)		16.78
Dali Bai Minority Region	47.29	9.15	7.20	10.67	18.67	19.00	20.31	22.27	27.38	(45)	51.58 (84)		61.30
Baoshan Prefecture	40.58	1.65	1.67	3.77	6.20	9.00	9.95	10.67	14.89	(29)	50.96 (99)		51.70
Dehong Dai-Jingpo Minority Region	—	0.01	—	0.10	0.03	0.13	0.83	1.04	0.85	(9)	0.85 (9)		9.58

Lijiang Prefecture	12.99	8.40	6.11	8.22	16.53	12.82	15.25	17.77	20.20 (59)	23.77 (69)	34.27
Nujiang Lisu Minority Region	2.33	2.31	2.00	0.80	1.40	0.13	0.24	0.19	3.78 (4)	11.00 (13)	87.66
Diqing Zang Minority Region	–	1.04	1.89	2.17	1.33	3.73	5.13	4.54	2.67 (18)	7.66 (51)	14.94
Lincang Prefecture	3.66	1.76	5.71	2.00	0.43	4.20	5.57	4.00	11.00 (13)	11.00 (13)	87.66
Yunnan Province											
Hybrids	494[a]	89	99	128	184	207	191	192	257 (27)	537.35[a] (57)	–
Total Corn (compiled)	1,087	1,087	1,048	1,019	975	920	937	953	945	945.08	945.08
Total Corn (official)	1,087	1,087	1,048	1,019	975	920	937	953	945	945.07	945.07

Note: Percentages indicate area in each prefecture sown with hybrids, and with all improved varieties (including hybrids), respectively, in 1988. Corn area is apt to be underestimated in compiled and official data, particularly in highland areas where it is cultivated on slopes not included among official cultivated area statistics.

[a] Refers to all improved varieties, including but not limited to hybrids.

Source: YZZLTM, 3, 20, 39, 68, 97, 126, 155, 184, 209, and Appendix tables thereafter. Sources of official data are cited in Table 3 – 8.

suggest that rapid dissemination of hybrids must have occurred even in these prefectures during the last few years.

The breeding system has not yet been adapted to the needs of many poor areas that face unusual environmental constraints, even though existing technology can considerably improve yields in such localities. These areas are lagging for a number of reasons, in addition to environmental difficulty and to shortcomings in research and extension.

The successful adoption of existing hybrid varieties is more apt to require the use of plastic sheeting in highland areas, and the returns are greatest when additional fertilizer is used. The allocation bias against poor areas for either of these complementary inputs can inhibit adoption. In most provinces, price subsidies are provided to the poorest counties, recognizing that farmers in such areas are less able to afford them at market prices. Most provincial governments, however, try to hold down their subsidy burdens, which results in low levels of allocations to poor counties.

The complementarity is even more pronounced with hybrid rice varieties which often achieve lower yields than the varieties they replace at low fertilizer application levels. The high price of hybrid rice seed makes the survival rate of seedlings, considerably increased with plastic coverings for seedbeds, an important consideration. In Fugong County (Nujiang Prefecture, northwest Yunnan), the survival rate averages 90 percent with plastic sheeting and 20 percent without.[45]

Guizhou Province has recognized the urgent need for plastic sheeting to facilitate yield-increasing hybrid adoption in its poor, mountainous localities. In 1989, 43.6 percent of Guizhou's plastic for agriculture was allocated to the province's 17 poorest counties. But total coverage amounted to only 33,800 hectares, a tiny fraction of the requirements.[46]

An even more fundamental problem for hybrid adoption in poor localities is the availability of hybrid seed. When hybrid seed is imported from other provinces, it usually costs the provincial seed corporation several times what it pays within-province farmers, and the same difficulties with increasing the extension of other expensive inputs to poor areas apply to seed. Yet while within-province production has increased considerably in most provinces, the more advanced areas where seed production is centered lay claim to a large share of the seeds produced. Furthermore, the inability of seed corporations to guarantee seed farmers adequate and assured quantities of grain at stable prices has inhibited specialization of seed production among seed-producing farmers and, consequently, has slowed down the growth of hybrid seed production area.[47]

The above discussion shows that in southern China, there are a variety of factors that contribute to the slower rates of technological adoption in the poorer areas. In China's case, difficulties other than farmer risk avoidance and low cash availability seem to be the most inhibiting. Yet the data show that despite these limitations, adoption of hybrid corn and rice is proceeding in poor southern counties.

Chinese Reforms and the Diffusion of Staple Crop Technology

The exceedingly rapid growth in foodgrain production during the latter part of the 1970s and the first half of the 1980s was predominantly the product of technical change: the result of gains from investment in first-stage technological transformation in the previous decades, including improved water control, development of research, breeding, and seed production, and extension of high-yielding and early-maturity staple crop varieties. Some returns on investment followed immediately, as improved varieties and better water control were made available, yet much fuller realization of the gains came with the elimination of the final constraint, the insufficient availability of soil nitrogen and phosphate. With the fulfillment of this last basic requirement, dating from the late 1970s, the difference between actual and potential yields from HYV staple crops quickly narrowed throughout China's major growing areas. Yield growth, calculated in terms of national averages, accelerated to high and unsustainable rates, and then, inevitably, slowed down.[48]

As the data indicate, some of the growth involved more complete extension throughout China of fertilizer-responsive and stress-resistant varieties; another part, especially for rice, can be associated with further varietal improvements on farming areas already planting HYVs. But the largest share of the gain was accomplished by significantly narrowing the gap, over vast regions of China's nutrient-deficient soils, between the nutrient requirements of HYVs and nutrients actually provided by soils, manures, and manufactured fertilizers.

Production progress for staple crops during the last fifteen years has consisted primarily of progress with yields, while sown area for staple crops as a whole and for most individual categories actually declined during the 1980s. The fastest growing yields have been those for sweet potatoes, white potatoes, and the principal Green Revolution crops (rice, wheat, corn, and sorghum). An examination of their yield trends in Figure 3-3 suggests four general observations: 1) the yield patterns of these crops are strikingly similar; 2) they reflect sustained and fairly rapid growth for almost three decades; 3) ignoring the poor weather years, 1959–61, there appear to be at least two and probably three important points of inflection for the major cereals (rice, wheat, and corn)—one between the late 1950s and the mid-1960s and another in the mid-to-late 1970s; 4) only the first point of inflection is relevant for sorghum and sweet and white potatoes; if anything, there is a slight deceleration of yield growth in the root and tuber crops in the mid-1970s; and 5) a third common inflection point, in this instance a deceleration, appears to have occurred between the early and late 1980s, generally after 1984.

When linear trends are fitted to this data, it is discovered that the inflection points marking the beginning of the fastest period of yield growth all predate the institution of the household responsibility system (early 1980s) and even the beginning of the reform period (1979). (Chapter 2 examines the agricultural reforms in China, particularly the household responsibility system.) The closest linear approximations are achieved when the breaking point is around 1972 for corn, 1973 for wheat, and 1978 for rice.[49] In fact, a linear trend is not really ideal for the 1970s: the data for rice, wheat, corn, and sorghum yields more closely describe a hyberbolic acceleration typical of technological change. Thus the causes of this acceleration are likely to be found among technical developments originating during the previous decade.[50]

Some analysts[51] point to the dissolution of the communes and the introduction of the household responsibility system as important factors in bringing about the 1980s' staple crop growth. The argument is made that farmers' incentives to produce were greatly increased by the establishment of household rather than collective accounting and the return to something akin to private farming. Unfortunately, the attempts at estimating these effects in a country as complex as China are still too crude to be relied on for aggregate quantitative accuracy. Further, the degree to which the current Chinese system resembles private farming without state control and the degree to which the former system could operate in complete disregard of local income incentives have been exaggerated in these accounts.[52]

There is no question that the responsibility system, initiated between the late 1970s and mid-1980s, was fundamental to rapid growth in nongrain foodcrops, noncrop farming categories, and nonfarming rural categories of economic growth. But the effect on foodgrain production, in and of itself, could easily have been, and probably was, negative. Fertilizer purchases in previous decades were constrained not by demand but by inadequate supplies.[53] Green manure cultivation on foodcrop land plummeted (see Figure 3–7), as many farmers were doing more immediately profitable things with their time in the winter. Large quantities of land were taken out of foodgrain production during the period — 10.5 million hectares, between 1978 and 1988,[54] a decline of 8.7 percent — and converted to more profitable economic crops, or retired as marginal land, or developed for construction purposes. Multiple cropping reductions occurred as individual farmers found the degree of foodgrain cropping intensity promoted by local authorities, particularly triple cropping, to be uneconomical. All of these trends can be linked to the responsibility system, related adjustments, and to greater decentralization of authority.

While the population continued to grow in rural areas, there was a massive withdrawal of hundreds of millions of people, occasioned by the reforms, from concentrated attention to staple crop farming. The argument is made that there was nevertheless a net increase in effective labor,

Figure 3-7.

Production and Imports of Farm Chemicals and Area Sown with Green Manure Crops, 1952-87

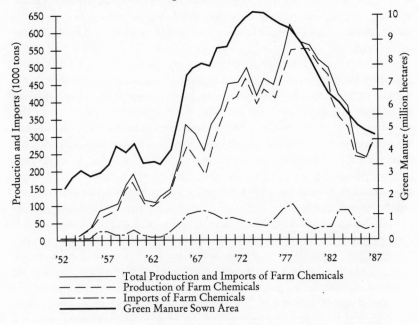

——————— Total Production and Imports of Farm Chemicals
— — — — Production of Farm Chemicals
—·——·— Imports of Farm Chemicals
——————— Green Manure Sown Area

Notes: According to two other sources, green manure area reportedly peaked at around 13.2 million hectares sometime in the 1970s, but the exact date was not mentioned. Also reported for 1980 were 9.961 million hectares, and 6.6 million hectares for 1987. These may refer to an expanded definition of green manure crop inclusion. Regardless of definition adopted, the general pattern of long-term rise and recent decline is certain.

Sources: Green manure: Zhongguo Nongyebu Turang Feiliaosi, "A Decade of China's Chemical Fertilizer Work," *Zhongguo nongbao* 17 (1959): 25; *Renmin ribao*, June 5, 1965; ZGNYNJ 1980, 96, 97, 349; ZGTJNJ 1981, 138, 141; ZGNYNJ 1981, 22; ZGNYNJ 1982, 81; ZGNYNJ 1983, 48; ZGNYNJ 1984, 83, 96; ZGNYNJ 1985, 143, 157; ZGNYNJ 1986, 176, 191; ZGNYNJ 1987, 208-209, 227; ZGTJZY 1988, 25; NYJJZL 1949-83, 133-39; "Land Sterility," *The China Daily*, May 15, 1988. Area data for 1966-69 are estimated from data for "other crops" for those years, including vegetables, melons, green manure, and green fodder crops. The proportions attributable to green manure crops are derived by linear interpolation using pre-1966 and post-1969 data. Data in notes are from "Land Sterility"; Zhang Xiaohua, "Tuiguang dong lüfei" [Extension of Winter Green Manure], ZGNYNJ 1981, 149; Sun Han, "Organic Farming—Growing Plants the Organic Way," in Sylvan Wittwer, Yu Youtai, Sun Han and Wang Lianzheng, eds., *Feeding a Billion* (E. Lansing: University of Michigan Press, 1987), 116.

   Farm chemicals: ZGNYNJ 1980, 40: AGTJZY 1988, 42, 87: NYJJZL 1949-1983, 293. PRC SSB, *China Trade and Price Statistics in 1987* (Beijing: China Statistical Information and Consultancy Service Center, 1987), 199-200.

because the intensity, duration, and quality of work improved with the responsibility system incentives.[55] But the critical question is whether foodgrain production in China was more constrained by shortages of labor or of fertilizers. On China's nitrogen- and phosphate-depleted soils,[56] with limited quantities and limited effectiveness of recyclable organic manures, the fertilizer-responsive varieties fundamentally lacked soil nutrients. A large part of this deficiency could only be addressed by manufactured fertilizers.

If technological change (including water control, HYVs, fertilizer use, and other techniques and industrial inputs) has been the principal basis for staple crop production growth in China, how has this process been affected by reforms? In addition to the household responsibility system and rural economic diversification, the reforms explicitly included: the institution of relatively free markets, supplementing the governmental marketing activity; a 20 percent increase in procurement prices, plus a 50 percent increase for over-quota deliveries; and regional reallocation of cropping specialization. To this list must be added various other institutional adjustments, including decentralization of financing for agricultural investments such as water control and extension systems and efforts to make such systems (including fertilizer deliveries) more financially self-supporting. These adjustments were made necessary by the immense food subsidy burden which followed the increases in procurement prices, foodgrain production, and urban populations (1979–84), without a commensurate increase in urban sales prices. The government's role as buyer of last resort for foodgrain products was formally eliminated in 1985, and state procurement was placed on a contract system which directly linked farmer deliveries of grain crops with government provision of specific fertilizers and other inputs.[57]

Regional Specialization
Regional specialization in cropping has had an important positive effect on economic crops. Along with foodgrain sales guarantees, higher purchase prices, tied fertilizer deliveries, and other measures, it has brought about a tripling of output in many economic crop categories between the mid-1970s and the late 1980s.[58] But aside from the large net loss of staple crop land to economic crops, the regional reorganization has had relatively little aggregate effect on foodgrain production. The principal increases have been for soybeans and several lower-valued coarse grains more suited to marginal areas, in which government-sponsored wheat and corn expansion had displaced them. Such adjustments have generally been sensible and important to local, often poorer, communities, particularly when accompanied by greater farmer choice in crop selection. Yet the aggregate impact has been relatively small and probably does not counterbalance the reassignment of higher-quality staple crop land to economic crops.

Price Changes

Price changes certainly helped to maintain incentives to concentrate sufficient labor and inputs, especially fertilizers, on grain crops, despite the liberalization of more profitable economic activities. Without price increases, the absorption of massive quantities of fertilizers required for the yield increases would have been much more difficult. Some of the most important price adjustments in promoting fertilizer application to staple crops were indirect ones, and were supported by market restrictions. Of particular significance was the tying together of deliveries at subsidized prices of a large amount of high quality fertilizer to grain sales.[59]

Adjustments in Markets

Price increases helped to maintain grain production incentives, but probably were larger than necessary and contributed to the budgetary problems which forced the government in 1985 to eliminate its role as guaranteed buyer of staple crops. For some lower-valued foodcrops, this had a depressing effect in surplus areas. In a single year the marginal rate dropped from a very high level to a very low level, inasmuch as local market prices in surplus areas were not adequately buoyed up for lower-valued crops,[60] and excess demand arose in deficit areas, owing to a low level of national market integration. This underdevelopment resulted from poor transportation and communication infrastructures, local administrative and policy barriers, and from lagging development of private marketing institutions.

The availability to farmers fulfilling their contract obligations of private market alternatives for more highly valued foodcrops undoubtedly had a positive effect on farmer incentives to produce them. Since yields were constrained primarily by inadequate fertilizer supplies, the appropriate interpretation is that the availability of private markets helped to maintain incentives to increase production in the face of rapidly rising availability of fertilizers and access to other income-earning activities.

Budgetary Adjustments

More importantly, the price increases were accompanied by major budgetary adjustments. State investment in agriculture declined from 10 percent of the capital construction budget during most of the 1960s and 1970s, and 14 percent in 1978, to 3 percent in the period 1985–88.[61] The decline was particularly significant for water control projects, which declined, according to official data, by 2.1 percent (1978–85).[62] While some regions and localities were able to handle the decentralization in financing, many, including the poorest areas, were not. These financial problems were exacerbated by the greater difficulty of organizing cheap or free farm labor to maintain irrigation systems. The pace of new irrigation construction

77

declined considerably, while deterioration and capacity reduction in existing systems accelerated, especially in poor areas (see Table 3-6).[63]

Investment in thirteen large-scale synthetic ammonia/urea complexes in the early 1970s made possible a rapidly increasing supply of nitrogen fertilizers in the late 1970s and early 1980s. But by the mid-1970s, national investment in new fertilizer production capacity had fallen precipitously. From 1979 to 1985, budgetary problems brought on by the price increases insured that investment in new capacity remained at low levels through the mid-1980s. Reliance on imports, requiring scarce foreign exchange, to maintain supply increases has kept distribution excessively focused on market-oriented areas where fertilizer use is already intensive and marginal response is relatively low.[64]

There were also important effects on fertilizer prices. The effort to reduce the budgetary drain from fertilizer subsidies in market-oriented areas led to high marginal prices for fertilizer delivered at above contracted quantities.[65] This was especially disadvantageous for middle-level and poor localities where fertilizer is generally scarce, and which are less linked into abundant high-quality supplies through the public farm product marketing system.

The task of the extension system was made considerably more complicated by the dissolution of collectives. Seed production and distribution were placed on a commercial basis. Although these organizations typically run large deficits, economic factors have led to a concentration on seed distribution for highly valued crops (including hybrid rice and corn seeds) for major commercial areas. Provision of improved seeds for non-maize coarse grains and for root and tuber crops in the poorer areas has clearly fallen further in priority. There is also evidence that economic factors, including the high price of hybrid seeds imported from outside the province, and the expense of providing guaranteed quantities of subsidized grain to within-province farmers specializing in seed production, have inhibited the rate of expansion of supplies of hybrid seed.[66] Despite these limitations, area under cultivation with corn and rice hybrids has increased, even in poor areas.

The foregoing suggests that the whole package of reforms, including budgetary adjustments, had divergent and complex effects on foodgrain production. The overall effect, net of higher prices and private market opportunities, was almost certainly negative. Even these positive measures must be viewed in terms of maintaining rather than creating incentives to purchase fertilizers and to apply them to foodcrops. As fertilizer supplies rapidly increased, rural economic activities were liberalized, and labor was withdrawn from staple crop production.

Grain Production Stagnation (1985–89)
How then should grain production stagnation be viewed? One can suggest in general that this should be viewed without too much alarm. Diversifica-

tion away from excessive concentration on staple crops was, after all, a specific goal of the reforms. Gross value of agricultural output, calculated at constant prices, even during these "stagnation" years, increased by an average of 4.4 percent per year.[67] Grain output value actually increased between 1984 and 1988 (even without considering adjustments for quality improvements within crop categories) and has set a record in total quantitative terms in 1989, despite economic retrenchment.

There are a wide variety of causes for the deceleration in grain production growth during the 1985–89 period. The most important is that the differential between potential and actual yields had closed substantially in China's major market-oriented foodgrain areas, as the required fertilizers had been supplied. Thus a significant deceleration from the unsustainably high rates of the 1978–84 period was inevitable. Further growth in foodgrain yields will depend on increased distribution of fertilizers to middle-income and poorer areas, continued technical change in all three basic categories throughout China, and (inevitably slower) improvements in the efficiency of these systems and in the quality of associated inputs. There is ample evidence that progress in these areas is continuing.[68]

Several special conditions also contributed to grain production stagnation during the 1985–89 period: a decline since the late 1970s in multiple cropping (recovering since 1985) and in irrigated area (recovering since 1986) due to financial retrenchment and decentralization (see Table 3–1); decline since the mid-1970s in fertilizer production capacity completions (recovering since 1985); massive dislocation in foodgrain and fertilizer markets (1985–86);[69] nationwide hybrid seed shortage (1988); a farm credit crisis (1985–89); failure of the government to pay cash for grain deliveries (intermittent throughout 1985–89);[70] net deterioration of foodgrain purchase prices (1985–88); periodic exclusion of grain from free markets (1986–89);[71] and an increase in the marginal price of several fertilizers (especially since 1986), hybrid seed, and plastic sheeting. Yet most of these problems have become less serious at the close of the decade.

China as a Source of Technology and Agricultural Innovation

Some of the world's earliest agricultural civilizations existed within the area of modern China. China is the genetic center of origin for numerous foodcrops of global significance, including rice, several millets, Chinese sorghum, soybeans, and other bean crops. China's size, geographic diversity, and its historic and present barriers to the movement of people and products have combined to allow the development of genetically diverse plantings of several other important foodcrops, such as wheat, corn, and sweet potatoes, imported centuries ago from other parts of Asia and the western hemisphere. China, in addition, enjoys a wealth of unusual varieties of medicinal herbs, fodder grasses and legumes, tropical fruits, tree crops, and edible roots. Thus, collection, taxonomy, and presentation of China's genetic resources and the continued development of genetic exchange with China is of considerable importance.

It is less well appreciated that China is an important innovator of agricultural technology, especially in applied research, development, and extension of simpler and inexpensive forms of imported technology, and with regard to sophisticated farmer practice under conditions of low capital/labor and low land/labor ratios. It is currently fashionable to point to the inefficiency of socialist systems, yet China's generation and diffusion of technology are worthy of closer study by the rest of the world. A partial listing of significant innovations may be useful.

Hybrid Rice

An area of research investigated and then dropped by scientists in Japan, the United States, and Europe during the first half of the twentieth century, hybrid rice development has been pursued aggressively in China since the 1960s. Several Chinese hybrids now have the highest per unit yield potential of all rice varieties. While reservations have been expressed regarding the economic viability of hybrids outside of China, continued research and development in China over the past fifteen years, and improvements in subsequent varieties, have ameliorated many of the shortcomings. The difficulty and expense of breeding work remains a limitation for some other national systems, but the greatest costs have already been borne by China, where breeding procedures are continually being streamlined.

HYVs for Other Cereals and Distant Crosses

Yield potentials of Chinese-bred varieties for wheat, corn, and sorghum, as well as on-farm yields in high-input regions, match the best in the world, while average-yield levels already surpass those of most developing nations and several developed countries. China is a center for work on distant crosses, including proven successes such as triticale, wheat-elytigia, and indica-japonica rice, as well as more exotic crosses like rice-sugarcane and rice-sorghum. Substantial work on upland rice varieties for North China is being planned.

Sweet Potatoes

Sweet potato research in the advanced countries has almost disappeared, along with cultivation, while the overworked breeding and research systems of countries where the crop is of greater economic and food security importance rarely allocate sufficient resources to sweet potato development. China has a large and active sweet potato research and breeding system and produces four-fifths of the world's output. This consists primarily of short-maturation period varieties, often planted in less hospitable seasons, with modest use of inputs and often on poor quality land. Yet mean yields for sweet potatoes in China are substantially above the national averages of other major producers. China is working with the International Potato Center on promising crosses between domesticated and wild species.

Varieties Resistant to Environmental Stress

Of particular interest to many regions of developing countries are the Chinese varieties tolerant of, or resistant to, various forms of environmental stress, including waterlogging, flash floods, hot winds, heavy rain and hail storms, low temperatures, various types of poor soils, insects, diseases, and, particularly, lodging and drought. A few significant breakthroughs occurred during the 1970s; since the early 1980s crop research and development on behalf of environmentally stressed areas have become an official priority of the Academy of Agricultural Sciences.

Significant improvements in varieties in the last few years have been extended to several poor regions. China's ability to marginally adjust cropping systems and seasonal timing, combined with varietal improvement aimed at minimizing losses from locally defined environmental stress, is an underappreciated contribution to improvements in stability and mean levels of grain production.

Rapid Application of Research Results

For new seed technology, China's system for moving research results through development, testing, and registration procedures and on to seed production and extension is perhaps the most rapid in the world. This involves between three to five years for wheat and rice in the fastest regional systems, as opposed to the seven to twelve years that is more typical internationally. During the 1950s and 1960s there were substantial penalties paid for overhasty extension, repeated on a smaller scale in the late 1970s and the early 1980s with hybrid rice and corn. But China has now substantially reduced the riskiness of the system. This has been an extremely important factor in prolonging growth in cereal yields in advanced regions where farm yields quickly approach experimental potential. In such regions, major varietal turnover may occur every two to three years, though the national average is twice this interval.

Plant Tissue Culture

The speedy turnover process is, in part, the result of aggressive development of tissue culture research, collapsing generational time requirements and increasing breeding precision. Such techniques are skilled-labor-intensive but require relatively inexpensive equipment, making them especially attractive to capital-poor countries with good educational systems in agricultural sciences. Important tissue culture results date from the early 1970s in China and now cover all major foodcrops, economic crops, fruit, vegetables, fodder crops, and medicinal herbs.

Intercropping

China, where the technique originated and first developed as a subscience, is still unquestionably the intercropping center of the world. The difficulties it presents for mechanization of on-field activities seem to have dampened interest in developed countries. Chinese farmers use intercropping as a way of maintaining soil health while generating greater output value per unit of land. Judiciously selected pairs of crops compete less for soil nutrients when planted in alternating rows. But the technique is also used for control of insects and disease transmission. As environmental problems and production sustainability issues receive greater attention, enthusiasm for the growing fund of Chinese research and farmer experience may increase. The potential attractiveness for less developed countries is especially clear.

Plastic Sheeting and Plastic Soil Mulch

Polyvinyl chloride and polyethylene plastic films used as seedling covers transmit sunlight for plant growth while at the same time protecting plants from cold and freezing temperatures, hot desiccating winds, and excessive rain and hail, all of which present problems in regions of China. Used primarily to protect high-priced vegetables and fruit in the West, plastic sheeting was first employed in China in 1958 as cover for rice seedling beds. By 1965, use had spread to selected localities throughout China[72] as a means of extending the growing season, reducing cold weather risk, facilitating increased crop intensity, and extending the range of several important crops to higher elevations and more northern latitudes. But it was not until 1979 that China's Agricultural Inputs Corporation began to supply plastic sheeting on a large scale. Within two years, sheeting covered an area of 2.2 million hectares. In 1989, 300,000 tons of plastic sheeting were supplied to farmers.[73] This provides for an incremental coverage of 0.8-2.0 million hectares, depending on the thickness of plastic provided.

Plastic sheeting is now widely used on a variety of field crops during the early stages of plant growth. A recently developed Chinese product is capable of blocking or diffusing intense sunlight but intensifying weaker sunlight. The price, supply, and product durability of standard types of plastic sheeting now rival the quality and quantity of fertilizer and hybrid seed, in terms of farmers' input concerns in temperate rice-growing regions. While supply to many poorer regions is inadequate or nonexistent, plastic sheeting is almost ubiquitous in most rice regions, is becoming widespread in highland areas in order to extend hybrid corn, and is frequently observed elsewhere.

A logical extension of plastic sheeting for conserving resources is the construction of plastic greenhouses, not only for high-priced fruit and vegetable crops, but also for rice seedlings in areas with cold spring weather. Even Guizhou, one of China's poorest rice growing provinces, had in 1987 plastic greenhouses for rice seedlings covering 11,300 hectares, and 26,700 hectares by 1989.[74]

Plastic soil mulch was introduced from Japan during the 1970s for use on municipal vegetable gardens, and its use spread quickly: from 5,000 hectares in 1980 to 1.3 million hectares in 1984, primarily on cotton (64 percent), peanuts (12 percent), and vegetables and fruit (10 percent). During the latter half of the 1980s, its use has increased on corn, potatoes, and sugar crops so that application in China is now more varied and extensive than anywhere in the world.[75]

Soil mulches, like sheeting, increase and stabilize soil temperature and are useful for raising production by allowing earlier planting of longer-season, higher-yielding varieties, or the substitution of shorter-season varieties. These mulches can facilitate the cultivation of an additional crop within the year and limit soil desiccation in arid areas. Mulches are also used increasingly in advanced areas for weed control, as rising opportunity costs for labor combine with poor factor mobility to reduce traditional hand weeding. Weed control is particularly important because of the quantities of fertilizers applied, at a time when herbicide supply remains limited, uncertain, and expensive.

Biological Control of Diseases and Pests

From the mid-1960s to the late 1970s, the development of biological plant protection techniques was given emphasis as research-intensive control mechanisms that would obviate the need for industrial and imported inputs. Much of this emphasis dissipated in the early 1980s as the new leadership embraced internationally popular chemical products to improve soil fertility and control pests and diseases, just as alarm over farm chemical use was growing in the rest of the world. Nevertheless, China banned DDT and BHC on edible crops in 1978, finally enforcing a total ban, complete with import controls and moratoriums on supply of basic chemicals to factories in 1982–83. China purchased additional biological technology from several American firms that went bankrupt from the expensive registration procedures matching those for chemical industry products at the time. But despite an apparent decline in output from factories, as reflected in official data (Figure 3–7), more potent and dangerous farm chemicals were imported or produced illegally, causing serious problems in China in the mid–to–late 1980s.

Research and development emphasis on biological controls has reintensified, and China already is one of the world's leaders in both variety of techniques and extent of farm coverage. One type or another of control now covers twenty million hectares — roughly one-fifth of Chinese farmland.[76] The most broadly extended technique is the mass breeding and release of predatory and parasitic insects, such as Trichogramma wasps. Others include the fabrication of insect and disease resistant natural pollens, bacterial and viral control, techniques for flooding combined with innovative use of frogs and ducks, and the use of beneficial insect varieties.

Organic Manures and Other Soil Treatments

China is by far the world's leader in the application of organic manures, as measured by the quantities and varieties applied, extent of adoption and technical sophistication of the average farmer, and by scientific research. The almost ubiquitous use of organic manures is one of the principal reasons growth in nitrogen use and average yields have increased so rapidly during the 1970s and 1980s. This also explains why Chinese soils can be farmed so intensively and productively on a sustainable basis. The total use of organic manures is estimated at 25–30 million tons of nutrients annually, or around ten tons of materials per cultivated hectare.[77]

In sophisticated farming areas, techniques for storing, fermenting, disinfecting, and applying manures have improved, partly as the result of the development of cheap but effective biogas generators. While the biogas fad flourished and then disappeared throughout much of the world, China reached extension levels of approximately twelve million family-size units concentrated in Zhejiang, Hunan, and Sichuan, where climatic conditions are favorable, and developed a few large and successful municipal units. Predictably, the extension efforts failed in areas outside the optimal climatic zones.

As with other areas of research, China has continued with biogas development and is successfully extending the practical frontier, now enclosing all central and southern provinces, and even much of North China.[78] Biogas digesters not only furnish cheap energy for household and modest production uses, but also provide hygienic anaerobic housing for wastes, limit the spread of disease, reduce nitrogen volatilization losses from manures, and add absorbable proportions of other nutrients through fermentation gains.

Traditional Chinese green manure crops such as sesbania, astragalus, alfalfa, clovers, legumes, and vetches have suffered substantial area losses during the 1980s as a result of greater individual control over cropping decisions, closer links between farm production value and farmer income, and higher food and economic crop prices (see Figure 3-7). But China remains one of the principal areas of research and on-farm use of azolla and nitrogen-fixing algae, which have not experienced on-farm declines. China also is an important source of research, development, and practical experience involving a variety of soil additives and inorganic soil treatments.

Fresh Water Aquaculture
Japan is the unquestioned technological and production leader in marine aquaculture, yet China reigns in fresh water fish farming and has done so for most of recorded history. Treatises on the construction of ponds, collection, hatching, and growth augmentation techniques date from at least the fifth century B.C. Integrated aquaculture development, exploiting the ecological and symbiotic relationships among varieties within a single system, is most closely identified with the Ming Dynasty some five hundred years ago.

During the People's Republic period, most of the popular edible carp varieties were domesticated, and considerable research and development on new feed materials, artificial breeding, and interregional crossbreeding were carried on. Aquatic product yield in the most productive Chinese areas exceeds ten tons per hectare, with average yields around 750 kilograms nationally.[79]

During the 1980s, simplified aquaculture techniques, developed during the previous decade, were extended to new regions with little or no farmer experience with aquaculture. Economic liberalization and commercial expansion within China's prime aquaculture areas (Guangdong, Hunan, Hubei, and Jiangsu) and other southern and central provinces, coupled with briskly rising rural incomes, created a boom in supply and demand for aquaculture products. This increased from an annual average of only 755,000 tons per year (1975–78) to 3.90 million tons in 1988. Even marine aquaculture products rose from a stagnant 420–460,000 tons (1977–81) to 1.42 million tons in 1988.[80]

Now that much of the Chinese population has reached the diversification stage of food consumption, the demand for fish will continue to grow rapidly with rising incomes. With continued depletion, eutrophication, and pollution of Chinese coastal and natural freshwater resources, already advanced and practically irreversible in major population regions, the dependence on aquaculture will increase as will emphasis on continued development of cheap, easily extendable, and increasingly productive technology.

Other Areas of Innovation
Chinese innovations indirectly related to agriculture, or related to farming more broadly, include acupuncture and moxibustion for animals, decentralized energy development, and hydraulic engineering aimed at overcoming various kinds of special water-related problems.

International Transfer of Chinese Technology
The listing above is only partial but indicates the variety and dimensions of China's ongoing contribution to technical development in agriculture. Does the rest of the world appreciate and profit from this development?

To a certain extent the answer is yes. The Food and Agriculture Organization (FAO) has sponsored exploratory studies in a number of the above areas. Nine of the thirteen institutes that comprise the Consultative Group for International Agricultural Research have cooperative activities with China, some of which are extensive. The International Bank for Plant Genetic Resources and the International Potato Center have established program offices at the Academy of Agricultural Sciences in Beijing. The cooperative activities of the International Rice Research Institute (IRRI), Centro Internacional de Mejoramiento de Maiz y Trigo (CIMMYT), Centro Internacional de Agricultura Tropical (CIAT), and International Food Policy Research Institute (IFPRI) are considerable and long standing. Most of these institutes exchange genetic materials with China and undertake other forms of technological cooperation. IRRI and IFPRI conduct cooperative economic research on Chinese technology and related issues.

IRRI assisted in establishing the China National Rice Research Institute in Hangzhou, modelled in conception, if not realization, after IRRI. An International Freshwater Aquaculture Center has been established in Hunan, with FAO's cooperation. There has been, in some areas, commercial interest: both Japanese and American companies are now working with China's hybrid rice. IRRI has had a hybrid rice research program for most of the decade, and there exists experimental hybrid rice cultivation in India and in the Philippines.

There is university-based technical cooperation between North American, European (especially German), and Japanese universities and Chinese counterparts. Foreign governmental organizations, notably the Australian Center for International Agricultural Research (ACIAR) and the German Technical Assistance Organization (GTZ), have funded numerous technical research projects in China. The flow of technology, however, is primarily toward China, although non-Chinese have the opportunity to work on Chinese problems in a Chinese setting and become more familiar with Chinese approaches.

Yet it is difficult to avoid the conclusion that too little use has been made of China as a generator of technology. And it is important to ask ourselves why that is so. There are several obvious reasons. Relatively few Chinese speak English or other foreign languages with any degree of facility. Chinese is a difficult language and few non-Chinese speak it. China has been open to relatively easy foreign contact only recently, and this opening is still incomplete. Chinese research and development institutions are highly compartmentalized and geographically dispersed, and information flow among them is inefficient, making it difficult to understand the state of the art or the degree and experience of extension of technologies. But there are additional problems which warrant consideration.

Although south-south interchange between China and other developing countries is not unknown, it rarely gets very far. Occasional technical delegations are organized, but there is too little follow-up. Developing countries evidently do not have the resources and technical manpower to devote to low-priority activities such as interchanges with other developing countries. China's advanced position in agricultural technology is poorly appreciated within that community.

Among industrialized countries, there appears to be an approach-avoidance problem with respect to China. Western enthusiasm for and interest in China, culturally and economically, is cyclical. A similar pattern can be detected with technological research, even within international organizations. There have been several waves of enthusiasm with and interest in particular aspects of Chinese agricultural technology which are invariably followed by the discovery of limitations to the technology. The conclusion is drawn that particular items are not very practical or applicable to the rest of the world. Yet, in instance after instance, Chinese scientists and institutions continue to work on these technologies, and in many cases problems are resolved and the limitations are substantially reduced. Western countries still maintain their outdated evaluations as a result of the failure to follow-up and monitor developments in China. Hybrid rice is an excellent example, but there are others for which valuable time has been lost, or is still being lost, by other countries for whom Chinese technologies could prove useful.

There is generally little Western technical or commercial interest in Chinese innovations, outside the relatively small community which specializes in work related to developing countries. The participation of donor and other international organizations associated with developing countries is relatively limited. This lack of interest in the West is particularly related to differences in factor proportions. Most Chinese innovations are particularly appropriate for countries with low capital-to-labor and low land-to-labor ratios. Several of these innovations also require for their development a relatively large and sophisticated research community and a fairly well functioning extension and monitoring system. The absence of these capabilities in a number of developing countries hinders their receptivity to Chinese technological models.

Summary

China has entered a new stage of food consumption development, as the current consumption of basic staple crops for the large majority of the population has reached adequate levels. Progress is now more appropriately focused on dietary diversification and improvements. Thus growth in agricultural output value, which has continued at a reasonable pace, even during the recent years of staple crop production stagnation, is a more appropriate indicator of success.

Yet further growth in staple crop production continues to have strategic importance in China for a variety of reasons. China has now entered a second stage of technical transformation of its agricultural sector, with further yield progress in advanced areas depending increasingly on improvements in efficiency and quality of inputs and services related to farm productivity. Continued attention has to be paid to bringing China's poorer areas through the first-stage transformations, with an emphasis on basic irrigation and flood control, and adequate HYV and fertilizer availability. This process for less-advantaged areas will remain important for the foreseeable future, despite necessary efforts to diversify poor-area income sources away from excessive dependence on agriculture and to liberalize factor and product markets.

The process of diffusion of basic technical change for staple crop products in China's poor regions and localities has always lagged behind progress in wealthier areas, and more obstacles to this diffusion process have arisen in the 1980s. Yet progress in supplying needed fertilizers throughout such areas has increased considerably in the 1980s. Supplies of appropriate HYV staple varieties have increased in many poorer counties and complementary plastic sheeting has been introduced in some. Water control has suffered, however, with new facilities opening in only a few localities, while capacity has deteriorated in most of China's poorer areas.

China is an important source of technological innovations related to agricultural productivity. Yet international mechanisms are weak in evaluating and transferring those technologies for the benefit of other developing countries that are characterized by low capital-to-labor and low land-to-labor ratios. An exception is the increasing inclusion of Chinese varietal diversity into international banks for genetic resources. As the world approaches the twenty-first century, China's experience will provide an increasingly important source of knowledge and of unrealized potential for facilitating agricultural progress in developing countries.

Notes

1. For a review of the theoretical elements of this strategy, see John W. Mellor, "Agriculture on the Road to Industrialization," in *Development Strategies Reconsidered,* U.S. Third World Perspectives no. 5, ed. John W. Mellor and Valerina Kallab (New Brunswick: Transaction Books, 1986). For a summary of the relationship of this body of theory to China's agricultural development, see Bruce Stone, "Chinese Socialism's Record on Food and Agriculture," *Problems of Communism* 35 (September–October 1986): 63–72.

2. Classic 1960s treatments quantifying developments in Asian countries include Shigeru Ishikawa, *Economic Development in Asian Perspective* (Tokyo: Kinokuniya, 1967); and John W. Mellor, *The Economics of Agricultural Development* (Ithaca: Cornell University Press, 1966).

3. See Shigeru Ishikawa, "China's Food and Agriculture: A Turning Point," *Food Policy* (May 1977): 90–102; and Reiitsu Kojima, "Possibility of Expansion of Scale of Farm Operations," *The China Quarterly* 116 (December 1988).

4. For a full discussion of these stages, see Bruce Stone, "The Next Stage of Agricultural Development: Implications for Infrastructural, Technological and Policy Priorities," a paper presented at the Colloquium on Agricultural Reform and Development in China, held in conjunction with the Annual Meetings of the American Society of Agronomists, Las Vegas, October 18–19, 1989 (publication forthcoming, 1990).

5. Bruce Stone, "Chinese Socialism's Record on Food and Agriculture"; Bruce Stone, "Foodcrop Production and Consumption Performance in China and India," a paper prepared for the Annual Meeting of the American Association for the Advancement of Science, Chicago, February 15, 1987.

6. Bruce Stone, "Developments in Agricultural Technology," *The China Quarterly,* no. 116 (December 1988): 767–822; see also Anthony M. Tang and Bruce Stone, *Food Production in the People's Republic of China,* Research Report no. 15 (Washington, D.C.: International Food Policy Research Institute, 1980).

7. For detailed treatment, see Stone, "Developments in Agricultural Technology," 771–90; and James E. Nickum, "Dam Lies and Other Statistics: Taking the Measure of Irrigation in China, 1931–1988," a paper prepared for the International Food Policy Research Institute, Washington, D.C., November 1989.

8. "Foodgrains" (*liangshi*) include rice at paddy weight, wheat, corn, sorghum, millet, other minor cereals, soybeans, broad beans, mung beans, peas, and other minor bean crops, and, valued at one-fifth fresh weight, sweet potatoes and white potatoes. Calculations are based on Statistical Yearbook of China, Chinese edition, 1989 (hereafter, ZGTJNJ), 198.

9. Bruce Stone and Gunvant Desai, "China and India: A Comparative Perspective on Fertilizer Policy Requirements for Long-Term Growth and Transitional Needs," in *China's Rural Development Miracle,* ed. John Longworth (St. Lucia: University of Queensland Press, 1989).

10. Ibid.; and Bruce Stone, "Chinese Fertilizer Application in the 1980s and 1990s: Issues of Growth, Balance, Allocation, Efficiency, and Response," in *China's Economy Looks Toward the Year 2000,* ed. U.S. Congress Joint Economic Committee (Washington, D.C.: U.S. Government Printing Office, 1986).

11. In this paper, Hainan Island, which has recently been accorded independent provincial status, is treated as part of Guangdong Province for the entire period.

12. For detailed analyses of the 1980–86 period, see the sources cited in n. 7. This subsection updates and summarizes that treatment.

13. Based on review of materials on Chinese wheat varieties organized and summarized in Bruce Stone, Charles Greer, Tong Zhong, Clark Friedman, Mary McFadden, and Melanie Snyder, "Agro-Ecological Zones for Wheat Production in China: A Compendium of Basic Research Materials," a compendium prepared for the International Center for Maize and Wheat Improvement (CIMMYT), International Food Policy Research Institute, Washington, D.C., 1985.

14. Information provided by Zhou Guorong and Cao Bingyi, Director and Vice-Director, Yunnan Province Seed Corporation, Kunming, January 9, 1990.

15. Information provided by Hong Ceyu, Agricultural Technical Extension Station, Guizhou Provincial Bureau of Agriculture, Guiyang, January 2, 1990.

16. Guojia Tongjiju Nongcun Shehui Jingji Tongjisi [State Statistical Bureau, Division of Rural Social and Economic Statistics] (eds.), *Zhongguo fenxian nongcun jingji tongji gaiyao, 1980–1987* [Statistical Abstract of China's Rural Economy, by County, 1980–1987] (Beijing: Zhongguo tongji chubanshe, 1989).

17. Li Yuecheng et al. (eds.), *Yunnansheng shuidao zaipei jishu guifan huibian* [Yunnan Province Official Compilation of Paddy Rice Cultivation Technology] (Kunming: Yunnansheng jingji weiyuanhui nongyechu, Yunnansheng nongye kexueyuan keji kaifachu, 1987) (hereafter YSZJGH).

18. Yunnansheng Nongyeting, *Yunnansheng Zajiodao Zaipei yu Liyong Tuiguang Mianji 1978–1988* [Yunnan Province Hybrid Rice Cultivation Use and Extension Area] (Kunming, 1989) (hereafter, YZZLTM); also discussions with Li Yuecheng, Yunnan Academy of Agricultural Sciences, Kunming, January 12 and 14, 1990.

19. Zhou Guorong and Cao Bingyi; according to a 1986 survey of hybrid rice areas in 47 counties, covering 42.2 percent of the provincial total, 29 percent of surveyed area averaged yields between 5.25 tons/ha and 6 tons/ha, 60 percent averaged more than 7.5 tons/ha, and 38 percent averaged more than 8.25 tons/ha. This development has helped to pull up the provincial average for all rice (including hybrids) from 4.2 tons/ha (1982) to 4.536 tons/ha (1988). Agricultural Yearbook of China, Chinese edition, 1983 (hereafter, ZGNYNJ), 37, and ZGTJNJ 1989, 194 and 202.

20. YZZLTM, 206; Zhou Guorong and Cao Bingyi.

21. Discussions with Guizhou Province Agricultural Bureau staff, Guiyang, August 1989; with Hong Ceyu, Agricultural Technical Extension Station, Guiyang, January 2, 1990; and with Li Jiaxiu, Grain Production Institute, Guizhou Academy of Agricultural Sciences, Guiyang, January 5, 1990.

22. YSZJGH, 26–68; and discussions with Li Yuecheng, Kunming, January 14, 1990.

23. YSZJGH, 109–135.

24. YZZLTM, 206.

25. Discussions with Li Yuecheng, Kunming, January 12 and 14, 1990; and with Zhou Guorong and Cao Bingyi, January 9, 1990.

26. Zhou Guorong and Cao Bingyi.

27. Although the varieties produce many shoots from each plant, the kernels themselves have low weight. Average per-hectare yields in some areas are higher, and in some, lower, although superior disease and cold resistance protects against large shortfalls. Also, separation of the grain from the plant is more difficult unless accomplished by machine, impeding farmer acceptance in Yunnan where separation is normally done by hand (Li Yuecheng).

28. Zhou Guorong and Cao Bingyi.

29. YZZLTM, 208.

30. See, for example, Bruce Stone, "Relative Foodgrain Prices in the People's Republic of China," in *Agricultural Pricing Policy for Developing Countries*, ed. John W. Mellor and Raisuddin Ahmed (Baltimore: Johns Hopkins University Press, 1988).

31. Discussions with Yunnan Province Poor Area Development Office staff, and various officials in Fugong County, Gongshan County, and Nujiang Prefecture governments, northwestern Yunnan, September 1989.

32. Director, Agricultural Development Research Group, Yunnan Province Bureau of Agriculture, Kunming, January 9, 1990.

33. Nicholas Menzies, Director of Beijing Office, Winrock International.

34. Charles Gitomer and Bruce Stone, "Sweet Potato and White Potato Development in China," a report prepared for the International Potato Center, Lima, March 1990.

35. Professor Wang Jun, Yunnan Normal University, Kunming, January 16, 1990.

36. Stone, "Developments in Agricultural Technology."

37. Gitomer and Stone, "Sweet Potato and White Potato Development in China."

38. Field notes, Nujiang Prefecture, September 1989, interview with Professor Wang Jun; and in January 1990.

39. Wang Jun.

40. Gitomer and Stone, "Sweet Potato and White Potato Development in China."

41. Peter Gregory, Masa Iwanaga, Ed French, Romeo Opena, Bruce Stone, and Charles Gitomer, *Sweet Potato Technology in China* (Lima: International Potato Center, 1987).

42. Niu Ruofeng, Director, Agricultural Economic Institute, Chinese Academy of Agricultural Sciences, Beijing, November 1, 1987.

43. Xiong Fengming, Hubei Seed Corporation, November 13, 1989; other field visits in South China, August 1989–January 1990.

44. Wu Sikai and Hong Ceyu.

45. Fugong County Vice-Chairman Fu, Nujiang Prefecture, September 1989.

46. Wu Sikai and Hong Ceyu.

47. Field visits in six provinces, August 1989–January 1990.

48. See Stone, "Developments in Agricultural Technology," and sources focusing on inputs and on varietal improvement for various foodcrops, cited therein.

49. For more detailed statistical treatment see Stone, "The Next Stage of Agricultural Development."

50. Stone, "Developments in Agricultural Technology."

51. For example, Justin Yifu Lin, "Farming Institutions, Food Policy, and Agricultural Reforms in China," included in this volume, and papers cited therein.

52. See, for example, Bruce Stone, "Fertilizer Marketing and Allocation in China," a paper prepared for the World Bank, June 1984; Stone, "Relative Foodgrain Prices in the PRC"; Scott Rozelle, "Village-Level Decision Making in Jiangsu," doctoral dissertation for the Agricultural Economics Department, Cornell University, 1990; Terry Sicular, "Ten Years of Reform: Progress and Setbacks in Agricultural Planning and Prices," *The China Quarterly* 116 (December 1988).

53. Stone and Desai, "China and India: A Comparative Perspective on Fertilizer Policy"; Stone, "Chinese Fertilizer Application in the 1980s and 1990s."

54. ZGTJNJ 1989, 192.

55. These ideas were developed by Jaroslav Vonek, *General Theory of Labor-Managed Market Economies* (Ithaca: Cornell University Press, 1970); the ideas were first applied to Chinese reforms of the late 1970s in Bruce Stone, "China's 1985 Foodgrain Production Target," in Tang and Stone, *Food Production in the PRC*.

56. Virtually all Chinese soils are deficient in nitrogen, and as of 1981–83, 73.4 percent were tested deficient in phosphate, of which the majority are seriously

deficient. There are growing potash deficiencies on 23–47 percent of China's farmlands, depending on the standard applied, and scattered deficiencies of micronutrients. Stone, "Developments in Agricultural Technology," 813 (table 9).

57. This system actually dated from the 1950s, but was formalized in explicit contracts beginning in 1984 with cotton, and in 1985 for staple crops.

58. These include cotton, peanuts, sesame, sugarcane, fruit, tea, and tobacco. Production quadrupled for jute and ambary hemp, rapeseed, and sugarbeets. Vegetable crop area has also grown rapidly. For details, see Stone, "The Next Stage of Agricultural Development"; or ZGTJNJ 1989, 200–201.

59. Stone, "Relative Foodgrain Prices"; Stone, "Chinese Fertilizer Application in the 1980s and 1990s"; Stone and Desai, "China and India: A Comparative Perspective on Fertilizer Policy Requirements."

60. This has been especially important in depressing production of root and tuber crops, although local governments stopped purchasing these crops as early as the late 1970s in some important producing provinces. Gitomer and Stone, "Sweet Potato and White Potato Development in China."

61. ZGTJNJ 1988 (English edition), 504.

62. ZGTJNJ 1989, 183.

63. For details see Stone, "Developments in Agricultural Technology," 771–90.

64. Stone, "Chinese Fertilizer Application in the 1980s and 1990s"; Bruce Stone, "Systemic and Policy Adjustment in the Administration of China's Fertilizer Development," a paper prepared for the World Bank, December 1986. Fertilizer production capacity decreased from 1.18 million metric tons (mmt) of nutrients per year (1976–79) to 0.32 mmt per year (1980–85) (ZGTJNJ 1989, 538).

65. Ibid.

66. Interviews with provincial officials in Guizhou, Yunnan, Hubei, Hunan, Jiangxi, and Guangxi, August 1989–January 1990.

67. Even including the stagnation period, the annual growth rate of agricultural output value, calculated in 1980 constant prices, averaged an impressive 7 percent per year (1980–88). Calculations are based on Robert Michael Field, "Trends in the Value of Agricultural Output, 1978–1988," a paper prepared for *The China Quarterly* Workshop on Food and Agriculture in the Post-Mao Era, Hong Kong, December 30, 1989–January 2, 1990, table 3A.

68. For the improvements in efficiency and quality, see Stone, "Chinese Fertilizer Application"; Bruce Stone, "Agricultural Production and Fertilizer in China (Parts I, II, and III), *Agro-Chemicals News in Brief,* October 1988, January 1989, and April 1989.

69. Sicular, "Ten Years of Reform"; Bruce Stone, "Chinese Fertilizer Sector Review, 1986/1987," a paper prepared for the World Bank, December 1987; Bruce Stone, "Fertilizer's Greener Pastures," *The China Business Review* 16 (September-October 1989): 46–55.

70. Sicular, "Ten Years of Reform"; *The China Business Review,* January-February 1985; for impact on fertilizer purchases, Bai Nansheng, "Guanyu nongcun zijin zhengci di jige wenti" [Several Issues Related to Rural Financial Policy], and Zhuang Musheng and Liu Chunbin, "Kongji nongcun xindai guimo yao qubie duidai zhangwo liangda" [Control of the Scale of Rural Credit Should Be Conducted on a Realistic Basis], Research Center for Rural Development reports, Beijing.

71. Field, "China: Trends in the Value of Agricultural Output"; and Sicular, "Ten Years of Reform."

72. "The Plastics Revolution," in *Feeding a Billion,* Sylvan Wittwer, Yu Youtai, Sun Han, and Wang Lianzheng, eds. (East Lansing: Michigan State University Press, 1987).

73. "Farm Ties Boost Growth" and "Sheeting for Farms Tops Production List," *The China Daily,* February 11, 1990, p. 4.

74. Tan Xiaohong, Plant Protection Dept., Guizhou Province Bureau of Agriculture, Guiyang, January 3, 1990.

75. "The Plastics Revolution," in *Feeding a Billion.*

76. "The War on Pests," in *Feeding a Billion.*

77. Zhongguo Nongye Kexueyuan, Turang Feiliao Yanjiusuo [Chinese Academy of Agricultural Sciences, Soil and Fertilizer Research Institute], *Zhongguo huaxue quhua* [China's Chemical Fertilizer Regionalization Plan] (Beijing: Zhongguo nongye chubanshe, 1986).

78. ZGTJNJ 1988 (English edition), 199.

79. Wittwer et al., *Feeding a Billion.*

80. ZGTJNJ 1989 (Chinese edition), 219.

CHAPTER 4

Dryland/Rainfed Agriculture and Water Resources Management Research and Development in India

R. P. Singh
Director, Central Research Institute for Dryland Agriculture, Hyderabad, India

Introduction

Water is the key input in agriculture. The progress in the farm sector of any country depends on how wisely water resources are managed and used. This is particularly the case for a large country like India, which is situated in the tropical belt and experiences extreme variations in climate and rainfall across the country.

It is estimated that the total precipitation in the country is approximately 400 million hectare meters (mhm) annually, of which 70 mhm is lost through evaporation. Of the remaining 330 mhm, around 150 mhm enters the soil and 180 mhm constitutes the runoff. For all the major and minor irrigation projects in the country up to this point, we have been able to utilize only 17 mhm out of the 180 mhm runoff, thus leaving about 160 mhm of precipitation that flows through rivers into the sea.

There is extreme variation in rainfall ranging from 10 centimeters (cm) at Jaisalmer in western Rajasthan to 1,000 cm at Cheerapunji in Meghalaya. Therefore, it is not surprising that floods and droughts can strike the country simultaneously at different places. Obviously for such a large country there can be no single strategy for management and utilization of water resources.

I am grateful to Dr. B. Venkateswarlu, Senior Scientist, Central Research Institute for Dryland Agriculture, Hyderabad, for the assistance provided in writing this paper. But for the generous help extended by the Smithsonian Institution and the permission accorded by the Government of India, it would not have been possible for me to participate in the colloquium.

Irrigation Development in India

India is blessed with many rivers and, therefore, great emphasis in large-scale development of surface irrigation has been given to dams and reservoirs. An amount slightly in excess of 152 billion rupees (Rs), or 9.5 billion U.S. dollars, was spent on irrigation between 1951 and 1985. By 1985-86 a total of 47 million hectares (mha) net irrigation potential was created. In other words, out of the 143 mha under cultivation, 47 mha, or 33 percent, has access to irrigation water. This irrigated area has played a key role in the increase in food production in India, a radical change often characterized as part of the Green Revolution. However, of late there have been serious problems with large irrigation dams. It costs today about Rs.27,000 to create an irrigation facility for a single hectare. Other problems arise in closing the gap between the potential created and that which is actually realized, in stemming high-level evaporation losses, and in overcoming extremely low irrigation water use efficiency (around 20 percent), waterlogging (i.e., rise in water table due to inadequate drainage), and salinity development.

Fallout of Large Irrigation Projects

The gap between the irrigation potential created after independence and that which is actually utilized is as large as 5.5 mha. Similarly, by 1980 waterlogging affected about 6 mha, and salinity about 7 mha, thereby forcing 13 million hectares out of cultivation. It is estimated that it costs about Rs.15,000 per hectare (ha) to reclaim these affected lands. There is also a problem of large-scale soil erosion in catchment areas that causes siltation of reservoirs (i.e., the depositing of sediments carried with runoff water), thereby reducing their storage capacity and depleting power generation. The efficiency of irrigation water use, in the final analysis, is so low that even with only a 10 percent saving in the efficiency, an additional 3 mha can be irrigated. Irrigation also has created regional imbalances in economic development.

Critical Issues Affecting Irrigation

Numerous studies and experiments have examined the problems arising from irrigated agriculture. Some of the issues are the following:

1. Priority must be given to realizing the irrigation potential already existing by improving its efficiency rather than creating new potential. This includes large-scale afforestation and soil conservation in the catchment areas (i.e., land area that contributes runoff to a given reservoir). For example, between 1951 and 1985 only Rs.27.23 billion had been spent on afforestation and soil conservation, which indirectly increase the availability of rainwater for agriculture at relatively lesser cost, as compared to the Rs.152.06 billion spent on direct crop irrigation projects. The former not only helps in the conservation of precious soil but also in preventing siltation. Greater allocations for "command area" development are needed, which would go a long way toward improved water management and higher irrigation efficiency. (Command area development refers to the entire range of activities related to land development, drainage, and cropping systems, etc., in the area affected by a given irrigation project.)

2. Work has to be done to identify crop patterns with high water use efficiency. Extensive research has been conducted in this area. It takes, on an average, 0.90 hectare meters (ha m) of water to irrigate one hectare by surface method, as compared with 0.65 ha m if it is from groundwater. Therefore, it becomes obvious that adequate attention has to be paid to the choice of crops in order to optimize irrigation. In general, crop mixtures use irrigation water more efficiently than discrete crops. The most appropriate cropping patterns have been determined for various projects based on experiments. However, the decision to shift a cropping system does not take place quickly as it is governed by choices of farmers and by socioeconomic conditions above and beyond net economic returns.

3. Conjunctive use of groundwater and surface water (e.g., canal water) leads to better irrigation efficiency. It is estimated that 40 million hectare meters (mha m) of groundwater are available in India today almost at no cost. Studies have been conducted on its potential. However, more emphasis needs to be given to groundwater utilization, in particular the recharging (i.e., refilling) of aquifers through better soil water conservation measures on watersheds. (An aquifer is a natural groundwater reservoir that is recharged as a result of yearly rainfall.)

4. Yet another issue is the provision of adequate drainage facilities from the very beginning of an irrigation project in order to avoid waterlogging and salinity development. These problems, unfortunately, affect some of the most fertile land of the country.

In view of the constraints on irrigation there is growing agreement in India to expand rainfed agriculture and the uses of water where it falls by means of appropriate water conservation. Extensive research has been undertaken to extend and stabilize the applications of water conservation in rainfed agriculture.

Rainfed Agriculture—Research and Development

In terms of the area covered and the population dependent on it, rainfed agriculture has become far more extensive in India than irrigated agriculture. Of the 143 million hectares (mha) of arable land in India, about 70 percent (100 mha) is currently rainfed. Most of the cereals, pulse and oilseed crops, and raw cotton are produced on rainfed lands. These lands, therefore, are important for the economy of the country today and will continue to be so in the year 2000 and beyond. The problems of these areas relate mainly to: low-level and erratic rainfall; impoverished soils; small and fragmented holdings; use of low-yielding local cultivars; the scarcity of fodder, fuel, and draft power; and poor infrastructure.

Concerted and well-directed research efforts for improving the productivity of drylands in India through the application of rainfed agricultural methods were initiated in 1970 with the establishment of the All India Coordinated Research Project for Dryland Agriculture (AICRPDA). These efforts were further strengthened with the setting up of the International Crops Research Institute for the Semiarid Tropics (ICRISAT) in 1972 and the Central Research Institute for Dryland Agriculture (CRIDA) in 1985.

Water Resources Management

A brief summary of the research and development work being carried out in India on water resources development in rainfed regions can be divided into three categories.

1. Cropping strategy, based on rainfall analysis and moisture availability periods.

2. *In-situ* moisture conservation technologies for optimum utilization of rainfall.

3. Rain water harvesting and use for crops at critical stress periods.

Crop Planning and Climate Analysis

Crop production on drylands depends upon the amount and distribution of rainfall. With the initiation of the dryland research, historical rainfall data of twenty-three representative locations in the country were analyzed with regard to: a) the dates of onset and termination of the rainy season and its variability, and b) the distribution of rainfall within the rainy season.

The information so generated was fit into the process of selection of efficient crops, varieties, and cropping systems. Later, the agroclimatological studies helped dryland research workers to: a) identify suitable crops and varieties for early, normal, and late commencement of sowing rains; b) identify and match intercropping systems with the rainfall pattern; c) determine optimum sowing periods for different crops and cropping systems; and d) assess the amount of inevitable runoff available for water harvesting and recycling in arid, semiarid, and subhumid regions of the country. All the data developed on efficient crops and cropping systems have been translated into packages of agronomic practices which are being disseminated by the state governments.

Weekly water balance computations have been carried out to determine the water availability periods for crop growth. Based on this information, regions that are suited for monocropping, intercropping, and double cropping have been identified. The date of commencement of sowing rains was observed to exercise considerable influence on the water availability periods for crop growth in dry farming tracts. Therefore, the drought vulnerability of rainfed crops was assessed, reflecting dates of commencement of rainy seasons, and threshold values of moisture availability for obtaining above-average yields were identified. In order to explain the productivity patterns of rainfed crops in relation to various dates of commencement of the rainy season, crop/weather models were developed using the concept of water requirement satisfaction of the crop during its growth cycle. (Water requirement satisfaction indicates the amount of soil water available for the crop in a given season in relation to the water needed for its optimum growth.)

Both long-term and short-term strategies for mitigating the effects of droughts in dry farming areas have been worked out and documented. A contingent crop production strategy has been worked out as a result of these experiences and has become a set of guidelines for managing weather aberrations in rainfed farming.

Rainfed/dryland farmers generally grow long-duration local varieties of crops that do not exactly fit into the growing season. Under such circumstances, introducing a suitable crop or cultivar that fits into a particular water availability period not only minimizes the risks but also results in a net yield enhancement. Based on the research conducted by AICRPDA, a number of cropping systems have been identified that effectively utilize the rainfall resources of a given region and provide a stable income over the years.

In-Situ Moisture Conservation

The second approach is to utilize the water where it falls by means of appropriate land treatments and *in situ* (i.e., at the same place) moisture conservation practices.

Some of these include off-season tillage, mulching, dead furrows, key line cultivation, compartmental bunding, graded border strips, and inter-plot water harvesting. Off-season tillage helps the rainwater to enter into the soil profile more effectively and, in addition, helps in weed control. Such practice in alfisols (i.e., highly leached red brown soils) of the Telengana region in the state of Andhra Pradesh increased the sorghum yield by 43 percent. Off-season tillage, however, is not suggested for aridosols (i.e., sandy soils of the desert regions) as this would accelerate wind erosion. Deep ploughing (i.e., up to 22 cm), once every two or three years, also helps to increase crop yield in soils with a hard subsoil below the plough layer.

Mulching is a well-known practice for minimizing the movement of moisture from the soil into the atmosphere. Poor infiltration of rainwater is a problem in vertisols (i.e., heavy black soils), which often leads to water stagnation. Vertical mulching (e.g., placing sorghum stubbles in trenches 40 cm deep, 15 cm wide, and protruding 10 cm above the ground level) has been found to enhance available soil moisture by 4–5 cm and to increase the grain yield of sorghum by 40–50 percent in vertisols at several locations in India. The making of "idle furrows," also called "dead furrows," at each 3.6 m interval helps in improving water retention. Such treatment at Anantapur in South India was found to increase the grain yield of groundnut by about 10 percent.

In alfisols, crops such as sorghum and pigeonpea can be grown as intercrops on slopes, and ridges are made later that help in controlling soil and water erosion. Such simple practices enhanced the seed yields by 15–20 percent, as compared to sowing on a flat surface. Broad bed and furrows (BBF) is another system eminently suited to vertisols. The basic objective of this system is to drain out excess water. A broad bed of 100 cm alternated with a 50 cm shallow furrow having a depth of 15 cm is useful in improving the moisture regime and draining excess water in places where water stagnation is a problem. This situation arises in high rainfall vertisol areas. ICRISAT conducted extensive experiments on this practice. On-farm trials at Akola in India showed that sorghum yield can be increased by 25 percent, as compared to flat sowing. Graded border strips of 130 × 11 m with a 0.1 percent grade are effective in deep alfisols with medium rainfall. Finger millet yield was increased by 42 percent as a result of this treatment at Bangalore in South India.

Ridge-and-furrow *in-situ* water harvesting is yet another promising system for the inceptisols (i.e., soils with poor horizon development as in alluvial soils) of subhumid areas. Maize is planted on the ridges and rice in furrows, thus meeting the varying water requirements of crops. The water requirement of rice is met by the water that is harvested into the furrows. Yield increases of about 18–21 percent for both crops can be obtained by this system, as compared to flat sowing.

The interrow water harvesting system is a practice suitable for light textured soils found in the arid region. Significant yield advantages have been recorded with the pearl millet crop by adopting this practice, in combination with the recycling of the water for supplemental irrigation.

Runoff Harvesting and Recycling

Rainwater can be utilized by collecting in small dugout ponds excess runoff during high-intensity rainfalls and then recycling it for supplemental irrigation at critical stages of crop growth. This water also can be used for pre-sowing irrigation of a rabi crop in potential double-cropping regions. A rabi crop is a crop grown during the post-rainy season (i.e., October–March) on the basis of stored soil moisture. Extensive studies have been undertaken on these aspects both in arid and semiarid areas. Experiments on catchment size and slope, size of the pond, effective sealants, water lifting devices, and choice of crops have been conducted both in alfisol and vertisol regions.

Existing water harvesting systems suffer from the fact that the donor catchment (i.e., actual area that is contributing the runoff) does not benefit from the runoff water. In a modified system with small dugout ponds, the water can be used for the donor catchment. Studies have shown that appropriate pond size varies with rainfall, ranging from 200 cu m to 3,000 cu m. Seepage losses pose a major problem in these dugouts. Though natural silting minimizes seepage losses in large tanks, it causes a reduction in storage capacity in small dugouts. Among the sealants evaluated, cement plus soil in a 1:8 ratio was found to be reasonably efficient and cost effective. But an ideal sealant has not been found yet that is both efficacious and cost effective.

For lifting water (i.e., taking out water from the pond and adding it to the cropped area), our experience has shown that for small ponds of 200 cu m, manual methods are more suitable. Only for big ponds of 3,000 cu m is it feasible to use mechanical pumps.

Benefits of Supplemental Irrigation from Stored Water

A number of experiments have been conducted on the criteria for using stored rainwater. For a number of crops, e.g., sorghum, pearl millet, cowpea, and tobacco, it has been found that maximum payoffs in terms of yields can be obtained if irrigation is applied at flowering. For post-rainy-season crops such as wheat and barley, the crown root initiation stage was found to be the most appropriate. Experiences at Bellary in South India have shown that a single application of 10 cm of water increased the yield of cotton by 76 percent in a subnormal year. In an ICRISAT experiment the sorghum yield in a vertisol region was 2,570 kilograms/hectare (kg/ha) without supplemental irrigation, whereas a single irrigation of 5 cm from runoff water boosted the yields to 3,570 kg/ha. Even greater benefits were apparent by supplemental irrigation in the aridisol regions of North West India. Experiments conducted at Jodhpur on light textured sandy loams showed that an irrigation of 5 cm to a pearl millet crop at a critical stage increased the yield by 35 percent. Application of a modest dose of fertilizers further enhanced the yield.

The effects of supplemental irrigation have been studied on a number of short- and long-duration crops in both the kharif season (i.e., rainy season, June–September) and the rabi season (i.e., post-rainy season, October–March). Short-duration, shallow-rooted crops like sorghum and pearl millet responded better than deep-rooted crops like castor. The latter crops needed relatively more water for a significant yield response. Scheduling of irrigation by the moisture depletion approach was also attempted for wheat in the post-rainy season. Irrigation at 50 percent depletion in two installments gave the best results. As compared to grain crops, higher economic returns for vegetable crops such as chilies, brinjal, and beans can be obtained if they receive the water from a dugout pond. The principle is to sow the crops in the late rainy season and supply water at the reproductive stage.

The cost of initial construction of a farm pond is high for a water harvesting system, and it is one of the principal constraints in the spread of this technology. Planting a horticultural crop such as ber (*Zizyphus numularia*) helps in quick repayment. Recently, efforts have been made to introduce pisciculture to optimize the returns.

Among the water application methods tried, an irrigating alternate furrow system was found to be more effective than use of the furrow method and flooding. Despite the clear demonstration of benefits of *in-situ* moisture conservation and runoff recycling in both the experimental plots and the operational research projects, these practices have not yet been applied on a wide scale by the farmers. There are many constraints, both financial and technological, but the most critical constraint is the fact that farm holdings in India are very small and fragmented. The average size of an operating farm is about 1.8 hectares, which limits the application of conservation methods. Therefore, it is now realized that water conservation development projects should be undertaken on a watershed basis. The impact of water resource development can be better seen when improved practices are adopted in a watershed as a whole (i.e., a unit of land and a drainage area contributing runoff water to a common collecting point).

Watershed Development Program

The principal components of a watershed development program are: a) improvement of water resources; b) *in-situ* soil and water conservation;

c) increased cropping intensity; and d) alternate land-use systems for efficient use of lands. Alternate land-use systems refer to all land-use practices other than growing regular arable crops. These include agroforestry, horticulture, pastures, and tree farming.

The Government of India in its Seventh Five-Year Plan has launched a national development program of rainfed agriculture on a watershed basis. By 1984–85 work was launched on 4,400 micro watersheds covering an area of 4.2 million hectares. Forty-seven model watersheds are being monitored by the Indian Council of Agricultural Research (ICAR) with field-level implementation by the state governments. The initial results have been quite encouraging. At Mittemari in Karnataka State in South India there has been significant improvement over a three-year period in crop yields, water resources development, and in the socioeconomic status of the people in the watershed, as compared to the outlying villages. At Tejpura in Uttar Pradesh there has been a marked improvement in the water table following the implementation of soil conservation programs. Significant improvement in crop yields and cropping intensity also has been recorded. In some watersheds it has now become possible to plant a double crop. During the last three years watershed management projects have won national productivity awards for significant contributions to farm productivity in rainfed regions.

Of late, nongovernmental organizations also are taking an interest in the concept of watersheds as the organizational units for long-term development of rainfed regions. These organizations are voluntary, or social work agencies, financed by public donations and trusts, or partly supported by the government. The Government of India trains hundreds of personnel annually to work in watershed development programs. Village development plans prepared by banks and other credit institutions are now being established on a watershed basis. Since there is an acute shortage of fodder and fuel wood in rural India, their supply has become a component of alternate land-use systems that have been introduced on a watershed basis.

Many of these water resource management technologies are being disseminated as a result of the operational research projects involving watersheds. However, unless a total package is adopted, individual components by themselves will not contribute to visible improvements in crop yields. The watershed concept, it is hoped, will go a long way in persuading farmers about the importance of comprehensive watershed resource management.

Considering the severe limitations on the future expansion of irrigation and the fact that groundwater exploitation cannot continue endlessly, there is little choice other than the efficient utilization of rainwater for a country like India, where the population is heavily dependent on agriculture.

India's Experiences in Rainfed Agriculture: Lessons for Other Countries

Many developing countries in West and South Asia, the Middle East, and Africa have problems of rainfed agriculture somewhat similar to India's. The technologies and experiences of India can be beneficially utilized by these countries.

For example, the technologies of water harvesting in sandy soils of arid and semiarid regions can be used with appropriate modifications in the nations of West Asia that have an arid climate and light textured soils. In fact, technical cooperation in water resource management already is being undertaken by the Central Arid Zone Research Institute (CAZRI) in Jodhpur, India, to train experts in many countries in arid land management to combat desertification.

Land degradation, low productivity, erratic rainfall, and problem soils are constraints shared by India and a number of African nations. India over the years has gained rich experience in soil and water management technologies applicable to semiarid and subhumid zones. Of importance is the Indian experience in watershed development for rainfed agriculture, in particular our development of methodologies for surveying and planning watersheds, monitoring hydrological changes, and identifying the various constraints. This experience can be useful for rainfed regions of Africa.

India also has developed a series of alternate land-use systems, including agroforestry, agrihorticulture (i.e., planting of fruit trees), silvi-pasture (i.e., grass and legume coverage), and alley cropping (i.e., tree plantings as hedges), with extensive research conducted over the past eight years. Some of these practices can be productively adapted in African countries that have low rainfall, adverse climatic conditions, marginal lands, and a high-density human and livestock population.

Policy Issues in Rainfed Agriculture

For a number of obvious reasons, the Government of India has laid heavy emphasis during the last thirty years on irrigated agriculture. Yet with the lessons learned from a heavy reliance on the large dams, the government has begun to emphasize the importance of rainfed agriculture, beginning with its Sixth Five-Year Plan (1980–81 to 1984–85). A comprehensive national watershed development program was launched in 1984. However, due to a number of technological and socioeconomic constraints, rainfed agriculture has not benefitted sufficiently from these limited policy initiatives.

To strengthen the research and development of rainfed agriculture, I put forward the following proposals.

1. Undertake a significant shift in investment from irrigated areas to rainfed areas, with a major emphasis on afforestation and soil conservation projects organized on a watershed basis.

2. Investment in soil conservation practices, including creation of appropriate infrastructure as well as water harvesting systems such as farm ponds, has to be undertaken on a village-by-village basis. This expenditure will only be a fraction of what the government already is spending on irrigation. Otherwise, without such government investment the high cost and the time delay in realizing immediate benefits will prohibit farmers from engaging in rainfed agricultural practices.

3. Weather aberrations continue to plague dryland farmers. Since seed is the primary input in the adoption of improved farm technology, seed banks must be established with government support in order to help farmers adopt contingent strategies whenever the weather becomes aberrant.

4. Draft power is a serious constraint in dryland agriculture. Individual farmers cannot afford to purchase mechanical implements such as tractors. Therefore, a system of custom-hiring in the villages would help farmers to complete their operations in a timely way at an affordable cost.

5. One of the principal factors explaining the nonadoption of improved crop production technologies is the element of risk involved in rainfed farming. Therefore, the availability of crop insurance for drought protection involving selected dryland crops would go a long way in instilling confidence in farmers and in stabilizing crop production.

6. Since farm holdings already are excessively fragmented, further division of lands should be minimized by means of weaning away some population from agriculture. This can be done by encouraging the development of small-scale, agro-based industries and services in the rainfed regions. In fact, agro-based industries are synergistic in their effects. For example, in the Indore area of Madhya Pradesh, a chain of soybean processing industries backed by high-level marketing and adequate price supports has served as a catalyst in the rapid improvement of soybean yields, both through the expansion of plantings and the rise in productivity.

7. In addition to low productivity in dryland areas there is also an acute scarcity of fodder. Silvi-pastoral systems on marginal lands should be encouraged through liberal financing, and fodder banks should be established to cope with scarcity during drought years.

The foregoing account highlights the crucial importance of judicious management of water resources both in the rainfed and irrigated areas for sustaining yield improvements in food crops. This will be absolutely necessary to feed a growing population in India which is expected to reach one billion people by the year 2000.

Readings

A Decade of Dryland Agricultural Research in India: 1971–80. 1982. Hyderabad, India: CRIDA.

Kanwar, J. S. ed. *Water Management—The Key to Developing Agriculture*. 1988. New Delhi: Agricole Publishing Co.

Randhawa, N. S., and R. P. Singh. 1983. "Fertilizer Management in Rainfed Areas: Available Technologies and Future Potential." *Fertilizer News* 28 (September): 17–32.

Singh, R. P. "Crop Production under Rainfed Conditions in India." Paper presented at the FAO Regional Expert Consultation on Rainfed Agriculture, Bangkok, Thailand, 29 November–2 December 1988.

Singh, R. P., and S. K. Das. 1988. "Strategies in Water Conservation and Planning for Dryland Agriculture." Proceedings of Second IWRS Symposium on Water Conservation for National Development, 11–12 December, 1988. Bhopal, India: IWRS.

———, and B. V. Ramana Rao. 1988. *Agricultural Drought Management in India*. Technical Bulletin no. 1. Hyderabad, India: CRIDA.

———, K. Vijayalakshmi, G. R. Korwar, and Mohd Osman. 1987. *Alternate Land Use Systems for Drylands of India*. Research Bulletin no. 6. Hyderabad, India: CRIDA.

Vohra, B. B. 1985. *Land and Water—Towards a Policy for Life Support Systems*. New Delhi: Indian National Trust for Art and Cultural Heritage.

CHAPTER 5

The Diffusion of Agricultural Research Knowledge and Advances in Rice Production in Indonesia

S. W. Sadikin
Director General Emeritus, Indonesian Agency for Agricultural Research and Development, Bogor, Indonesia

Introduction

I would like to refer to some of our experiences in Indonesia where four essentials have contributed significantly to accelerating the application and diffusion of agricultural research knowledge in enhancing food and agricultural production during the past twenty years. Specifically, they are: national stability, political commitment, a growing research and extension capacity, and a motivated farming community. I shall refer also to the cardinal requirements in promoting the diffusion of new information and new agricultural technologies to farmers and policy makers. In dealing with these factors, I shall feature the history of Indonesia's successful effort to achieve self-sufficiency in rice production.

Country Profile
To many people, Indonesia is a small island country south of the Philippines. People tend to confuse the Republic of Indonesia with the island of Bali.

Indonesia is, indeed, not an economic giant, but in terms of popula-

---

I gratefully acknowledge the Winrock International Institute for Agricultural Development, and its president, Dr. Robert Havener, for their continuing support of the preparation of a manuscript on the history of agricultural research in Indonesia. This paper both draws from and contributes to that manuscript. I also wish to thank Dr. Edwin B. Oyer for his assistance in the preparation of the paper.

tion, with its 179 million inhabitants, it is the fifth largest country after China, India, the Soviet Union, and the United States. The archipelago nation, which consists of the big islands of Sumatra, Java, Kalimantan, Sulawesi, and Irian Jaya, plus 13,000 smaller islands, when superimposed on the world map stretches from London to the Ural Mountains or from the west to east coast of the United States. In the past twenty-five years the Indonesian economy has been transformed from a very low level to a fast-growing middle-income economy.

Agricultural Background

Conforming to the general trend in developing countries that have rising per capita incomes, Indonesia's agricultural sector population declined from 70.5 percent in 1965 to the present 54.5 percent. Most farmers own less than half a hectare of land and seek additional jobs and income in other sectors of the economy. Agriculture's contribution to the gross domestic product is, therefore, proportionally low, and it declined from 58.75 percent in 1965 to less than one-quarter today, mainly due to the oil boom in the mid-1970s and to the rapid growth of the service and manufacturing sectors. Exports for 1988 totaled about $20 billion. Primary and value-added agricultural products accounted for 17.4 percent of the total.

Agriculture, nevertheless, has been a major contributor to Indonesia's economic growth in the past twenty years and is expected to continue to play a significant role in the economy of the country. At the center of Indonesia's agriculture is rice, the nation's food staple. Rice provides 68.1 and 61.9 percent of the daily caloric and protein intakes, respectively. Annual per capita consumption is 133 kg and is expected to increase by 2.3 percent annually in the next decade. Rice is a key commodity in the Indonesian economy, and a shortfall in supply is considered a threat to economic and political stability. Self-sufficiency in rice production, therefore, has been a long-cherished goal. It is my conviction that without the favorable environment of national stability and political commitment, our efforts to achieve this goal would not have been successful.

National Stability

In the second half of the 1940s Indonesia's neighboring countries had mobilized their resources for the enormous task of national reconstruction and the clearing up of the economic and social ruins of the Pacific War of 1942–45. Indonesia, on the other hand, harnessed its energies to win the physical fight for independence up until 1950, when the United Nations recognized the country as a sovereign state. The post-independence era of the 1950s and 1960s, however, was witness to political turmoil, insecurity, economic stagnation, and social unrest. The political upheavals that peaked with the communist rebellion in 1965 were accompanied by an economic crisis that plagued the country with shortages of food, clothing, and essential goods; with poor public services; and with an inflation rate of 650 percent. The transportation and telecommunication infrastructure, the irrigation system, and health services were in a dilapidated condition. Factories, plantations, and mines for extracting oil and minerals were in serious neglect.

By 1967, strategic actions had been taken by the government to stabilize the economy. The inflation rate was reduced to 120 percent in 1967 and 85 percent in 1968. Rice production showed a sharp increase from a low level of 9.7 million tons of milled rice in the drought year of 1967 to 11.6 million tons in 1968 and 12.2 million tons in 1969. Production of food and agricultural export commodities, textiles, and oil also showed encouraging improvements. Indonesia's export earnings improved and its imports showed a healthy shift to capital goods and basic materials for industry.

In 1968, the New Order government, which placed technocrats rather than politicians in the cabinet, was formally established. It pledged strict adherence to the 1945 Constitution and committed itself to uphold political and social stability by fostering economic growth and improved income distribution. The government was successful in maintaining peace and establishing order and in creating a stable political climate in which economic development could be initiated. The first Five-Year Development Plan (FYP) was launched in 1969 with agricultural growth as the central thrust. Law and order gave the people protection and a sense of security. The general election held in 1972 was only the second after twenty-seven years of independence, the first having been held in 1955.

In retrospect, it is amazing how quickly the New Order government in the late 1960s won control over internal security, political turbulence, and runaway inflation, and how vigorously and effectively the economic recovery program was launched. In the agricultural sector, the nation's leadership demonstrated its determination by seizing upon the opportunity to increase rice production. This was done by utilizing modern rice varieties (MVs) developed by the International Rice Research Institute (IRRI) and the accompanying technologies with a speed and vision commensurate with the nation's pressing demand for political and economic change.

Political Commitment

There is no lack of political will in Indonesia to fight poverty, hunger, and malnutrition, as illustrated in the official Guidelines of State Policy that emanate from the country's highest sovereign body, the elected People's Consultative Assembly. What was lacking during a quarter of a century after independence was political and social stability and security — a favorable environment for development. The Guidelines of State Policy, in which agriculture has traditionally been accorded top priority, opened opportunities to remove or mitigate various existing obstacles to agricultural development. The emphasis given to agriculture has not changed much since 1973, except for the fact that the 1988 guidelines establish both agriculture and industry as top national priorities.

The first Five-Year Plan (FYP) and the subsequent plans of 1973, 1978, and 1983 adopted an agriculture-oriented strategy with three underlying themes: 1) creating and nurturing healthy and dynamic national stability; 2) promoting economic growth, particularly in the rural and labor-intensive sectors; and 3) fostering equity in the distribution of the rewards of development, across all twenty-seven provinces of the republic, as well as across all social groups. Economic growth was accompanied by an increase in the budget for repair, maintenance, and expansion of the irrigation network, improvement of farm-to-market roads, and for the upgrading of the transportation and communication infrastructures.

Improvements in Infrastructure

Tremendous progress has been made in the last twenty years in the upgrading, maintenance, and expansion of transportation facilities to advance the flow of goods and services and the mobility of people. Agriculture has benefitted through improved distribution of agricultural supplies such as fertilizers, seed, and pesticides on the main islands, especially on Java, where 60 percent of the population resides, and throughout the archipelago. Farm-to-market transportation of agricultural produce also is much improved.

Improvements in the irrigation system contributed to yield and production stability and assured the effectiveness and impact of the application of technological innovations in rice and agricultural production. An improved water supply to households and the generation of hydroelectric power are additional benefits.

Assuring the Supply of Agricultural Inputs

Government policies encouraged the development of agricultural processing, seed, and agrichemical industries. The availability of natural gas, for example, has pushed domestic nitrogen fertilizer production from 85,000 tons in the early 1970s to almost four million tons of urea at present, thereby lessening the risks of insufficient or untimely imports.

The distribution of fertilizers to the rice and agricultural production centers in the four large and the numerous smaller islands outside Java, where transportation and communication facilities are less developed, poses continuing problems. In these areas higher transportation and storage costs have led to increases of 40 to 60 percent in the price of fertilizer, placing outer-island farmers at a disadvantage in applying modern inputs, as compared to their colleagues in Java. In order not to stir political and social sensitivities, the government has absorbed the price differential and has a one-price policy for fertilizer throughout the archipelago.

A similar policy decision was taken in the early 1970s, when the Ministry of Agriculture opted for the use of safer chemicals by farmers, chemicals that are less harmful to the environment but are more expensive than the very effective though highly toxic chlorinated hydrocarbon pesticides. The government provided a pesticide subsidy to lessen farmers' expenditures caused by the switch to less toxic chemicals.

With these subsidies and the improved transportation, fertilizer consumption increased rapidly from about 500,000 tons in 1970 to almost five million tons in 1988, and the use of pesticides more than quadrupled during the same period to 11,400 tons at present. The amount of credit extended to small farmers increased from 1.03 billion Rupiah in 1970 to over 402.6 billion in 1988. Subsidies for rice production and for agriculture in general are a current issue of national concern. The situation was aggravated in 1985–86 by the decline in oil prices, which placed constraints on the government's development budget. Steps now are being taken to gradually reduce and eventually eliminate the subsidies.

There are encouraging developments in this respect. Transportation and storage facilities on the outer islands have improved substantially. Fertilizer and pesticide formulating plants are operating more efficiently. Experience gained in integrated pest management and in early warning systems has led to a more efficient application and an overall reduction in the use of pesticides. Field experiments in the main rice-producing centers where relatively high dosages of chemical fertilizers have been applied in the past fifteen to twenty years demonstrate that a build-up of phosphorous has occurred to warrant a significant reduction in the application of this nutrient.

Growth in Research and Extension Capacity

The agriculture-oriented FYPs also have supported the strengthening of agricultural research and extension. The first FYP in 1969 explicitly emphasized that the search for and research on new high-yielding rice varieties must be pursued vigorously. The continuing need to foster agricultural research, extension, training, and the support of rural institutions has been stressed in every succeeding FYP.

Building on Experience

Experience gained in the research institutes through the release and application of improved Indonesian varieties in the 1950s paved the way for a smooth introduction and a rapid spread of the IRRI MVs in the 1960s and 1970s. There existed in the country a capability to conduct large-scale adaptive trials of new introductions, to organize demonstration plots, produce the necessary stock and extension seed for farmers, and introduce the new MVs supported by packages of recommendations. Agricultural extension personnel had experience in identifying optimal target areas in which suitable physical and social infrastructure and the responsiveness of farmers to agricultural innovations would give the best assurance of success.

In the late 1960s planners and policy makers were baffled by a projected doubling and tripling of domestic fertilizer consumption following the nationwide introduction of the modern rice varieties. The first national fertilizer study, which was conducted in 1970, provided pertinent data for planning future imports and domestic production, distribution, trade, and pricing of fertilizers. As stated earlier, domestic production of urea fertilizers increased from 85,000 tons in 1970 to four million tons at present.

When rapid acceptance of the MVs by farmers led to shortages of high-quality seed, thereby adversely affecting actual yields of the MVs, the research institutes were quick to provide basic information in 1972 for the creation of a national seed system to promote the production, distribution, trade, and proper supervision of certified seed. This effort stimulated a continuous flow of new crop varieties into the production system.

The diffusion of research-based knowledge to farmers as well as to policy makers and the use of new technologies was accelerated in the 1970s and 1980s. This resulted from government policies and actions that brought about: the rehabilitation and expansion of the irrigation network; improved rural roads; the supply of agricultural chemicals, tools, and machinery; the provision of attractive rural credit; the stabilization of rice prices; and the strengthening of agricultural research, extension, and training.

Fostering a Research Capacity

The contribution of research to food production and agricultural development became even stronger when the agricultural research effort was consolidated under the Ministry of Agriculture, following the issuance of a presidential decree in 1974 on the reorganization of ministries. In 1975, the research institutes and stations on rice and various food, horticultural, and industrial crops, forestry, fisheries, animal production, veterinary medicine, soils, agricultural economics, as well as the National Library of Agricultural Sciences, were brought under one body: the Agency for Agricultural Research and Development (AARD).

The director-general of AARD was appointed the chairman of the management board of the semi-autonomous estate crops research institutes. This carried the responsibility of supervising research on rubber, coffee, cacao, tea, cinchona, oil palm, and sugar, and strengthening the capacity of the research institutes to provide support to the big estates and plantations as well as to the smallholders. AARD seized the opportunity to build a solid research infrastructure, strengthen the human resource base, and broaden the research agenda and its coverage, enabling the new agency to increase its support for development.

When the nation's struggle for independence was over in 1950, there were no Indonesian scientists to run the institutes. When all the research institutes of the Ministry of Agriculture were brought under the management of AARD in 1975, only 33 of the 446 research staff had received formal training in research. By 1988, however, the total research staff had grown to 2,244, and one-third held Ph.D. or M.Sc. degrees. Scientists at the research institutes in many instances also serve as resource persons and advisors in planning and implementing development projects in the provinces. A growing number of research staff are also moving into responsible positions relating to policy, planning, and supervision in the Ministry of Agriculture, where they serve a linkage function for the diffusion of research-based knowledge to policy- and decision-makers. Most of the existing 27 national research institutes, 42 research stations, and 154 experimental farms have been renovated or are newly built. All are relatively well equipped.

Delivering Technological Innovations

Agricultural extension also has been strengthened. There are at present 15,500 field extension officers supported by 450 extension subject-matter specialists, 3,750 village rural bank units, 6,455 village unit cooperatives, 18,730 rural retail warehouses for storage of production inputs, and 211,008 farmer groups to spread new information and technologies. The diffusion of information and research knowledge has proved successful as a result of the support given to existing rural institutions. Agricultural extension work via radio and television also has become standard practice.

Sustaining a Continuous Flow of Technologies

The institutions to generate or adopt technologies, to adapt them to local agricultural environments, and to demonstrate and introduce them to farmers have been established and have proven their ability to respond well to pressing problems of the farming community. When the brown planthopper and its biotypes ravaged rice fields, a nationwide monitoring system was established to support an integrated pest management effort. As a result, serious outbreaks of the pest have not occurred in the past five to seven years.

When farmers complained about the reduced selling price of the once very popular MV IR36, due to a high percentage of green and chalky grains, rice scientists determined that the early-maturing, high-tillering IR36 variety, when planted in the rainy season, would produce immature grains in the late tillers at harvest time. The Indonesian Cisadane variety was recommended as a replacement for IR36 in this season. While yields were not as high, farmers received a premium for its better grain quality and favored taste.

Improvements in the diffusion of research knowledge to farmers were not restricted to rice. The introduction in the mid-1970s of high-yielding clones of rubber, coffee, and tea and of dwarf coconuts and oil palm, along with relevant packages of recommendations on cropping practices, promoted the rehabilitation of these export crops. The research institutes also have been in the forefront of the modernization of the dairy, poultry, egg, fish, and shrimp industries and the expansion of agricultural lands in the outer islands. The Research Institute for Freshwater Fisheries, for example, was highly commended in late 1980 for containing and controlling a severe outbreak of a fish disease that had caused great damage to production of carp in West Java and in the southern tip of Sumatra.

The growing demand for research support calls for a broadening of the research agenda to include issues affecting the great variety of food and agricultural commodities, pressing problems of the environment, post-harvest technology, agribased industries, and biotechnology. Furthermore, the bulk of the present agenda is directed to adaptive research. The need to sustain the flow of research knowledge to farmers and policy makers calls for increased investments in enhancing the capabilities not only in adopting and adapting technologies, but also in generating new knowledge and technologies.

Consequently, with all the progress made in staff development and the strengthening of the research infrastructure in fostering research-extension-farmer-policymaker linkages and in broadening the research agenda, we are still only halfway to our goal of building a solid, viable, and self-sustaining national agricultural research network. Staff development, streamlining the research organization, advancing interinstitutional linkages, and improvements in program, project, and financial management call for yet further improvements.

Motivating the Farming Community

The cardinal ingredients for the rapid adoption of technological innovations by farmers are: economic and social incentives; a reliable supply of production inputs such as water, seed, chemicals, and equipment; availability of credit; access to information; sufficient numbers of trained people; ample processing and storage facilities; adequate farm size; and a favorable transportation infrastructure.

Indonesia's agriculture-oriented development process, implemented in an environment of peace and security during the past twenty years, has furnished these ingredients for development and motivated farmers to apply modern practices. However, for farmers who own very small plots of land (e.g., 0.25 hectare), it may not be worth their trouble and the perceived risk to embrace the new technologies and apply the modern inputs, even if these can be shown to double or triple their yields. This has posed a problem because in Indonesia 85 percent of the farm holdings are small, less than one hectare, and more than 50 percent are less than 0.5 hectare.

Group Farming

The rice production program has overcome the constraint of small farm size by introducing the practice of group farming. Groups of fifty to one hundred farmers in a unit area are encouraged to operate as a common organizational unit. Group decisions determine which rice variety should be planted by the unit, when to start land preparation and lay out a joint seedbed, what amounts and types of agricultural chemicals and equipment should be used, and how the water supply, drainage, and repair and maintenance of the farm-level irrigation system should be organized.

Another form of group farming is the "nucleus estate-smallholders scheme," in which a government or private estate of approximately 3,000 hectares of rubber or oil palm trees serves as the organizational core for 10,000 contiguous hectares of smallholdings of two hectares each. Land clearing, land preparation, and the initial development of the young rubber or oil palm trees are executed by the core estate. When the crops have passed their uneconomic stage (after five to six years for rubber), ownership of the two-hectare plots and the responsibility to nurture the young trees is transferred to the individual smallholders with support in the form of loans provided by local banks. The core estate will continue to provide paid services for the processing and marketing of the produce.

Experience has shown that group farming has led to the active participation of small farmers, has greatly improved farming efficiency, and has reinforced the aims of government policies involving the supply and pricing of modern inputs, guaranteed floor prices for rice, and the provision of a rural credit system. The potential value of investments in irrigation and drainage facilities, in rural transportation and communication systems, and in agricultural research, training, and extension, is greatly expanded. This has led, in turn, to a fuller expression of the potential of modern production technologies.

Rural Welfare

Indonesia's agriculture-oriented development strategy also brought schools and public health clinics to rural communities. Basic education has been extended significantly. The number of children attending primary school has doubled from thirteen million in 1974 to twenty-six million in 1987. Attendance at junior and senior high schools has quadrupled and quintupled, respectively, during the same period. Participation in primary schools and in junior and senior high schools is now 92.0, 74.8, and 47.3 percent, respectively.

Health care has improved. The number of public health clinics has increased and continues to increase substantially throughout the country. The impact of this increased attention on health care is reflected in the fact that infant mortality has dropped from 138 to 93 deaths per thousand live births from 1965 to 1986. The improved access to primary health care and the educational opportunities in rural villages engender a sense of well-being among farmers and stimulate their interest in increased food and agricultural production and in better income.

The Path to Rice Self-Sufficiency

Great efforts were made during the two decades after independence to step up food and agricultural production in the country. But the absence of one or more of the above-mentioned ingredients of development rendered a number of projects ineffective.

Plans in the late 1950s to increase agricultural production by means of modern inputs ground to a halt when available supplies could not meet the rapidly growing demand for agricultural chemicals, and transportation and storage facilities failed to support the distribution system. The campaign to attain rice self-sufficiency in the late 1950s through the use of the Indonesian improved varieties and the intensification of production met with only limited success, because public security in the main rice production centers such as West Java, South Sulawesi, and East Java was poor, and irrigation systems and transportation infrastructures were in a dilapidated condition.

The plans for the expansion of agricultural land and rice production areas into the tidal swamps of Kalimantan, and into the upland rainfed environments in Sumatra, Kalimantan, and Sulawesi, were virtually a failure since they depended on the use of heavy equipment. The poor infrastructure caused the transport, maintenance, and repair of the equipment to be difficult and costly.

The ambitious "Eight-Year Overall National Development Plan," promulgated by the People's Consultative Assembly in 1961, in which agriculture and the increased production of food were given an important place, failed in practical terms to be implemented. The nation lacked political stability, a necessary condition for development in the country. Cabinets were reshuffled frequently and ministers moved in and out with rapidity. There was no consistency and continuity in planning or operations. Nor was the budget adequate for implementation.

Indonesia was losing ground with regard to food self-sufficiency. Rice imports, which on the average were less than 300,000 tons per year during 1950–55, rose to an average of 810,000 tons during 1956–60 and exceeded one million tons per year in the 1960s. In the late 1970s and in 1980, Indonesia became the biggest rice importing country of the world, with imports as high as two million tons per year (see Table 5-1).

An encouraging sign in rice production emerged in 1963–64 when students at the Bogor Agricultural University, using a demonstration area of fifty hectares, proved that rice production could be nearly tripled if the recommended packages of technologies for use with Indonesian improved varieties were properly utilized. An important lesson emerged: improved production depended on a secure supply of agricultural inputs and on face-to-face communication with farmers. The experiment led to the creation in 1965–66 of the BIMAS (i.e., "mass guidance") program to increase rice production by means of encouraging and enabling farmers to take full advantage of technological innovations.

The Initial Breakthrough

In 1966 and 1967, rice yields at adaptive trials and on farmer's plots, planted with the IRRI modern varieties, were found to be impressive as compared to yields of the popular Indonesian improved varieties. The cooking and eating quality of the MVs was rated low, but farmers were very much attracted by their vigorous growth, high yields, and early maturity.

An appeal went out from the Ministry of Agriculture to experimental farms, extension centers, provincial and district agricultural officers, and farmers to save and produce as much seed as possible from the first harvests of the MVs. The ministry mobilized considerable resources to secure a sufficient supply of fertilizers and pesticides to support a national campaign of introducing the MVs, with the ambitious target in 1968 of planting 150,000 hectares.

Hands-On Experience with the New Varieties

A crucial factor was the need for extension and agricultural officers as well as researchers to gain hands-on experience with the MVs. Rice production training courses were conducted in the application of the new varieties and technologies and in the realities of rice farming. The governors of South Sulawesi, West Sumatra, and East Java gave prominence to the rice production training by organizing a special training package for "Bupatis," the influential heads of the district-level governments. This, again, demonstrated the government's commitment to development and provided a welcome boost to the national rice production effort.

Within five years, the areas planted with the MVs increased to over three million hectares. After 1972 farmers also planted Indonesian MVs, which have cooking and taste qualities favored by Indonesians and produce fewer green chalky grains when planted in the rainy season. The area now planted annually with the Indonesian and the IRRI MVs is 7.78 million hectares, or 85 percent of the total harvested rice area.

This national undertaking in applying technological innovations did not proceed without obstacles and setbacks. It was thought in the early

Table 5 – 1.

Indonesia: Imports of Milled Rice, 1954–87 (Thousand Tons)

Year	Import	Year	Import
1954	260	1971	490
1955	130	1972	730
1956	820	1973	1,660
1957	550	1974	1,070
1958	920	1975	670
1959	890	1976	1,280
1960	890	1977	1,960
1961	1,060	1978	1,850
1962	1,020	1979	1,950
1963	1,040	1980	2,030
1964	1,010	1981	530
1965	200	1982	300
1966	310	1983	1,160
1967	350	1984	380
1968	630	1985	0
1969	600	1986	0
1970	960	1987	0.05

Source: National Logistic Agency (BULOG). The table was prepared by AARD in August 1989.

1970s that everything necessary and feasible had been done to get agriculture and rice production off the ground. There was confidence that a conducive policy environment could be developed to encourage resource-poor rice farmers to adopt the MVs and to apply the new technologies to increase production. In the eagerness to attain quick results, the rice production scheme was launched as a crash program, and this led inevitably to problems in the overall management.

Dealing with Realities

The program expanded too rapidly, particularly in areas in which farmers had limited access to the services of a small number of extension personnel and rural bank units, and in which transportation and irrigation facilities were less favorable. This resulted in shortcomings in the application of the recommended packages of technology as well as in the management of the supply of farm inputs and in the recovery of production credit. In certain areas returns to the additional inputs were marginal, yields were lower than expected, and debts owing to production credit were mounting.

Nevertheless, aggregate rice production increased faster than the population. As a result of the general improvement in income, however, rice consumption per capita also increased substantially, with the effect that rice imports continued to increase. At the end of 1972 the nation experienced a depressed food supply due to increased demand and to a drop in rice and agricultural production resulting from a severe drought that hit South and Southeast Asia. That was a tremendous blow to our prestigious BIMAS program, and criticism ran high. Fortunately, rice production in 1973 and 1974 returned to a rapid growth pattern, and efforts were made to improve the planning, implementation, monitoring, and evaluation of the program (see Figure 5-1 and Table 5-2).

Environmental Stresses — Weather and Insects

Another serious problem emerged in the form of an insect infestation involving the brown planthopper. An outbreak of the hopper in 1974–75 destroyed crops planted with the popular Indonesian MVs (Pelita I and Pelita II), affecting an area of 240,000 hectares. Losses in 1974 and 1975 ranged from 400,000 to 500,000 tons of milled rice each year, enough to feed more than three million people for each of those years. The outbreak continued in 1976 and 1977. Many observers and practitioners expressed the view that the rice intensification program was largely responsible for the outbreak of this pest, and that the effectiveness of the BIMAS program was leveling off. Researchers, nevertheless, remained committed to their belief that the new rice varieties and technologies had not yet fully expressed their potential due to the varied environmental stresses such as the brown planthopper and the occasional droughts, as well as management short-comings of the BIMAS program.

A decision was made to introduce, on a large scale, the IRRI IR26 rice variety, which had a high degree of resistance to the planthopper. However, while this was accomplished, another biotype of the brown planthopper (biotype-2) evolved, which eventually destroyed the IR26 variety. The response was to quickly replace the IR26 with the IR36 variety, which was resistant to biotype-2. A countrywide monitoring system for the brown planthopper and an integrated pest management scheme were vigorously implemented in order to avoid an outbreak of a new biotype and to cope with it if and when it did arrive.

After we learned to live in peaceful coexistence with the brown planthopper, the MVs yielded another stream of benefits. Rice production jumped by 9 percent in 1978, from 15.8 to 17.5 million tons of milled rice. Modest drought intervened in 1979, but production increased again in 1980 and 1981 to unprecedented levels of 20.1 and 22.2 million tons, respectively. In 1982, drought again caused a decline in the harvested rice area, and a new

Figure 5 – 1.

Harvested Area and Production of Milled Rice in Indonesia, 1965–88

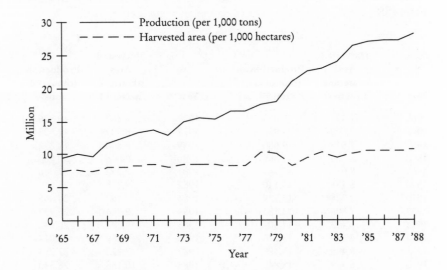

Source: Compiled from data on production and on harvested areas, furnished by AARD, August 1989

biotype of the brown planthopper emerged in North Sumatra, which caused rice varieties resistant to biotype-2 to break down. Large-scale ground and aerial spraying of pesticides was undertaken and the situation was monitored closely. Varietal screening to identify resistant lines showed that two Indonesian varieties and an IRRI variety carried some resistance to the "North Sumatra biotype." However, there was not enough seed available domestically to plant these resistant varieties. Twenty-one tons of IR56 seed, delivered from IRRI and from the Philippine Seed Growers Association, had to be airlifted for immediate relief.

Reaching the Goal

As these environmental obstacles were removed, the diffusion of technological innovations to farmers gradually and substantially accelerated. The national research capacity to support food production and agricultural development and to help solve technical, social, and economic problems continued to expand. The number of extension personnel and specialists with competence to help the eighteen million farm households in Indonesia was growing rapidly. Improved irrigation and drainage facilities

Table 5 – 2.

Harvested Area and Production of Milled Rice in Indonesia, 1965–88

Year	Harvested Area (thousand hectares)	Production (thousand tons)	Year	Harvested Area (thousand hectares)	Production (thousand tons)
1965	7,327	9,463	1977	8,360	15,876
1966	7,690	9,945	1978	8,929	17,525
1967	7,515	9,680	1979	8,803	17,872
1968	8,020	11,666	1980	9,005	20,163
1969	8,014	12,249	1981	9,392	22,286
1970	8,135	13,140	1982	8,988	23,037
1971	8,324	13,724	1983	9,162	24,006
1972	7,898	13,183	1984	9,764	25,932
1973	8,403	14,607	1985	9,902	26,542
1974	8,509	15,276	1986	9,989	27,014
1975	8,495	15,185	1987	9,922	27,253
1976	8,369	15,845	1988	10,138	28,340

Source: AARD, August 1989

provided a more secure base for ensuring yield and production stability. Improved communication and transportation smoothed the flow of agricultural inputs and credit. The National Logistic Agency had gained experience in implementing a sound government price stabilization policy to purchase the increased rice production at a guaranteed floor price and to sell rice in times of pressing market demand.

There was a growing awareness and understanding among policy makers, legislators, and development professionals at the national, provincial, and district levels about the way to solve problems in the agricultural sector. As a result, rice production rose sharply to reach a production level of 25.9 million tons of milled rice in 1984. This achievement, along with the presence of government-held reserves of two million tons at the end of the year, allowed the government to call a halt to rice imports, marking a historic turning point in Indonesia's quest for self-sufficiency in its staple food commodity.

Complacency, a relaxation of efforts in the main BIMAS regions, and declining profitability of rice farming caused production to stagnate in 1986 and 1987. Corrective measures had to be taken to push production up again in 1988 and 1989. Policy adjustments have been necessary to enable the National Logistic Agency to relieve swelling national stocks through rice exports and to supplement shortfalls in production with imports during bad years.

Concluding Remarks

Under the volatile political conditions of the 1950s and 1960s, it would have been very difficult, if not impossible, for Indonesia to initiate and sustain an intensified rice production program of great magnitude. Contrary to the critics' concerns that the government's stabilization effort would stifle change and dynamism, the two decades of political stability have enabled us to pursue appropriate policies, take strategic actions, and provide dynamism with stability that stimulated the diffusion and application of technological innovations leading to higher food and agricultural production.

In a favorable agricultural development environment in which production inputs are secure, credit is available, and incentives and supporting rural institutions are in place, farmers are quick to adopt technological and managerial innovations that result in improved agricultural productivity. However, pushing modern technologies into areas where the cardinal requirements for modernization are not yet in place is likely to result in disappointment.

The Power of Successful Examples

Successes achieved in the intensive use of the modern rice varieties and appropriate technology packages, and institutional experience gained in launching countrywide development programs, have led to new initiatives in food and agricultural production. Renewed efforts have been made to step up the production of corn and soybeans, modernize the poultry, dairy,

Table 5 – 3.

Indonesia: Production of Major Agricultural Commodities, in 1966–67, 1976–77, and 1986–87, in Thousand Tons

(Numbers in parentheses are indexed to a baseline of 100 in 1966–67)

Commodity	2-Year Mean 1966–67	2-Year Mean 1976–77	2-Year Mean 1986–87
Milled Rice	9,704 (100)	15,861 (164)	27,234 (281)
Maize	3,309 (100)	2,858 (94)	5,507 (181)
Cassava	10,990 (100)	12,340 (112)	13,896 (126)
Sweet Potatoes	2,310 (100)	2,421 (105)	1,998 (87)
Soybeans	417 (100)	523 (125)	1,214 (291)
Groundnuts	253 (100)	375 (148)	583 (230)
Fish	1,192 (100)	1,510 (127)	2,600 (218)
Meat	n.a.*	377	894
Eggs	n.a.*	120	464
Milk**	44 (100)	60 (136)	224 (509)
Rubber	718 (100)	815 (114)	1,121 (156)
Palm Oil	174 (100)	464 (267)	1,381 (794)
Copra	1,120 (100)	1,468 (131)	2,073 (185)
Coffee	151 (100)	191 (127)	348 (231)
Tea	72 (100)	77 (107)	147 (204)
Clove	14 (200)	29 (207)	56 (400)
Pepper	27 (100)	40 (148)	45 (167)
Tobacco	63 (100)	81 (129)	140 (222)
Cane Sugar	638 (100)	1,343 (211)	2,011 (315)
Logs***	3,929 (100)	21,569 (549)	29,246 (744)
Sawed Lumber and Plywood***	n.a.*	620	13,490

* not available
** in million liters
*** in thousand cubic meters

Source: Compiled from data supplied by AARD, August 1989

and fish industries, and accelerate the rehabilitation of plantations and the expansion of oil palm plantations. This has led to new plantings of coconut, rubber, coffee, tea, pepper, and oil palm, and has spurred the shift in export from primary to value-added products. (Table 5-3 shows the progress achieved in the production of major agricultural commodities.)

The government recently reported that during the past eleven years, twenty-four million people have been raised above the poverty level. Nevertheless, some 30 million, almost 17 percent of the total population, still do not have enough to eat to sustain a healthy and productive life. The successful drive to attain self-sufficiency in rice and to advance overall agricultural production has, indeed, lessened the problem of hunger and malnutrition, but it has not eradicated it. More comprehensive government interventions, attacking underemployment, poverty, and hunger, are called for. Indonesia's agricultural development officers and research scientists have a good understanding of the political, social, and economic dynamics of rural areas. Given proper incentives and institutional commitments, they will play an even more assertive role in the future in the fight against poverty and hunger.

Readings

Afiff, Saleh. 1988. *The Role of Agriculture in the Changing Structure of the Indonesian Economy.* Jakarta: The Indonesia Institute of Management Development.

Ministry of Agriculture, Republic of Indonesia (R.I.). 1987. Round Table: Indonesian Agricultural Development for REPELITA V. Jakarta.

Ministry of Information, R.I. 1988. The State's Policy Guidelines for Development. Jakarta. (In Indonesian.)

Ministry of Information, R.I. 1989. The Fifth Five-Year Development Plan 1989/1990–1993/1994. Jakarta. (In Indonesian.)

Mosher, A. T. 1965. *Getting Agriculture Moving: Essentials for Development and Modernization.* New York: The Agricultural Development Council.

Sadikin, S. W. 1982. "The Role of Cropping Systems in Increasing Food Production and Farmer Prosperity." Workshop on Cropping Systems Research in Asia. Los Baños, Philippines: The International Rice Research Institute.

———. 1984. "Agricultural Research Program Review and Evaluation." Workshop on Research Program Evaluation. Dhaka: International Service for National Research/Winrock International Institute for Agricultural Development/ Bangladesh Agricultural Research Council.

———. 1986. "Indonesia: From Rice Self-Sufficiency to Greater Food Security." The World Food Day Symposium. Tokyo: Japan-FAO Association.

———. 1986. "Institutionalizing Review and Evaluation in National Agricultural Research Systems." Workshop on Evaluation in National Agricultural Research. Singapore: International Development Research Center/International Federation of Agricultural Research Systems for Development.

Ward, W. B. 1985. *Science and Rice in Indonesia.* Washington, D.C.: U.S. Agency for International Development.

CHAPTER 6

The Iringa Integrated Nutrition Program in Tanzania: Research and Development

Calister N. Mtalo
Coordinator, Joint WHO/UNICEF Nutrition Support Program, Iringa, Tanzania

Introduction

The purpose of this paper is to explore the Iringa Nutrition Program in Tanzania in the context of research and development.

To understand this program it is necessary first to gain insight into the status of health and nutrition in Tanzania as a whole and then examine this in relation to the situation in Iringa and the Iringa program.

From the very conception of the program, research and development aspects have been built into the program and its components in order to allow for flexibility and refinement of the implementation methodology as community needs evolve and research expands. The emphasis has been on operational research, whereby new findings could be made available for immediate utilization.

The integrated multisectoral approach to hunger, malnutrition, and infant mortality was, at its inception, a new concept not only for Iringa but for Tanzania. The traditional approach had viewed nutrition from a unisectoral perspective, in which malnutrition was equated simply with a lack of food. The other causative factors were not given much consideration.

Background

The Iringa Nutrition Support Program in Tanzania is one of eighteen Joint Nutrition Support Programs (JNSP) sponsored by the World Health

Organization (WHO) and the United Nations International Children's Emergency Fund (UNICEF). The programs were conceived in November 1980 with the objective of making improvements in the nutritional and health status of women and children and reducing the incidence of malnutrition and infant mortality. Several meetings were held with WHO and UNICEF staff that resulted in a draft program adopted in December 1981 and approved in May 1982. A grant of $85 million from the Italian government made it possible to launch the program immediately after official approval.

A look at some basic health and nutrition data in Tanzania will explain the reasons for the program and its objectives.

The Republic of Tanzania has a land area of 945,000 square kilometers (sq. km.) and considerable agricultural potential (see Figures 6-1 and 6-2). The total population (1988 census) is 23,174,000, out of which 11,327,000 are males and 11,846,000 females. Life expectancy at birth for male/female is 50/53 years, respectively. The population growth rate is 2.8 percent, and the average household size is 5.2 persons.

The nation is sparsely populated with an average of 25 people per sq. km. Most of the population, an estimated 86 percent, reside in rural areas and are organized in a village system. Fourteen percent reside in urban areas, with the highest population concentration existing in the capital, Dar es Salaam, which has a population of 1,360,000 people, or 5.9 percent of the country's total. Children under the age of five years, who are the program's target population, represent 4.7 million, or 18 percent of the entire population.

Tanzania embarked on a Universal Primary Education System in 1977, with the goal of ensuring that all children of school age receive a primary school education. As a result, 86 percent of the school age children have been enrolled in primary schools. However, enrollment in secondary schools lags far behind enrollment in primary schools. The ratio of secondary school enrollment for males and females is 5.5/3.2, respectively. The country has embarked on a literacy program to ensure that all adults are literate. The male/female adult literacy ratio in 1986 was 93/80.

Health and Nutrition in Tanzania

Tanzania is among the developing countries that have high rates of early child mortality and morbidity. The data in Table 6-1 show trends in infant and child deaths; though a decreasing trend is evident, average rates remain high.

National efforts to deal with the problem have taken many forms, including the provision of basic social services such as education, health, and water resources to communities. Efforts have been underway since the 1970s to shift the delivery of social services from urban to rural areas, and this has encouraged people to stay together in the villages, which number about 8,300. The villages, therefore, constitute the primary basis for improving the conditions of people. They are the centers of development and mobilization of local resources to complement the national efforts.

Malnutrition is a serious problem for children under the age of five. An estimated 48 percent of the under-five population suffers from malnutrition, with the great majority manifesting mild to moderate malnutrition, and a smaller number, severe malnutrition. Malnutrition is a result of a combination of factors, some of which have to do with the condition of the mother during pregnancy and after delivery. One indicator of the problem is the percentage of babies born with low birth weight (i.e., under 2.5 kg.), which stands at 14 percent.

The Iringa region is divided into 6 districts, which have 31 divisions,

Figure 6 – 1.

Tanzania

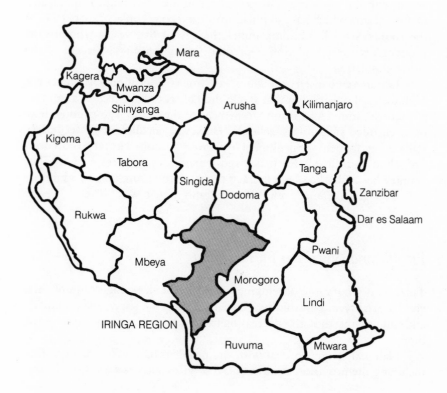

Figure 6 – 2.

Iringa Region (JNSP Areas)

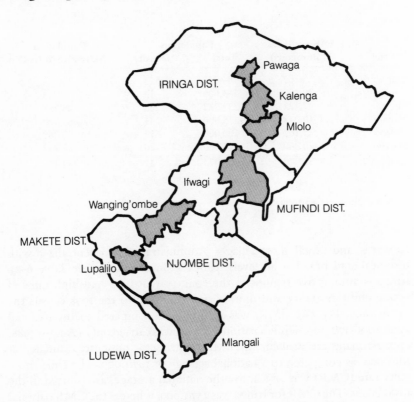

Table 6 – 1.

Infant and Child Mortality in Tanzania, 1957–88

Year	Infant Mortality Rate (IMR)	Child Mortality Rate (CMR)
1957	190	—
1967	160	260
1978	137	231
1988 (estimated)	107	179

Source: Population Census 1957, 1967, 1978, 1988

Table 6 – 2.

Population and Area of Iringa Districts

District	Area (square kilometers)	Population Total	Population Density	Population Under Five Years Old
Iringa (urban)	162	84,802	523	16,974
Iringa (rural)	28,457	363,605	13	72,764
Mufindi	7,122	229,732	32	45,758
Njombe	10,241	315,000	31	63,100
Ludewa	5,167	100,000	19	20,088
Makete	5,800	115,480	20	20,732
Total	56,949	1,209,973	21	239,416

Source: Population Census 1988

113 wards, and a total of 610 villages. Administration is decentralized with technical staff based at all levels from region to village (see Table 6-2). Iringa is among five regions in the country that have had high rates of young child mortality and morbidity. According to the 1978 census the infant mortality rate (IMR) was 152/1,000, as compared to the national average of 137/1,000. While a national census was carried out in August 1988, only estimates are available: the IMR for Iringa is presently estimated at 101/1,000, as compared to a national average of 107/1,000. The child mortality rate (CMR) was also above the national average, as reported in the 1978 census. The CMR for Iringa was 257/1,000, whereas the CMR national average was 231/1,000. Estimated figures for 1988 show that the CMR for the Iringa region and the nation declined to 160/1,000 and 179/1,000, respectively.

As regards malnutrition, Iringa seemed to be worse off than the national average. According to the Harvard standard, the percentage of Iringa children with moderate malnutrition was 48 percent, as compared to a national average of 42 percent. Of the children having one form or another of malnutrition, 6.5 percent were found to be severely malnourished (see Table 6-3).

Iringa Nutrition Program

The Iringa Region was chosen to implement the Nutrition Program for the following reasons: a) it is one of the few regions in which nutrition surveys

Table 6 – 3.

Demographic, Health, Nutrition, and Education Data, Tanzania and Iringa Region

Land area	Tanzania 945,000 sq. km.	Iringa 56,949 sq. km.
Demographic indicators		
Total population	23,174,000 (1988)	1,210,000 (1988)
Population density	25/sq. km.	
Population 0-15 years	11,600,000	
Population 0-4 years	4,700,000	243,000
Life expectancy at birth (years)	52	52
Male/Female (M/F)	50/53	50/53
Fertility rate/1000 pop.	7.1	
Crude birth rate/1000	50	50
Crude death rate/1000	15	21.8
Urban population (% of total)	14	10.8
Population annual growth rate total	2.8	2.7
Male population	11,327,000	565,241
Female population	11,846,000	643,673
Average household size	5.2	4.8
Education indicators		
% Primary enrollment	78 (1987)	86
Secondary enrollment ratio (M/F)	5.5/3.2	—
% Children completing primary level (entering 1979)	70	—
Adult literacy ratio (15 + years) M/F	93/88 (1986)	
Health and nutrition indicators		
IMR/1000 live births	107	101 (est.)
Mortality rate/1000 of children under 5 years old	179	160
Infant and child malnutrition (%)	48	50
% Weight for age — mild/moderate malnutrition	42 (1984)	48
Severe malnutrition	6	6.5
Babies with low birth weight (% < 2.5 kg)	14 (1984)	16
1-year-olds (% fully immunized)		
Measles	78	85
BCG	95	90
DPT	81	88
Polio	80	92
All 6 diseases	76	86
% pregnant women immunized (tetanus)	58	70
Mothers breast feeding (% at 3/6/12 months)	100/90/70 (1984)	100/95/85

Source: Population Census 1984, 1986, 1988

have been conducted, and the frequency of malnutrition and child deaths was found to be quite high; b) it includes a range of agroecological and economic zones that are found in many other areas of Tanzania, and this would facilitate program replicability in other regions; and c) the infrastructure for training and nutrition work in Iringa was judged to be relatively well developed.

To ensure a realistic implementation schedule and the achievement of intended outcomes, Iringa authorities proposed an intensive area concentration, selecting 7 of the 31 divisions in the region as focal points for the program. Approximately 25 percent of the Iringa region's total population resides in these areas. There were 28 wards and 168 villages implementing the program as of 1984. The total target population of "under fives" in the program area is estimated at 46,000.

In the course of implementing the program in the pilot areas villagers and officials living outside the pilot areas demanded that the program be expanded to cover the entire region. Regional and district authorities, in turn, expressed a willingness to use their resources to cover the additional costs involved. In response to this need, during 1987, it was decided that the Iringa Nutrition Program should be expanded to cover an additional 432 villages in the region.

The objectives of the Iringa Nutrition Program are: a) reduction of infant and young child mortality and morbidity; b) improved child growth and development; c) improved health and nutrition of mothers; and d) improvement in the capabilities at all levels of society to assess and analyze nutrition problems and to design appropriate actions.

Support for the Iringa Nutrition Program is derived from the national government of Tanzania and the governments of the Iringa region, along with support from WHO and UNICEF (the latter played a key role in the channelling of funds and technical support). Additional support came from a grant of the Italian government for a period of five years. Local support for the program also proved decisive. The local contribution over a five-year period is estimated to be US$ 500,000, consisting of finance, staff time, and labor contributed by the village communities. The community contribution is two-thirds of the total local contribution, whereas the remaining one-third derives from the district and regional governments (see Figures 6-3 and 6-4).

Implementation Strategy

The program, conceived in 1982, was affected by the conditions of economic austerity that prevailed in the country. In order to cope with this situation, the participation of the village communities was given high emphasis in the program design. A preparatory team was formed, comprising members from key ministries and institutions to provide a multisectoral approach. From the beginning, the team involved leaders at various levels as well as villagers in identifying the priorities of the program.

The conceptual framework underlying the program seeks to identify all the causal factors affecting child mortality, ranging from immediate and underlying causes to basic causes. This is the common framework used as a basis to discuss and analyze problems and seek possible solutions (see Figure 6-5).

The principle used to operationalize the conceptual framework is known as the "Triple A" approach. This approach of analysis, assessment, and action provides an ongoing and continuous process of evaluation at all levels to generate a situational analysis of the nutritional problems and the solutions available to address them (see Figure 6-6).

The combination of the conceptual framework and the "Triple A" approach has facilitated resource mobilization for child survival and hence the emergence of a social mobilization strategy (see Figure 6-7).

Figure 6 – 3.

National Inputs to JNSP Activities, 1984-87, in Percentages and Value of Funding Support, in Thousands of 1987 Shillings (TSh)

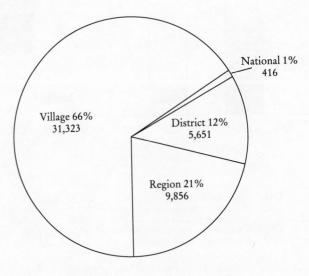

Source: Iringa Nutrition Support Program (JNSP)

131

The strategy focuses on the level where resources are available and will be put to use, namely, the household and the village community. The community level is particularly important for two reasons: to enable individual households to obtain access to production inputs and outputs; and to serve as a resource base for communal activities that can be allocated for child survival and other program tasks. The resources at the national, regional, and district levels have been used mainly to mobilize resources at the community level.

The principal strategy to ensure participation of all levels is the inte-

Figure 6 – 4.

Village, District, and Regional Inputs, by Functional Activities, Selected JNSP Activities, 1984-87

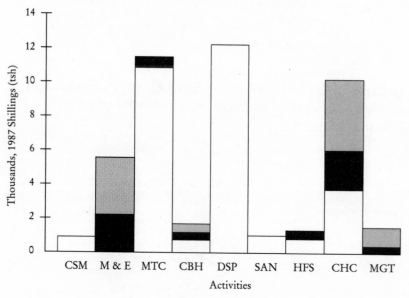

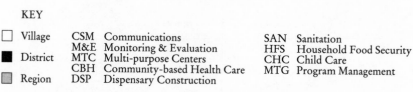

KEY

☐ Village	CSM	Communications	SAN	Sanitation
	M&E	Monitoring & Evaluation	HFS	Household Food Security
■ District	MTC	Multi-purpose Centers	CHC	Child Care
	CBH	Community-based Health Care	MTG	Program Management
▨ Region	DSP	Dispensary Construction		

(Thousands, 1987 Shillings (TSh)

Source: Iringa Nutrition Support Program (JNSP)

132

gration of the program with the existing government and party structure (see Figure 6-7).

Program Development

The following summary describes the program components and the research work undertaken for each component.

Figure 6 – 5.

A Conceptual Framework: Causes of Young Child Deaths

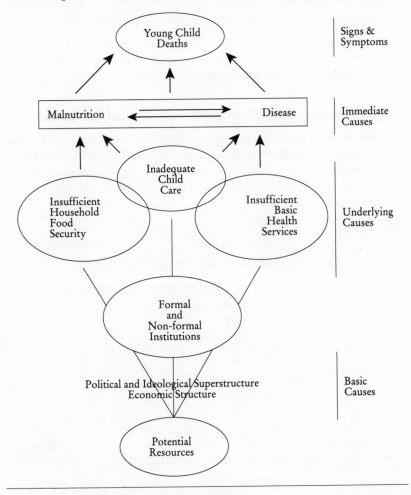

Source: Iringa Nutrition Support Program (JNSP)

Program Component 1: Systems Development and Support

Objective: To increase and sustain the capability to plan, implement, and monitor child survival and development actions in Iringa.

Research: An assessment of the monitoring and evaluation component of the program, which examines nutritional status and the risk of child death. This research is done by a specialist from the Tanzania Institute of Nutrition.

Program Component 2: Maternal and Child Health

Objective: To expand and improve health services in the program area, with special emphasis on controlling those disease factors that are responsible for maternal and child malnutrition and infant mortality.

Research: Survey and analysis of diarrhea/disease incidence and the associated factors, and of the changing patterns of knowledge, attitudes, and practices of villagers who have undergone training.

Program Component 3: Water and Environmental Sanitation

Objective: To improve the environment of the household, with special reference to the child, in order to reduce disease-related risk factors. This is to be done by establishing a capability in the program areas to construct afford-

Figure 6 – 6.

The Iringa Model: Assessment – Analysis – Action

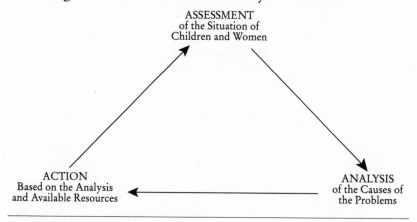

ASSESSMENT
of the Situation of
Children and Women

ACTION
Based on the Analysis
and Available Resources

ANALYSIS
of the Causes of
the Problems

Source: Iringa Nutrition Support Program (JNSP)

134

able pit latrines and promoting an understanding of the role of sanitation education in sustaining good health.

Figure 6 – 7.

Social Mobilization Strategy of Iringa Program

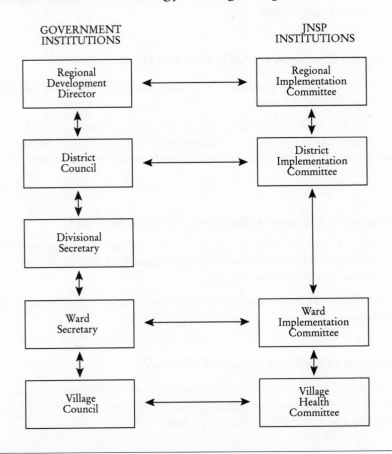

Note: At subdistrict level, the divisional and ward secretaries act as program coordinators. These secretaries are both Party and government functionaries, which has enabled them to play a very important role in program implementation. Village Health Committees and Village Health Workers are responsible for program implementation and follow-up. They compile on a quarterly basis growth monitoring and child death information and discuss these reports with the Village Councils, which then take action within their power to solve the problems that have been identified. The reports are then sent to higher administrative levels and serve as a basis for decisions regarding the allocation of resources.

Source: Iringa Nutrition Support Program

Program Component 4: Household Food Security

Objective: To improve household accessibility to food throughout the year by promoting drought-resistant crops, home gardens, labor-saving devices, simple techniques for food preservation, small-animal keeping, and improved weaning practices.

Research: Examine feasibility and effectiveness of a "household food security card." This is based on a study in Ilula that examines marginal families and malnutrition.

Program Component 5: Child Care and Development

Objective: To improve child care, especially through the regular and frequent feeding of children.

Research: Study of child feeding and rearing practices undertaken by the Muhimbili Medical Centre in collaboration with the Iringa program; in particular, the relationship of feeding and rearing to infant and child mortality.

Program Component 6: Income-Generating Activities

Objective: To support women's groups in their efforts to start up income-generating activities, thereby increasing household income for use on improving family and child welfare.

Research: Operational research on the management of income-generating activities.

Program Component 7: Nutrition Research

Objective: To strengthen national nutrition research capabilities through the coordination of research meetings, participation in scientific meetings, and direct support to relevant research studies.

Achievements Resulting from the Iringa Nutrition Program

The implementation of these program objectives began after a massive nutrition education campaign was conducted in all 168 villages to create nutrition and health awareness in the village communities. The earliest activities included weighing all children under five years and creating a growth monitoring system; establishing village health committees; immunizing all children; providing health education on the prevention of endemic diseases such as malaria and diarrhea; and demonstrating the preparation and uses of weaning food to reduce dietary bulk by means of germinated cereals and the technology known locally as "power flour."

A number of achievements have been observed in the course of implementing the Iringa program. The program ultimately seeks to change attitudes and behaviors of the target populations by means of education, training, and the offering of incentives to households and to villages to make the desired changes. These desired changes ultimately depend on persuading both the husbands and the wives to become partners in child care and rearing, whereas in the past women have been the predominant providers of child care. Further, it has been important to persuade both husbands and wives to transform their households into more cohesive economic units, with a greater sharing of work and income-generating activities. Once this is accomplished, the task has been to convince households to participate in the nutrition and health education programs; and to cooperate with JNSP staff and with government authorities in implementing the programs of child-growth monitoring, food preparation and proper feeding, immunizing children against diseases, etc. Much progress has been made on all these fronts.

1. Improvements in Diet and Nutrition

Improvements in diet and nutrition have been made, resulting from the establishment of a village-based growth-monitoring system with quarterly reporting by village health workers. The community-based system has the advantage of sustainability and easy follow-up. The villages have established rehabilitation units to care for severely malnourished children. Mothers are less likely to have to leave their families behind when children require rehabilitation. Overall malnutrition rates have decreased from an average of 50 percent (1984) to 38 percent (1988). Severe malnutrition has decreased from an average of 6.5 percent to 1.3 percent.

2. Raising Nutrition and Health Awareness and Mobilizing Villager Participation

Awareness of nutrition and health needs at all levels, from villagers to regional officials, has increased. Decision makers now recognize the growth and development of children as a high priority. Popular participation in implementing program objectives is high. Nutrition awareness has increased by means of advocacy programs utilizing films, newsletters, and songs, and by means of training in new practices. The information derived from ongoing program monitoring is utilized to mobilize further the households and village communities.

The following are some of the areas in which communities have generated resources for improved nutrition and health: creating day-care and child-feeding systems in all villages in the program area, with the use of paid day-care attendants and health workers; the formation of village health committees to discuss nutrition and health needs, and to coordinate action; and the use of labor for construction of dispensaries, training centers, and village health posts.

Other achievements include: the expansion of immunization coverage to nearly the entire target population (e.g., an increase from 50 percent in 1984 to 96 percent in 1987), resulting in the decrease of diseases preventable through immunization; establishment of income-generating activities among women's groups to enable women to have greater access to income and resources, resulting in improved household health and nutrition; integration of the program with government and party structures, and providing allocations from regional budgets for program activities, thereby facilitating program sustainability and expansion; and the decision by the national government to utilize the Iringa experience as a model in seven other regions and in Zanzibar.

In implementing the Iringa program certain constraints and problems have been observed, which have required attention and corrective adjustments:

(1) Seasonal trends in malnutrition and child deaths have been observed. They appear to be higher in the first six months of the year, coinciding with the agricultural and rainy seasons, in which mothers work full-time in the fields and therefore have less time to care for their children.

(2) Diarrhea and malaria remain the major killer diseases, particularly in the seasons mentioned above.

(3) There is a need for additional resources in the villages for child survival to sustain the process and support marginal families.

(4) Lagging investment at the national level in social services requires other resources, such as local councils, to fill in the gaps.

(5) Certain weaknesses have been identified in program implementation, which highlight the critical importance of social mobilization and income-generating activities to the overall success of the program. Research has identified these weaknesses and new priorities and modifications have been undertaken to correct them.

Conclusion

The Iringa nutrition program already has undergone a Phase I evaluation in 1988, following a midterm review in 1986.

The evaluation report contains a number of recommendations for the region and the nation, including the following:

a) The multisectoral approach to nutrition programs, as used in Iringa, has proven to be successful in dealing with nutrition and health problems; hence the need for consolidation and expansion into other areas within the Iringa region and in other regions in Tanzania. Phase II of the program is under preparation and will include consolidation and expansion.

At the national level, efforts to adopt the Iringa model have begun in eight other regions. A national coordinating committee has been formed to coordinate child survival efforts and to share information, resources, and expertise.

b) Program sustainability and expansion will depend on the generation of additional resources, particularly at the district and village community levels.

The experience of the Iringa Nutrition Program shows that an appropriate social mobilization strategy is a prerequisite to enabling the community to understand their nutritional problems and to take action. However, some amount of resources is needed at the district and regional levels to facilitate and sustain the mobilization process in the villages.

Start-up costs might seem to be high, but since they are spread over a long period, they do not need to be repeated. Operating costs are critical in sustaining the activities, particularly those that support management supervision and coordination.

Readings

JNSP Iringa Annual Reports, 1985–88.
JNSP Iringa Midterm Review Report, 1986.
The JNSP Iringa Nutrition Campaign Report, 1984.
JNSP Iringa Plan of Operations, 1982–88.
JNSP Iringa, 1983–1988: Evaluation Report. October 1988. Dar es Salaam, Tanzania: Government of Tanzania.
Mtalo, Calister N. 1989. "Community-based Health Care Project — Case Study of Iringa JNSP," paper presented to symposium in Nairobi, Kenya, 1989.
Quarterly Nutritional Status Reports from JNSP Villages, 1984–88.
Situational Analysis of Women and Children in Tanzania, UNICEF/Tanzania.
Tanzania Population Census, 1967, 1978, and 1988.

CHAPTER 7

Agricultural Development and Technology: The Growth of Chile's Fruit and Vegetable Export Industry

Anthony Wylie
Director General, Fundación Chile, Santiago, Chile

Introduction

This paper examines developments in Chile's fruit and vegetable export industry and the agribusiness structures that support its growth. A lesson derived from this case study is that the appropriate and timely evaluation of the nation's comparative production and/or marketing advantages, undertaken by Chile's agricultural sector, played a key role in the industry's development. This evaluation encompassed research into Chile's production capabilities, the needs of various consumer markets, the special niches that arise in markets and present opportunities for the industry, and, finally, the optimal combinations of investment, business know-how, and technical skills.

Market-oriented policies, which evolved slowly in Chile, performed a critical role in the growth of the fruit and vegetable industry. Entrepreneurs and investors responded over time to these policies and provided the drive and thrust that was needed for growth, as would be the case with any economic development process.

The private sector in Chile played a significant role in the growth of the fruit and vegetable industry, the origins of which date back to the mid-1950s, when the earliest entrepreneurs identified market niches and built the foundations of the nation's agricultural production. This sector's growth, however, was relatively slow-moving, despite government policies during the 1960s that were intended to stimulate the process. Accelerated growth in the fruit and vegetable export sector became achievable only after the mid- to late 1970s, at a time when congenial macroeconomic, political, and institutional conditions had arisen.

In the intervening years, many of the conditions that eventually generated the industry's growth were certainly present. Among these were agricultural, ecological, and market conditions, the advantages of off-season production, the technological know-how, and entrepreneurial capacity. Perhaps, then, the missing incentives for growth prior to the 1970s were related to the fragile political and economic environment — the instability, economic uncertainty, and the continuous threats to private property and to investment during that period.

This paper will describe the historical linkages in the fruit and vegetable industry's evolution, in particular the combination of economic policies and other key elements of technological and institutional capability that explain the industry's dynamic growth.

The Economic Environment in Chile

The economic policy reforms implemented during the past fifteen years have been crucial to the evolution of the agricultural sector and, specifically, to the fruit and vegetable industry.

Probably the single most important pillar of government policy affecting the long-term investments required for fruit production has been the guarantee of the right to private property, a necessary condition for any investment to make economic sense. Prior to the economic reforms, property rights had been challenged and undermined as a result of radical land reform programs and the accompanying uncertainty that discouraged major investments in this field.

In addition to the safeguarding of property rights, the Chilean government had implemented a liberalization program for the entire economy. The Chilean economy was opened to international trade, with access to a diversified market; protectionism was reduced through the removal of quantitative restrictions and the establishment of a uniform tariff structure at reasonably low levels; and along with the prevalence of a relatively high real exchange rate, all were important features of economic policy from the point of view of the agricultural sector's development.

The conditions that influence socioeconomic systems include many other factors besides economic policy. These range from worldwide recessions such as those that occurred in the mid-1970s and early 1980s, to unintentional acts that affect the extremely sensitive dynamics of consumer markets such as the problem with Chilean grapes in the U.S. market in early 1989. In both situations, negative results were produced in the entire economy as well as in specific sectors, even though the overall economic framework had been extremely appropriate for growth and development. Two major recessions have adversely affected Chilean agriculture's performance during recent years. The first one was market related, consisting of the oil recession that resulted in a decline in international market prices for agricultural and fruit products during the 1975–76 period.

The second resulted from an ill-timed combination of a market depression, high real interest rates, and overvaluation of the local currency. In fact, the nominal exchange rate had been fixed from 1979 to 1982 while internal prices continued to rise, leading to an overvaluation of the Chilean peso, which gradually curtailed the country's share of international markets for agricultural products. This set the stage for growing farm indebtedness as a result of a deterioration of farm income-generating capacity, which itself was exacerbated by the recession. The overvaluation of the local currency led farmers to prefer loans denominated in U.S. dollars, and, consequently, the immediate impact of the unavoidable devaluation of the Chilean peso was a widespread debt crisis, which was compounded by the high real interest rates that prevailed during the period.

The 1982 recession affected the entire Chilean economy, as it did other Latin American economies. The severity of the impact depended to a large extent on whether a country was a net oil exporter or importer. In the case of Chile, which is a net oil importer, the severity of the recession was increased by the exchange-rate problem mentioned above, and the economy experienced a drop of about 14 percent in Gross Domestic Product (GDP). In relative terms, agricultural GDP had a smaller-than-average drop (2 percent vs. 14 percent), which persisted through 1983 when GDP dropped again, this time by 3.6 percent.

Between 1980 and 1983, the agricultural sector's performance was quite poor in terms of overall GDP growth (0.3 percent on average). As mentioned above, the problems confronting the sector were mainly related to low agricultural prices, high outstanding debt, high real interest rates, and a drop in the real exchange rate. The latter is illustrated in Figure 7-1, which presents the evolution of the real exchange rate between 1974 and 1988.[1]

The difficult situation faced by Chilean agriculture in the early 1980s led to pressures for stronger protectionist measures. As a result, specific price-support programs (price bands linked to import prices) were established for wheat, milk, sugarbeet, and other commodities, and in some cases these were complemented by government entities that performed purchasing, storage, and marketing activities. The fruit growers had their difficulties as well during this period, but these were somewhat offset by the considerable natural advantages for fruit growing in Chile. There were bankruptcies among major producers and suppliers, mainly due to debt-related problems. The factor that had the largest influence in increasing agricultural prices relative to non-agricultural prices was not the increase in

Figure 7–1.

Evolution of Real Exchange Rate, 1974–88, in Chilean Dollars and U.S. Dollars (Ch $/U.S. $)

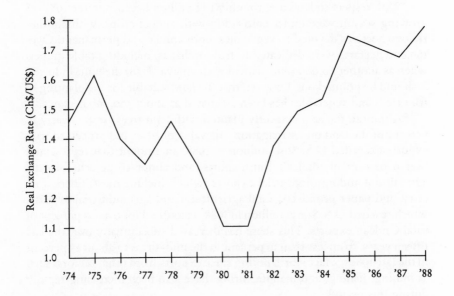

Source: Central Bank of Chile

protection awarded to agriculture, but rather the increase in the real exchange rate, which took place at that time.

At this point, it is necessary to underscore the complementarity that exists between the macroeconomic setting and other crucial factors such as an adequate provision of services, infrastructure, communications, and transportation; the existence of a relatively efficient capital market; a responsive bureaucracy; and the confidence that a sound economic policy instills in investors.

The Chilean Agricultural Sector: An Overview

The total area of continental Chile (islands and Antarctic territorial claims excluded) comes to nearly 756,000 sq. km (i.e., 75.6 million hectares, or 187 million acres). According to official figures, nearly 33 percent of this area (about 25.1 million hectares) is classified as suitable for cultivation, livestock, and forestry. Of this total, 20 percent is tillable land, 34 percent is suitable for pastures and livestock, and the remaining 46 percent is classified as available for forest development. The remaining 50.5 million hectares consist of either barren or nonproductive land such as mountains and deserts.

With respect to land use, roughly 1.12 million hectares in the 1987–88 growing season were under cultivation with annual crops, with another 110,000 hectares devoted to vegetables, both annual and permanent. Over 160,000 hectares were dedicated to fruit orchards, including table grapes, whereas another 60,000 were planted with vineyards for the wine industry. It should be pointed out, however, that the land suitable for the planting of fruit trees and vegetables has been estimated at about 500,000 hectares.

Although the area currently planted with fruit trees covers nearly 10 percent of the land under irrigation, the value of fresh and processed fruit exports exceeded U.S. $650 million in 1988, an amount that represented over 9 percent of total Chilean exports, and about 40 percent of total agricultural and agroindustrial exports (which include meat, fibers, forestry, and paper products). Total agricultural and agroindustrial exports, which reached U.S. $1,637 million in 1988, accounted for over 23 percent of total Chilean exports. This share has increased substantially over the last fifteen years, from less than 10 percent in the mid-1970s to about 25 percent in the late 1980s, a fact worth noting since exports from other sectors, such as mining, fishing, and manufacturing, have also been increasing rapidly during this period.

Thus, for example, over the 1974–88 period, total agricultural and agroindustrial exports in terms of 1988 U.S. dollars grew at a rate of 6.1 percent per year. Over the same period copper exports grew by 1 percent per year, while total Chilean exports grew by 2.7 percent per year.[2] When the 1983–88 period is considered, the average growth rates (in 1988 U.S. $) were 19.7 percent, 11.7 percent, and 12.5 percent for agricultural/agroindustrial, copper, and total exports, respectively. Thus, although growth in agricultural exports has been high, exports from other sectors have also increased dramatically during this period.

A broader perspective on the agricultural sector's importance within Chile's overall economy is found in Figure 7-2, which presents data on the rates of growth of the national and agricultural Gross Domestic Product and of agriculture's share in Chile's GDP.

It is interesting to note that although the agricultural sector's rate of growth maintained a fairly constant portion of total GDP, and growth over the period was approximately 8.4 percent on the average, its growth rate has not always been in line with that of Chile's overall GDP growth rate. This is evident by comparing the effect of the economy's slowdowns in 1973 and 1982 and the subsequent economic recoveries.

Figure 7-2 reveals two distinct periods in the time span considered:

one between 1974 and 1983 in which the agricultural sector was relatively stagnant; and another between 1983 and 1988 during which time the sector grew very rapidly. During the first period, agricultural GDP grew at an average rate of 3 percent per year, while during the second one it grew at a rate of 6.2 percent per year. In comparison, national GDP grew at rates of 3 percent and 5.2 percent, respectively, during the same two periods. The fact that the agricultural sector's GDP increased at a higher annually compounded rate than the overall economy during this second period indicates that the sector in recent years has performed more dynamically than the economy as a whole.

Perhaps the clearest picture of the agricultural sector's growth in recent years, particularly since 1983, is obtained by considering its balance of trade. These data are presented in Table 7-1, and illustrate the enormous increase in agricultural exports (i.e., roughly eleven times in real terms), the significant decrease in agricultural imports (i.e., roughly 80 percent in real terms), and the constant improvement in the balance of trade in agricultural

Figure 7–2.

Evolution of National and Agricultural Gross Domestic Product (GDP): Growth Rates and Agricultural Sector Participation (AgGDP), 1973–88

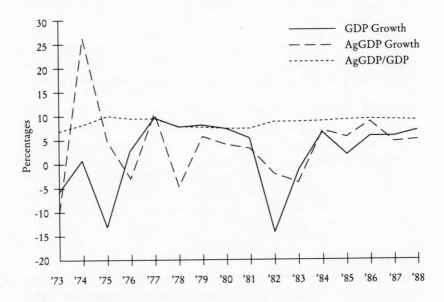

Source: Central Bank of Chile, National Accounts System

145

Table 7-1.

Agricultural Sector Balance of Trade (Exports and Imports), 1973–88 (Millions of 1988 U.S.$)

Year	Agriculture and Livestock Exports (1)	Forestry, Pulp, and Paper Exports (2)	Agricultural Sector Exports (1) + (2)	Imports (3)	Balance of Trade (1) + (2)-(3)
1973	58.6	86.1	144.7	1,405.3	-1,260.6
1974	120.0	250.4	370.4	1,182.4	-812.0
1975	263.7	213.3	477.1	915.4	-438.3
1976	249.9	283.5	533.5	733.8	-200.3
1977	331.8	331.0	662.9	702.5	-39.6
1978	356.5	380.2	736.8	747.6	-10.8
1979	417.2	538.1	955.3	772.5	182.8
1980	456.9	682.3	1,139.3	921.3	218.0
1981	407.4	447.3	854.7	820.4	34.4
1982	387.8	358.4	746.2	591.8	154.4
1983	343.6	335.8	679.4	528.7	150.7
1984	442.1	379.9	822.0	468.0	354.0
1985	521.1	329.2	850.3	254.4	595.9
1986	741.4	412.0	1,153.4	186.7	966.7
1987	816.2	570.8	1,387.0	221.0	1,166.0
1988	926.7	710.7	1,637.4	279.5	1,357.9

Source: Ministry of Agriculture and Central Bank of Chile

products. The improvement in the balance of trade can be attributed to several elements, chief among them the enormous growth in the area planted with fruit orchards that has transformed the fruit sector into one of the most dynamic sectors in the Chilean economy. The fruit sector will be considered in further detail, yet it is important to point out that during the same period other more traditional sectors of Chilean agriculture also evolved strongly; these increases also contributed to the improvement in the agricultural sector's balance of trade.

The increased value of the agricultural sector is the result of significant improvements in production technology and in management, as can be seen when one considers the increase in the average yields of the so-called traditional crops, as illustrated in Table 7-2.

Fruit Production

Chile's potential as a fruit-producing and -exporting country has long been recognized. The first exporting company was established in the 1930s, but the availability in the 1950s of technological improvements, such as refrigerated transport, signalled the concrete beginnings of what is today perhaps the largest fresh deciduous fruit exporting industry in the world. The initial steps were taken by entrepreneurs, whose efforts have been helped, and occasionally hindered, by the agricultural policies of the government in power at the time. For example, several administrations implemented positive development programs for the fruit-producing sector, whereas the agrarian reform policies implemented in the 1960s and early 1970s led to restrictions on growth in the agricultural sector as a whole and specifically in fruit production. Major growth in fruit exports occurred, however, over the last five to ten years, despite the fact that no specific government policies have been implemented for this sector.

As shown in Table 7-3, the industry's major emphasis has been on fresh fruit exports, with about half of the total production going to these markets, one-third to the domestic market, and the balance to processing. The major increase in plantings occurred during the late 1970s, as illustrated in Figure 7-3 and in Table 7-4. As shown in Table 7-4, the areas planted with fruit species have expanded at different rates, reflecting the response to market conditions, with major growth occurring in table grapes and kiwi plantings. This increase in cultivated areas has resulted in a continuous expansion in the volume of exports, as seen in Table 7-5.

The impact of fruit exports on Chile's economy, particularly its balance of trade, can be judged by the data presented in Table 7-6. It is interesting to note that when comparing the data for volume of exports

Table 7 – 2.

Annual Crops: Evolution of Average Yields for Periods 1974–83 and 1984–88 (Metric Tons/Hectare)

Crop	Average for Period 1974–83	Average for Period 1984–88	Percentage Change
Corn	3.56	6.49	+ 82%
Wheat	1.63	2.61	+ 60%
Barley	1.95	2.80	+ 44%
Rice	3.27	4.06	+ 24%
Beans	1.04	1.12	+ 8%
Potatoes	10.27	14.01	+ 36%
Rapeseed	1.37	1.68	+ 23%
Sunflower	1.41	1.83	+ 30%
Sugarbeet	37.12	44.54	+ 20%

Source: National Institute of Statistics, Santiago, Chile

Table 7 – 3.

Production and Uses of the Principal Fruits in Chile (1985)

Fruit	Production (tons)	Fresh Exports (%)	Processing (%)	Market Domestic (%)
Grapes	322,807	70	15	15
Apples	415,792	48	16	36
Pears	80,541	37	1	38
Peaches (fresh)	34,256	19	—	81
Nectarines	92,793	29	—	71
Plums	45,764	36	34	30
Cherries	9,702	12	25	63

Source: National Institute of Statistics

shipped with the dollar revenue, the latter has not increased in direct proportion to the former. As can be expected, the increasing volume of exports has affected prices in the major markets, with decreasing returns per unit shipped. This suggests that aggressive marketing techniques and significant efforts in improving quality and uniformity are essential in the years to come. This is doubly important since a large percentage of the

Table 7 – 4.

Evolution of the Area Planted with Different Fruit Species, 1973–88 (Hectares)

Species	1973	1977	1982	1988	Annual Compound Growth
Table grapes	4,150	8,405	20,300	45,450	17.3%
Apples	11,290	12,970	17,600	24,410	5.3%
Plums	1,685	2,310	5,500	9,225	12.0%
Pears	2,600	2,720	4,800	11,490	10.4%
Peaches	11,050	8,090	7,000	8,995	-1.4%
Nectarines	3,990	4,520	7,500	7,715	4.5%
Kiwi	—	—	95	9,000	—
Cherries	1,010	1,130	2,300	3,370	8.4%
Apricots	1,620	1,630	1,490	2,190	2.0%
Total Fruit Species	65,630	75,372	101,900	150,400	5.7%

Source: Ministry of Agriculture

acreage planted with fruit trees has not yet reached full production. Assuming favorable economic policies, the volume to be shipped in the coming years will continue to increase significantly.

Vegetable Production
The area planted with vegetable crops in Chile has remained fairly stable over the last twenty years at about 100,000 hectares, while significant changes in the crop mix have taken place. As Table 7-7 indicates, the value of vegetable crop exports has fluctuated over the years. However, taking into account the change in the crop mix toward export-oriented crops (e.g., asparagus, tomatoes, peppers, onions, etc.), a continued upward trend can be expected.

Investment in the Fruit and Vegetable Industry
Investment data, disaggregated by economic sector, are not available. However, a report on agricultural investment covering the period 1965–86, recently published by the Corporation for Production Promotion (CORFO), presents estimates of capital stock in the agricultural sector, which in 1986 reached approximately U.S. $2.24 billion. Of this amount $362 million (16 percent) corresponds to fruit tree plantations.[3]
As is the case with farm investment, statistics on investment in off-farm fruit-packing infrastructure are not available. This is also an area in which there has been explosive growth over the past decade; one partial

Table 7 – 5.

Volume of Fresh Fruit Exports from Chile, 1973–87 (Tons)

Species	1973	1977	1982	1987
Table grapes	13,375	20,262	109,244	273,178
Apples	24,545	63,140	181,661	331,422
Plums	590	1,321	3,048	24,671
Pears	4,051	9,540	25,630	44,892
Peaches	1,382	4,767	2,806	12,654
Nectarines	N/A	1,508	8,524	31,780
Kiwi	–	–	22	2,811
Cherries	208	379	672	2,050
Apricots	9	–	21	1,365
Total	N/A	100,917	331,628	724,823

Source: Ministry of Agriculture

indicator is the recent growth in cold storage capacity. Fundación Chile has conducted three surveys for the years 1983, 1986, and 1989, covering cold storage firms throughout the country. Table 7-8 summarizes the survey's results, showing the number of firms, the number of cold storage chambers, and total cold storage capacity.

All the indicators in Table 7-8 show impressive rates of growth, and, it is noteworthy, similar growth has occurred in the case of other facilities such as packing plants, fumigation chambers, controlled atmosphere chambers, and transport services.

With respect to agribusiness investment in general, available unofficial estimates indicate that the amount of capital invested in food industries jumped from about U.S. $235 million in 1977 to about U.S. $1.38 billion in 1988. During the period considered, there has been an increase of at least U.S. $1.15 billion in investment in the fruit packing and processing industry, without which the increase in exports of all fruit products of almost one billion tons could not have taken place. An estimate of the impact of improvements in fruit production and processing technologies can be obtained by relating the investment figures with the data on the total

Figure 7–3.

Evolution of Area Planted with Fruit Orchards, 1965–88

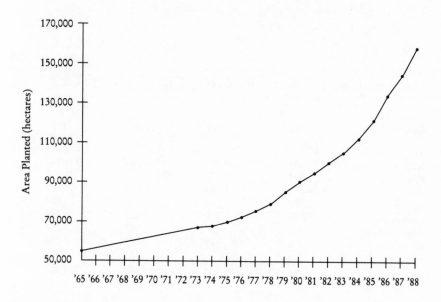

Source: Ministry of Agriculture

Table 7 – 6.

Expansion of Fresh Fruit Exports, 1974–88

Year	Fresh Fruit Exports (in millions of 1988 U.S.$)	Proportion of Total Chilean Exports (%)
1974	37.0	0.9%
1975	71.8	2.5%
1976	87.3	2.4%
1977	102.3	2.9%
1978	150.1	4.1%
1979	163.8	3.2%
1980	196.1	3.6%
1981	211.1	5.1%
1982	241.6	6.2%
1983	226.9	5.7%
1984	294.9	8.0%
1985	361.4	9.3%
1986	499.3	11.4%
1987	537.8	10.1%
1988	582.3	8.3%

Source: Ministry of Agriculture

annual export value of fresh and processed fruit and vegetables. Between 1977 and 1988 exports rose from U.S. $96 million to about U.S. $700 million. Based upon these figures, the export dollars obtained per dollar of invested capital in the fruit packing and processing industry alone increased from U.S. $0.41 to U.S. $0.51 over the period considered.

Table 7 – 7.

Vegetable Exports (Includes Fresh, Frozen, and Dried Vegetables, and Vegetable Crop Seeds), 1977–87

Year	Value of Exports (in millions of 1988 U.S.$)
1977	40.2
1982	20.5
1987	41.4

Source: Ministry of Agriculture

Macroeconomic Effects of the Fruit and
Vegetable Industry's Growth

The most obvious effects of the agricultural sector's economic vitality can be found in the acreage cultivated, the volume of agricultural products shipped, and the dollar returns of these exports, all of which have already been described in the previous section. Two additional elements, however, should be highlighted. The growth of agricultural exports as a whole has had an important impact upon the degree of diversification of the country's total exports. In real terms, agriculture and livestock exports have evolved from a mere 3 percent of Chile's total exports in 1974 to an average of about 15 percent over recent years, while copper exports over the same time have declined from 77 percent of the country's total to about 46 percent. Moreover, when forestry and paper products are included, agricultural sector exports accounted for over 25 percent of total exports in 1988, as compared to about 9 percent in 1974.

Secondly, although exports of fresh fruits and vegetables have in-

Table 7 – 8.

Evolution of Cold Storage Capacity in Selected Regions, 1983, 1986, and 1989[1]

Year	Total Number of Cold Storage Firms	Total Number of Cold Storage Chambers	Total Storage Capacity (Apple Boxes)[2]
1983	166	651	11,956,850
1986	215	805	20,684,100
1989	278	1,116	26,615,826
Growth 1983 – 86[3]	9%	7%	20%
Growth 1986 – 89[3]	9%	12%	9%
Growth 1983 – 89[3]	9%	9%	14%

[1] The figures for 1989 are available only for regions 3, 4, 5, 6, and Metropolitan. Thus, and for the purposes of comparison, only these five geographic regions are considered in the 1983 and 1986 figures. With respect to their relative importance, these five regions accounted for 82% of the firms and 66% of the total storage capacity in 1986.

[2] Original capacity figures for regions 3, 4, and 5 are expressed in boxes of table grapes. These figures were converted to apple-equivalent boxes, assuming that one box of table grapes occupies one-half of the space of a box of apples.

[3] Average annual compounded growth rates.

Source: Fundación Chile, National Survey of Cold Storage Capacity: 1983, 1986, and preliminary 1989 results

Figure 7-4.

Growth in Fresh Fruit Exports and Agricultural Sector's Balance of Trade, 1973–88

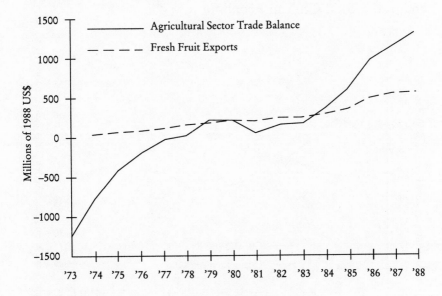

Source: Ministry of Agriculture and Central Bank of Chile

creased tremendously in both absolute and relative terms, exports from subsectors such as processed fruits and vegetables (i.e., frozen, dried, and juices/pulps) also have increased. This is readily apparent from Figure 7-4, which shows the even faster improvement in the agricultural sector's balance of trade as compared to fresh fruit exports alone.

Effects on Employment and Income

Despite the progress made with respect to the availability of employment statistics in Chile, it is still difficult to track the growth of labor force participation and employment within the agricultural sector. Data for the fruit and vegetable industry alone lag behind overall data that group together agriculture, fisheries, and forestry. The problem is further complicated by the fact that labor force data for the agricultural sector do not include off-farm fruit- and vegetable-packing activities, which have shown enormous growth over the last few years. Bearing in mind the limitations of the available data, Figure 7-5 shows that the agricultural sector's labor

Figure 7 – 5.

Agricultural Labor Force Participation, and Relationship between Unemployment Rates in Agriculture (U.R. Agric.) and in the Total Chilean Economy, 1975–88

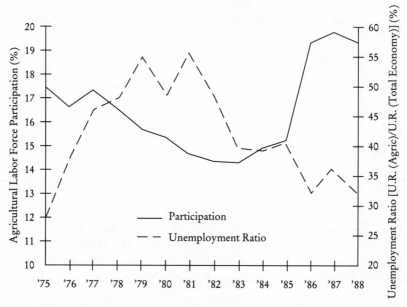

Source: National Institute of Statistics, Santiago, Chile

force participation not only did not decline significantly over the period but in fact has increased in recent years. Moreover, the rural-urban migration pattern common to developing countries and very noticeable in Chile up to the mid-1970s has actually been reversed in the last few years.

Another point to note in the data in Figure 7-5 is that, since 1982, the unemployment rate in the agricultural sector has diminished as compared to the overall unemployment rate, which also has declined. This is a clear indication that agriculture has been more dynamic than the economy as a whole in terms of its capacity to create new jobs.

Unfortunately, statistics on wages for farm workers are not available. These workers, typically, receive in-kind compensation, which makes it difficult to estimate overall income levels. An approximation of the growth of real wages for farm workers can be obtained, nevertheless, from the growth of real wages in the economy as a whole, as presented in Table 7-9. This approximation is limited, however, by the fact that the agricultural sector has a relatively small representation in this index.

In the case of skilled farm workers, the prevailing trend toward a higher technical level of farm operations has had an impact on the improvement of wages. Some evidence indicates that the figures presented in Table 7-9 provide only a lower-boundary estimate of the growth in wages over the last five years. For example, the rate of increase in real wages for specialized tasks such as cleaning grape bunches has been estimated at more than 120 percent during the period 1985–87, which may indicate an improvement in real wages that is double the figures shown in Table 7-9. These figures are, of course, consistent with the fact that the sector's capacity for job creation and labor absorption has been high, and one should expect that these expansion rates in the demand for labor would be coupled with increases in real wages.

Critical Factors in the Fruit and Vegetable Industry's Development

It would be overly ambitious and presumptuous to attempt to describe all the factors that have contributed to the development of Chile's fruit and

Table 7 – 9.

Evolution of Real Wages, 1974–88 (Base 1982 = 100)

Year	Real Wage Index
1974	55.17
1975	53.66
1976	59.47
1977	72.25
1978	82.57
1979	91.59
1980	99.47
1981	108.39
1982	108.71
1983	96.81
1984	97.05
1985	92.72
1986	94.65
1987	94.46
1988	100.67

Source: Central Bank of Chile

vegetable industry. Undoubtedly, a critical factor has been the favorable climatic and agronomic conditions for the development of export crops, coupled with the fact that these export-oriented fruits and vegetables can be produced and harvested off-season. It must be said, however, that when such favorable conditions are not reinforced by other critical factors, these alone are definitely not sufficient to create a viable industry. A brief analysis of some of the other factors critical to the industry's growth follows.

Economic Factors

There have been, overall, no specific sector-oriented policies aimed at subsidizing or favoring the fruit and vegetable production sector during the period being considered. One exception to this was the government's role during the crisis in March 1989, when, following a cyanide poisoning scare, Chilean grapes were recalled and consumers in the United States and in other markets were advised temporarily not to purchase Chilean grapes.

Perhaps the most critical factors — especially for the fruit industry, which is by nature a long-term investment — have been the overall stability in economic policy and the government's strong support for private property rights. Also of significance is the maintenance of a relatively high real exchange rate, which, combined with Chile's natural advantages for growing fruits and vegetables, has been a key factor in the sector's continued growth.

Institutional Factors

For positive policy changes to have the desired effects, a growth in services, communications, transport, and management skills also has to take place. These changes are neither spontaneous nor automatic and do not necessarily occur in the most desirable sequence, but they are, nonetheless, essential.

Some examples of significant transformations in Chile during the period being considered include activities as varied as domestic and foreign investment deregulation, banking and financial services development, communications and computer technology growth, simplification of customs procedures, favorable tax legislation, the development of efficient shipping and marketing services, and a streamlined bureaucracy at all levels. This is not to say that all these elements at present are problem-free. On the contrary, rapid export growth has created new demands and problems. Progress has been made in all these service areas, and this must continue.

Ecological Conditions

Chile's relative geographical isolation makes it comparatively free of certain pests and diseases. Natural borders, such as the Atacama Desert, the Andes Mountains, the Pacific Ocean, and Antarctica, to a large extent prevent the contamination that could occur by natural means. However, despite these barriers some agricultural pests and diseases exist in the country, a fact that poses problems for certain export markets.

These potential problems have led to cooperative efforts between the private and government sectors, which together have worked to facilitate the growth of fruit and vegetable exports. An example is the Ministry of Agriculture's plant protection services (SAG) agency, whose efforts have produced collaborative projects with major importing countries such as the United States, the European Community, and, most recently, Japan. These programs have been funded to a great extent by the exporters and growers, who are well aware of their importance.

As a result of the continuous exchange of information with consumer markets, all major exporters and growers are aware of the need to restrict pesticide usage for those products to be accepted in the importing countries and to maintain chemical residue levels within the limits of tolerance that have been established in each importing country. Fundación Chile is one institution that has pioneered work in this field and through its laboratory services has provided support to growers, exporters, and agricultural chemical suppliers.

Technological Factors

The adaptation and incorporation of advanced agricultural production practices in all aspects of the fruit and vegetable industry have played a highly significant role in the growth of this sector. The capacity and willingness of farmers, shippers, processors, etc., to search for and utilize proven modern technologies have played a big role in this process. Some examples of these technologies include: new plant varieties and horticultural practices; in-vitro propagation; cooling and storage techniques; advanced fertilizer and pesticide application procedures; as well as numerous examples of so-called soft technologies related to marketing, financing, and product promotion. It is important to point out that the similarity in species cultivated and in growing conditions in Chile with those found in the American states such as California, Oregon, and Washington, and other fruit-growing areas in the northern hemisphere has meant that the varieties and technologies available in these areas could be readily adopted and utilized in Chile. This factor alone has undoubtedly played a significant role in the industry's growth.

The achievement and maintenance of high quality standards as well as high yields at competitive costs have required a continuing emphasis on technological innovation. This has been achieved by a commitment on the part of leaders both in government and in the private sector. Gains have resulted from a variety of elements: from specific technology transfer projects such as the ones implemented by the Instituto Nacional de Investigaciones Agropecuarias (INIA), which has created and organized technology-transfer groups among farmers growing common crops in different areas; the existence of top-level training courses, seminars, and technical assistance programs such as those organized by Fundación Chile; the technical assistance provided to growers by the exporting companies; and last, but certainly not least, the aggressive search by the growers themselves for innovative technologies.

Human Resources

None of the preceding factors could have been effective without the appropriate human resources. These include farm workers with various skill levels, technical staff, farmers, and entrepreneurs. The Chilean agricultural labor force, for example, has proven to be receptive to new ideas and responsive in performing tasks and working with changing technologies. In particular, women in rural areas have been especially proficient in utilizing new fruit sorting, grading, and packing techniques. Manpower has been adequate, and workers have become specialized in appropriate ways in the various aspects of production.

Fruit and vegetable production, handling, processing, and exporting are capital-intensive activities in which considerable risks are faced both on the farm and in the international market. Chilean farmers and businessmen have shown a considerable capacity to manage this intricate process and to open new markets for their products. All the major exporting companies employ extensive technical staff, which often give assistance to growers who lack their own resources for keeping abreast of the latest technological developments. The staff involved in this process are highly trained graduates of Chilean universities and technical institutes. A large number of university graduates have gone on to postgraduate work, mainly in the United States, where they have obtained master's or Ph.D. degrees. These individuals then can supplement the graduate training in horticulture available in Chile. The availability of these skilled professionals has been critical in bringing Chile's fruit and vegetable industry to the forefront of technology. The evolution of the industry would certainly have advanced at a slower pace without this important resource.

Innovation and Technology Transfer

Societies exhibit varying degrees of acceptance of change and innovation. In general terms, developing countries are by nature less prone to change than more industrialized nations. This fact must be borne in mind when considering the best means of introducing innovations in food production, marketing, and distribution systems. The process of technology transfer, and how best to bring it about, constantly confronts this reality; perhaps the biggest challenge is to discover ways to overcome resistance to change. Undoubtedly, the most critical element in achieving technological innovation is in motivating the potential user. Once this has been established, and presuming the technology is appropriate, the transfer process itself is comparatively straightforward.

Fundación Chile's Experience

Fundación Chile was established thirteen years ago as a nonprofit organization by the Government of Chile and the ITT Corporation. An original endowment of U.S. $50 million was established, with each founding member contributing 50 percent of this amount over a ten-year period, after which no further endowments were contemplated. Management of Fundación Chile was entrusted to ITT for the first ten years. At present, it is an autonomous institution with half of its board of directors being nominated by each of the founding members. Funding for projects is provided by the sale of services, as well as from the interest on that portion of the endowment still in liquid assets.

Fundación Chile's objective is to transfer proven technologies to Chile's productive sectors, and its activities are presently centered in the fields of agribusiness, forestry, and marine resources, although other previous programs included telecommunications and electronics. Fundación Chile's approach to technology transfer is pragmatic and has been based to a large extent on its capacity to link technology to market forces and to provide knowledge of business opportunities for users of its projects. Motivating the users of a new idea, product, or production process is achieved by showing where and how strategic benefits leading to increased productivity can be obtained by implementing one or another innovation. The fact that, wherever possible, the costs involved in the transfer process are charged to the user makes the negotiation process more complex but guarantees the client's true interest.

Quality control, product and process development, marketing techniques, introduction of new species or varieties, as well as project evaluation, development and, if necessary, implementation, are among the methods that have been used in introducing new technologies. The formation of medium-sized companies with considerable technological input and in which Fundación Chile takes an equity share has also proven to be an excellent means of introducing new technologies. Producers will tend to follow the example of others who are successfully innovating and who are willing to invest their own funds in the projects they are promoting. Once these companies become operational and the benefits of technological innovations have been well established, Fundación Chile sells its share of the company to its original partners or to other investors.

Looking Ahead

One of the challenges in the future is to maintain quality and to expand export markets, given the fact that the amount of fruit for export that will be produced in orchards already planted will increase by about 50 percent over the next five years. The efforts required in shipping, marketing, promoting, and selling these greater volumes at reasonable prices in the world market will be considerable. A careful consideration of this situation should take the form of more stringent quality standards to ensure that existing markets are not lost due to a lack of uniformity of the products and that new markets can be opened. Consideration of alternative uses of fruits and vegetables in processed form will also have to be carefully evaluated. At the same time, as consumer concern for product safety increases, orchard management techniques, especially as they relate to pesticide usage, must be continually updated to ensure that each specific market's requirements are met.

An obvious and most desirable outcome of the country's development process over the next several years should be a steady and continuous increase in farm income and real wages. Higher labor costs will have to be offset by greater efficiencies in the productive process, the optimization of plant varieties, and higher yields. At the same time, it is reasonable to expect that as the cost of labor increases, the quality and productivity of farm labor will also improve, thereby maintaining a certain balance in the system.

A further challenge to be met by Chile's fruit and vegetable industry relates to technological innovation. So far, progress in this area has been achieved largely through the adaptation to Chile's conditions of technologies developed and proven in other countries. This process has been achieved most successfully and, as a consequence, the industry, from a technological viewpoint, is now essentially on a par with those of other leading countries. Having reached this stage—i.e., in the sense of having used up this technological backlog—and considering that some of the problems being faced today are specific to the Chilean situation, the time is fast approaching when local research and development efforts will have to provide specific and unique solutions for the industry's problems.

Thus, a continuous flow of technological innovations and solutions will become crucial to the industry's future development. The human resources for conducting this research and development are available in

Chile, but a continued effort to maintain training and specialization in this field is essential if this challenge is to be met. It should be pointed out that the continuing improvement of research facilities and in researchers' incomes and working conditions will require substantial investments, and the industry, growers, and shippers, as well as the relevant government agencies, will have to take the necessary steps to make this possible. Undoubtedly, the need for developing new technologies and maintaining aggressive marketing, in the presence of increasing costs in areas such as labor, pest control, shipping, etc., will narrow the profit margins for growers and exporters. However, there is no reason to doubt that the industry will continue to be a significant factor in the country's economy, especially given the major investments already made in new orchards which will reach their full production potential in the next few years.

Summary and Conclusion

The impact of Chile's economic policies on agricultural exports has been highly favorable over the last five or six years. The significant growth in fruit exports, combined with increased production of annual crops and with growth in forestry exports, has resulted over the last fifteen years in an aggregate improvement of the agricultural sector's balance of trade of more than U.S. $2.6 billion in real terms.

A major explanatory factor has been the existence of an appropriate economic policy framework. In this regard, trade liberalization policies have been crucial. In particular, the real exchange rate has been identified as a key policy variable that explains many of the ups and downs of agricultural performance during the period being considered. In general, the establishment of a market-oriented economy with emphasis on international trade and the government's strong support for private property have undoubtedly been critical factors behind the fruit and vegetable industry's accelerated growth. A key element in the whole process has been the confidence and credibility that these policies have instilled in investors.

A crucial complement to the policies has been the various innovations that have taken place in both technological and nontechnological areas. These include: the development of shipping and marketing services; the building of packing and processing plants; modernization and development of transportation and port services; communications; fruit production and postharvest technologies; local and foreign investment deregulation; modernization of banking and customs procedures; and tax legislation.

The private sector has played a key role in implementing the investments necessary for the process to take place and in opening up new markets for the industry's products. Government agencies have facilitated private-sector efforts through intergovernmental agreements that have made access to foreign markets easier.

An analysis of the impact of the export-oriented growth of the fruit and vegetable industry on rural employment indicates that the sector's dynamism has been reflected in a higher level of job creation than in the economy as a whole. At the same time, real wages have shown a marked upward trend, a situation that is expected to prevail and accelerate in the near future. The industry's positive impact on rural employment and on the level of economic activity in related services has been a major force in alleviating poverty.

Chile's human, technical, and institutional resources have played an essential role in the sector's evolution. The capacity to implement and adapt technological innovation and the mechanisms for the transfer of technology applied within the industry have undoubtedly contributed to this process.

Orchards established since 1985–87 will be coming into production over the next few years, thereby increasing the sector's GDP and the volume of fruit exports. This represents an important challenge in the future: to sustain an aggressive marketing program; to intensify technological innovation; and to step up the processing of an increasing volume of produce. The human, technological, and financial resources required for this are available and should be capable of responding to future needs, provided the present macroeconomic framework continues in place. The conjunction of all these factors will be critical in maintaining the kind of growth that Chile's fruit and vegetable industry has shown in recent years.

Notes

1. The real exchange rate (RER) is defined as: RER = NER × (USWPI/ChWPI), where NER is the nominal exchange rate (in Chilean \$/U.S.\$), USWPI is the U.S. Wholesale Price Index, and ChWPI is the Chilean Wholesale Price Index.

2. This assumes annual average compound growth rates, determined by using an exponential regression.

3. This includes only the value of fruit trees. It does not include capital invested in land, buildings, machinery, or other capital investment.

Readings

Central Bank of Chile. 1986. *Social and Economic Indicators 1960–1965*. Central Bank of Chile *Monthly Bulletin*.

Fundación Chile. *National Census of Cold Storage Capacity 1983, 1986, 1989.*
Hurtado, H., E. Muchnik, and A. Valdés. 1987. *A Comparative Study of the Political Economy of Agricultural Pricing Policies.* Washington, D.C.: The World Bank.
International Monetary Fund. *International Financial Statistics.*
Ministry of Agriculture. 1966. *Agricultural Statistics 1975-1987.*
Ministry of Agriculture. 1989. *The Chilean Agricultural Sector: Policy and Results.*
National Institute of Statistics. *National Agricultural Survey.*
National Institute of Statistics. *National Employment Survey.*

CHAPTER 8

A Colloquium Summary

Community-Based Development: A Cutting Edge for Innovation in the Nineties

Barbara Huddleston
Chief, Food Security Service, Food and Agriculture Organization, Rome, Italy

The individual who is asked to summarize a colloquium such as this one has a nearly impossible task, and I apologize to my fellow participants if I should happen to omit some important points or distort what has been said.

We have been addressing the theme of sharing innovation. Each of the presentations has brought a particular perspective to the problem of innovation with respect to agricultural and rural development. We have explored not simply innovations and the sharing of knowledge for development, but innovations for a development that will lead to sustainable food security for a growing world population.

One other common theme which I would like to draw out now, which was mentioned first by Dr. Aboyade, is that the development process that we have been discussing is synergistic. We are not talking about particular areas, or singular elements of action where there can be one quick fix. The idea that we can just select two or three action areas and focus in on those areas and succeed, I think, runs counter to the whole theme of this colloquium. For example, going only with a right policy, or only with a technical innovation which will somehow magically improve productivity, or only with a transformation of institutions which will somehow magically stimulate people to produce, will not be sufficient. All of the speakers have suggested in one way or another that we need all of these elements working together; none of them alone, even if the best in the world, will do the job.

However, speakers did refer to three general elements, that is to say, policies—economic policies in particular—technologies, and institutions in the broad sense as being the three central elements with which we have to work. Further, they have argued that whatever is done with respect to one of these three elements must be interactive with what is being done with respect to the other two. The actions in all three areas have to be coherent and consistent with one other.

Returning now to the theme of innovation, we heard in some detail from each of the speakers, some more on one element than another, about various frontiers which are facing us. Speakers have referred to several new areas of concern, where there is a cutting edge that requires our attention now.

I would like to discuss, first, the institutional element, because I think that some of the most interesting ideas emerged in this area. Dr. Aboyade described a very innovative institutional approach to planning and development at the community level, emphasizing the importance of people's participation and of determining the boundaries of a community so that each community would be homogeneous, yet would be of a sufficient size to permit a complex set of economic activities to grow up around an agricultural base. Although perhaps not fully developed in his paper, the concept of a viable community which can be a focal point for development is an interesting idea which merits more thought.

Dr. Lin described the Chinese experiments with different forms of communal rural organization, including communal organization at different size levels, and the successes and failures at each of these different size levels. Bruce Stone pointed out that the appropriateness of the organizational structures in China depended in part on the specific production goals and on the level of technological development at a given period of time. So we could conclude from his remarks, and I think from others as well, that there is no one ideal institutional framework, but rather that we have to be location specific and time specific in deciding what structures to encourage or adopt. This, I think, was also Dr. Aboyade's point.

Dr. Singh described the importance of introducing better resource management practices on an entire watershed basis. And here again, the organizational and institutional implications are a key feature. He was not talking only about technology, but also about the institutional environment within which an appropriate technology for dryland agriculture and rainwater management could be introduced.

Dr. Sadikin emphasized, among a variety of very interesting points, that in Indonesia, adequate farm size, which was achieved partly through group farming, had been an important precondition for success. Again, we see that the question of size was crucial. What is the appropriate size of a farm, or of an agricultural community? Is there a size that is too small? Is there a size that is too large? I think that we cannot really give a precise answer, but all speakers alluded to the importance of this point.

Dr. Wylie referred to the important role of private entrepreneurship in adopting new technology in Chile's fruit and vegetable industry. And Mrs. Mtalo's description of the Iringa integrated nutrition program in Tanzania clearly demonstrates the importance of community participation for the achievement of project goals.

A very interesting point which emerged from all of these different references to institutional organization and structure is that the institutions referred to by the speakers are mainly local, communal, household level, or private. And it has been emphasized more than once that response to incentive policies and receptiveness to new technologies depend on whether or not these institutions at the local level have the freedom and flexibility to act in accordance with their own perceived needs.

Mention has been made of the need for better public infrastructure such as, for example, transport, energy, and, particularly, for research networks as preconditions for a development program, yet we have heard rather little today about what public, governmental institutions should be doing or how they should be reformed. The emphasis has been almost entirely on communities, on households, and on individuals. And here, for me, thinking back over the years of discussion on these issues, it is quite a change to come to a colloquium and hear an entire day of discussion that does not offer many prescriptions as to what governments should do, nor many prescriptions about what official action should be taken at a local level. Rather, much of the discussion focused on the possibilities for institutional innovation outside the public sector. I think this is a cutting edge for development that has emerged from this discussion, and one that we can pursue.

The one public sector role which has been discussed is that of economic policy. Whether at the macroeconomic level of exchange rates, trade policy, public resource allocation, or at the microeconomic level of price policy, there does seem to be a general perception that governments do have a role in policy formation even though the movement may be in the direction of letting markets determine prices. There was a recognition that wages, interest rates, prices of production inputs, agricultural output prices, and prices of consumption goods must all be aligned with one another.

No speaker really argued for a deliberate policy of producer price incentives beyond what the market would naturally offer. However, I think there was a recognition, certainly by some of the speakers, that public policy to assure that agricultural producers are not disadvantaged through overvalued exchange rates or low urban wage rates is important. There was less attention given to consumer price policy, but I think it is fair to say that the speakers in general felt that the public sector has a legitimate monitoring role over prices and perhaps a limited intervention role, depending on the case.

An adequate supply of credit and adequate supply of inputs for the traditional Green Revolution technology—i.e., fertilizer, seeds, and water—were regarded by the speakers as essential. Subsidized prices for these inputs were credited by some of the speakers with having helped in the dissemination of new technology in the early phases of agricultural development, especially in China, India, and Indonesia. However, there seemed to be a general feeling that perhaps the availability of inputs and of credit, rather than the price, is the more crucial constraint in the coming decade.

These inputs—credit, fertilizer, seeds, and water—reflect the first stage of technological development through which the Asian countries already have passed and which at present African nations are grappling with. Drs. Aboyade and Odhiambo argued that Africa could not simply replicate or adopt the Green Revolution technological package which was made available for wheat and rice, but instead would require a new technology specifically adapted to its own ecological potential and its own dietary patterns. Dr. Aboyade saw the development and adoption of such a technology as a two-stage process, drawing on what exists in the short term and introducing new practices and new technologies in the longer term.

Following the presentation by Dr. Singh, there was a considerable discussion of the importance of water resource management and of different possible approaches to this important problem. While the speaker focused mainly on techniques for making better use of natural rainfall or for collecting, storing, and irrigating with rainwater, various discussants felt that groundwater and riverine irrigation would continue to be needed. Dr. Lipton queried the role of the public sector in financing water resource management. For major irrigation projects large capital investment is clearly needed. However, many of the techniques suggested for improving water resource management for dryland agriculture are, on the contrary, appropriate to the community-size development process alluded to earlier. Nevertheless, even though smaller in scale, the introduction of these techniques probably also requires an external resource input. How much, what kind, and the bureaucratic process by which to move external resources to community-level development activities, as opposed to activities where the bureaucracy itself manages them, all remain to be determined.

Reforestation, soil conservation, and the integration of mixed cropping systems with animal husbandry were regarded by the colloquium speakers as areas requiring priority attention. There were several references to the need for technologies which would sustain the environment by combining improved production practices with soil conservation techniques. Finally, small-scale innovations which improve the productivity of women, coupled with improved nutritional practices, were demonstrated to be a viable means of directly improving food security of undernourished children and their families in the short term.

The process that emerges from all of this is complex. And in the view of today's speakers, the management of it has to be decentralized. Thus, to be effective, the conclusions of this colloquium need to be addressed not only or not even primarily to governments, but to individuals, both within the donor community and within the countries directly engaged in the development process. For it is above all the effort of the individual workers who are struggling with the effective integration of the interacting elements discussed today that is the *sine qua non* of development. From the perspective of the participants in this colloquium, improving performance at the local level, based on individual and group effort, is the challenge for the nineties which innovation for food, agriculture, and rural development must address. Thank you.

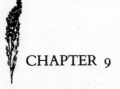

CHAPTER 9

Thoughts on the Global Issues of Food, Population, and the Environment

Robert F. Chandler, Jr.
Founding Director, International Rice Research Institute, Manila,
The Philippines

Introduction

It is a pleasure to return to the Cornell campus where as a faculty member I spent twelve satisfying years, from 1935 to 1947. In speaking to an audience much better informed than I am on recent developments I realize that I shall not provide any new information on the subject I have chosen. Rather, I shall express my views on some aspects of the important issues of food, population, and the environment, with the hope that they will stimulate an interesting discussion on this broad topic.

Food

Undoubtedly, greater progress has been made in the past twenty-five years in meeting the food grain needs of the world than in any similar period in the past. Of the many factors responsible for this advance, by far the most decisive was the development by agricultural scientists of the short, stiff-strawed, fertilizer-responsive, heavy-tillering varieties of rice and wheat,

This paper was originally presented on September 20, 1989, at a Cornell University seminar on international agriculture. This slightly revised version is included with the permission of the author and of Cornell University's Program in International Agriculture. Copies of the original paper have been circulated by Cornell University.

which have more than doubled the yield potential of mankind's two most important food crops.

For centuries until the mid-1960s, the typical rice plant of the tropics was tall, with long, drooping leaves. Developed to survive under prevailing conditions of inadequate insect, disease, weed, and water control, and the nonuse of chemical fertilizers, its yields were dependable but low. When, in an effort to increase yields, fertilizer was applied, the plant became even taller and leafier, and lodged (i.e., fell over) before harvest. The larger the amount of fertilizer applied, the earlier and more severe the lodging. Thus the tropical rice farmer was faced with a dilemma: if he did not apply fertilizer, yields would be low because of poor plant nutrition; yet if he tried to boost yields by applying fertilizer, he obtained little or no increase in grain.

The response of the traditional wheat plant to fertilizer and to modern management methods was essentially the same as that of the rice plant; the same improvements had to be made if yields were to be lifted above the rather static levels that existed before 1960.

As is well known, the work on tropical rice improvement on a global scale was sparked by the International Rice Research Institute (IRRI), which began its research program in 1962 in the Philippines, and on wheat by the International Maize and Wheat Improvement Center (CIMMYT) in Mexico, an outgrowth of the Rockefeller Foundation's Mexican Agricultural Program, which became an international center in 1966. The work of these two organizations, along with that of many cooperating national programs, doubled the yield potential of the traditional rice and wheat varieties and triggered the upsurge in production of these two crops that is commonly referred to as the Green Revolution.

Because it has been told many times, there is no need to go into detail as to how scientists created these new varieties and the appropriate technology to produce maximum yields. Rather, I shall portray recent trends in production and make some predictions of what lies ahead. More attention will be given to rice, a crop with which I am especially familiar, and one that is the staple food for about 2.5 billion people, nearly half the world's population.

Approximately 90 percent of the world's rice is produced and consumed in Asia. Table 9-1 shows the production of rough rice in those seventeen countries that are now harvesting over one million metric tons of rice annually, comparing the production in 1960 with that twenty-five years later (1985), and indicating the percent increase during that period.

Even though there has been a 114 percent increase in Asian rice production during the twenty-five-year period, four countries had less than a 15 percent increase and two are harvesting less rice today than they were in 1960. Briefly, the reasons for the slow-down in production in those countries are as follows.

In Taiwan and Japan all arable land is fully used, population pressures are intense, and as urbanization and industrialization expand, agricultural land is converted to other uses. Furthermore, as incomes have risen in these two countries, per capita rice consumption has decreased. Rice yields in both countries are already high (5.05 tons/hectare [t/ha] in Taiwan and 6.2 t/ha in Japan). Undoubtedly, rice production in Taiwan and Japan will continue to decline.

Kampuchea's 10 percent loss in production is a consequence of a decrease in area planted to rice and of almost constant low yields. The country's lack of progress can be attributed to the civil war that has ensued since the late 1960s.

Nepal's situation is the result of limited land resources suitable for rice production. Its 4 percent increase reflects a modest rise in yield (1.9 t/ha to 2.05 t/ha) but with little change in area devoted to rice. With an expansion in

Table 9 – 1.

A Comparison of Rough Rice Production in 1960 and in 1985 of Asian Nations Producing over One Million Tons Annually (Thousand Tons)

Country	Production in 1960	Production in 1985	Percent Increase
Bangladesh	14,507	22,650	56
Burma	7,199	14,317	100
China	62,235	171,416	175
Taiwan	2,504	2,847	14
India	51,861	96,306	86
Indonesia	12,814	39,033	205
Japan	16,740	14,578	– 13
Kampuchea	2,335	2,100	– 10
Korea (DPR)	1,535	5,800	277
Korea (Republic)	4,117	7,655	86
Malaysia	935	1,953	109
Nepal	2,690	2,804	4
Pakistan	1,545	4,357	182
Philippines	3,705	9,097	145
Sri Lanka	897	2,661	196
Thailand	7,635	20,120	163
Vietnam	9,167	15,897	73
Total	202,421	433,591	114

Source: The data in this table, and other rice statistics cited in this paper, were taken from the 1988 issue of *World Rice Statistics* published by the International Rice Research Institute.

irrigation systems and the use of more fertilizer, Nepal should be able to increase its rice production by close to 100 percent.

The substantial advance in rice production during the twenty-five-year period was due mostly to an increase in yield (82 percent) rather than to an increase in area planted to rice (12 percent). The area, yield, and production of rice in Asia are shown graphically in Figure 9–1. It is evident that there has been no consistent gain in area planted to rice since about 1977. The only Asian country that has shown a continuing expansion of land planted to rice during the past decade is North Korea (DPR). Average yields are already very high (7.0 t/ha), and if production is to continue to rise it can come only from an expansion in the area planted to rice.

The story for wheat is similar to that for rice except that the relative gains in production and yield have been much greater for wheat. In Figure 9–2 are plotted the index numbers (1961–65 = 100) for area, production, and yield in Asia (excluding the Middle East). Although the expansion in area planted to wheat since the 1961–65 period was relatively higher than for rice (40 percent as compared to about 12), the increases in yield (over 200 percent) and production (about 320 percent) were much higher than the corresponding figures for rice, which, as shown earlier, nearly doubled during the same period. The important fact to note in Figure 9–2 is that,

Figure 9 – 1.

Area, Yield, and Production of Rice in Asia, 1960–88

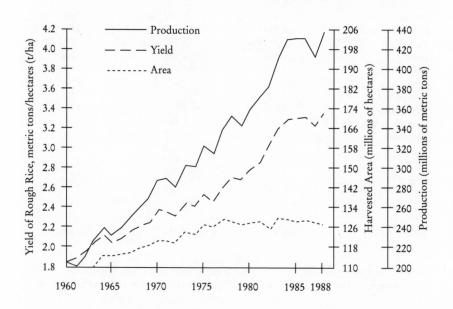

Figure 9-2.

Index Numbers for Area, Yield, and Production of Wheat in Asia (excluding Middle East), 1966–87

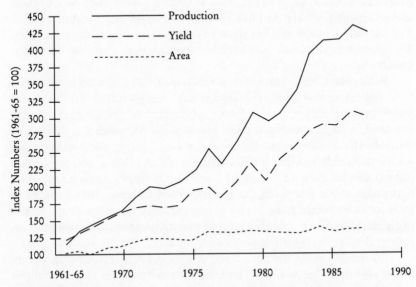

Note: Index numbers are derived from metric tons of production, metric tons/hectare of yield, and hectares of area.

here again, as with rice, there has been only a slight gain in area planted to wheat in Asia since the mid-1970s, which indicates that most of the land available for wheat production is being used for that purpose.

Although I am not sufficiently familiar with wheat to predict the potential for increased production in Asia, it would seem possible, with additional irrigation and fertilizer, to raise yields from the current 2.2 t/ha to at least 3.0 t/ha during the next two decades.

The United States, Canada, and Argentina will continue to supply much of the wheat for the developing nations of the world. Unfortunately, many of these poorer countries are so burdened with external debts that they lack the foreign exchange with which to purchase food grains and are forced to rely on food aid and other concessions to feed their burgeoning populations.

Let us reflect further on the prospects for continuing increases in rice production in Asia. Barker, Herdt, and Rose state in their book, *The Rice Economy of Asia*, that Asia can be self-sufficient in rice through the start of the next century if it will provide and utilize sufficient fertilizer and irrigation and if it enacts and enforces government policies favorable to increased production. I agree with their view, but we must remind ourselves that the next century is only a decade away.

Let us take a closer look at China and India, which together produce 61 percent of the rice in Asia and 56 percent of the rice in the world. China irrigates essentially all of its rice, uses abundant quantities of both organic and inorganic fertilizer, and has boosted its average rice yield to 5.4 t/ha. The harvested area of rice has shown no increase for more than ten years. Therefore, we can expect only a modest increase in rice production in that country.

India, like China, has shown no increase in area planted to rice since 1977, indicating that all suitable land is now being utilized; yet its current yields average only 2.2 t/ha. About 42 percent of the country's rice is irrigated, most of it during the wet season only. Although it is difficult to estimate the amount of fertilizer used on rice alone, the best available information indicates that India is applying about 35 kilograms per hectare (kg/ha) of nutrients (i.e., N, P_2O_5, and K_2O) to rice, which, by comparison, is about one-tenth the quantity used in Japan. If India were to increase its area of irrigated rice by 50 percent and triple to quadruple its use of chemical fertilizer, probably it could maintain its per capita rice production at current levels for the next twenty years.

Looking beyond that period and at Asia as a whole, the prospects are not at all bright. Since all land suitable for rice in Asia now essentially is being utilized for that crop, further increases in production will have to come from such measures as using more fertilizer, expanding irrigation systems, practicing better insect and disease control, developing varieties with higher yield potential and, in the tropics, growing two or three crops a year. Regarding the latter practice, I might mention that IRRI's experience of growing rice continuously in the Philippines on the same land for over twenty years resulted in a decline in top yields in spite of using the best management methods known today. Thus, sequential cropping of rice has its limitations.

Plant breeders will continue to develop better varieties with a higher yield potential, but it must be realized that the greatest gains in varietal improvement have already been made. There are limits not only to the amount of arable land and to fresh water supplies for irrigation but to the genetic improvement of plants. It is impossible at this stage to predict what advances in yield potential will come from genetic engineering and from other areas of biotechnology. My guess is that the impact will be largely through increased stability of yield, brought about by greater tolerance to adverse environmental conditions and to insect and disease attack. In estimating future yield potentials we should remember that we cannot increase average world precipitation or the quantity of solar radiation, the two most important factors limiting crop production.

Top average national yields today range between 6 and 7 t/ha, which is double the current mean yield in Asia and triple that in many of the individual countries. With the exception of Japan, China, Taiwan, the two Koreas, and Indonesia, countries that have attained rather high yield levels, all the other Asian nations have the potential of increasing average rice yields by a factor of 1.5 to 2.0, provided they use more inputs and their governments establish appropriate pricing policies and other socioeconomic incentives.

In my view it seems extremely unlikely that average Asian rice yields will ever exceed 6 t/ha, which is double the current level. Yet demographers estimate that world population will at least double before it becomes stabilized, and some predictions even place the ultimate population at twelve to fifteen billion. If such forecasts prove correct, global food production resources will be strained to the limit and, as I shall emphasize later, the environment will be severely damaged.

Population

Prior to about 1750, world population had remained rather constant for centuries, its growth limited by frequent famine and widespread disease. However, as the Americas became settled by Europeans, world population started to grow rather rapidly, although high mortality rates kept it under considerable control until the twentieth century. Then, because of better health care, it grew rapidly reaching a peak growth rate in 1970. Table 9-2, derived from estimates by the United Nations (as reported by Worldwatch Institute, 1988), shows the world population from 1950 to 1985, with projections to the year 2000.

The data reveal that although the population was expanding by only forty million annually in 1950, by the beginning of the twenty-first century over ninety million people will be added each year. This is in spite of the fact that the annual population growth rate is expected to decline from about 1.7 percent today to 1.5 percent by the year 2000. Hence, as the world struggles to control its human population, the number added each year continues to grow.

Discouragingly, the growth rate is much faster in the developing countries than in the industrialized ones. This is shown in Table 9-3, which gives for selected slow-growth and rapid-growth countries the 1988 population, the current rate of annual increase, and the projected stabilization levels as estimated by the World Bank. ("Stabilization level" refers to the population of a country when it attains a zero population growth rate. Demographers predict that world population will become stabilized by the last half of the twenty-first century.)

As the table indicates, the more prosperous, industrialized nations will add only 10 to 30 percent to their populations before stabilization levels are reached. Even China, still underdeveloped, will experience a population increase of no more than 50 percent. The other poorer nations, however, may increase their populations by 200 to 500 percent before reaching a state of zero population growth.

Bangladesh is an example of severe overpopulation. The country now has an estimated population of 113 million, which is increasing at the rate of about 2.4 percent annually. The density is 2,028 people per square mile, 80 percent of whom live in rural areas. The land area is about 55,000 square miles, roughly that of the state of Georgia, which, by contrast, has a population of 6.2 million and a density of 106 per square mile.

Earlier this year I participated in a workshop in Bangladesh helping to analyze the agricultural sector. Considering the frequency of floods and cyclones and the scarcity of arable land per capita, we estimated that if Bangladesh could irrigate twice as much land as at present and if it could triple the amount of chemical fertilizer applied, it possibly could increase its rice production by 85 percent during the next two decades. The additional area under irrigation would permit the country to produce more rice in the dry season and would allow the farmers to use supplemental irrigation during the monsoon season when precipitation is variable and unpredictable.

All major development projects in Bangladesh are financed by foreign aid, and the country has to import large quantities of food grain, most of it

Table 9 – 2.

World Population, 1950–85, with Projections to the Year 2000

Year	Population (millions)	Annual Growth Rate (percent)	Annual Increase (millions)
1950	2,516	1.6	40
1960	3,019	1.8	54
1970	3,693	2.0	74
1980	4,450	1.8	80
1985	4,837	1.7	82
1990	5,246	1.6	91
2000	6,122	1.5	92

Source: Data derived from United Nations, *World Population: Prospects, Estimates and Projections as Assessed in 1984* (New York, 1986) and as reported in Worldwatch Institute, *State of the World 1988*

through foreign aid rather than by purchase with national funds. Annual per capita income in Bangladesh is the equivalent of only U.S. $113. The literacy rate is 33 percent and attendance in primary school is listed as 23 percent. Sadly, nine out of ten girls who start primary school soon drop out. This decreases the likelihood that women will be employed outside the home and reduces the chances of a declining fertility rate. Only 4 percent of the appropriate age group attends high school and, of course, only a few go on to a college or university.

Bangladesh is already seriously overpopulated. It needs to make huge investments in education and take major steps to create off-farm employment opportunities. More than half the rural population is landless and is severely underemployed. Over 70 percent of the farms are less than one hectare in size. I cannot conceive of Bangladesh supporting the 342 million people predicted by the World Bank. This would then mean that the

Table 9 – 3.

Population in 1988 of Selected Countries and Their Projected Population at Stabilization

Country	Population 1988 (millions)	Current Rate of Population Growth (percent)	Population Size at Stabilization (millions)	Ratio*
Slow-Growth Countries				
China	1,069	1.0	1,571	1.5
Soviet Union	287	0.9	377	1.3
Japan	123	0.7	128	1.1
United Kingdom	56	0.2	59	1.1
United States	247	0.7	289	1.2
West Germany	61	−0.2	52	−0.9
Rapid-Growth Countries				
Kenya	23	3.8	121	5.3
Nigeria	112	2.8	529	4.7
Pakistan	107	2.6	423	4.0
Bangladesh	109	2.4	342	3.1
India	817	1.8	1,698	2.1

*Population size at stabilization divided by the population size in 1988.

Source: *World Almanac* (1989) and World Bank data reported in Worldwatch Institute's publications, *State of the World 1988* and *1989*

population density, when stabilized, would exceed 6,000 per square mile, far denser than in any other country or state today.

India, although much larger than Bangladesh, also faces severe population problems. Assuming its present population to be 820 million and the current growth rate to be 1.8 percent, one year from now there will be 14.7 million more people in the country than there are today. At this rate India will soon surpass China as the world's most populous nation.

Although Africa's population is growing faster than that of any other continent, it is likely that Asia will reach crisis conditions earlier. Asia has 29 percent of the world's land surface and 60 percent of its population, while Africa has 20 percent of the land area but only 12 percent of the global population. Yet Africa is in serious trouble today. Its per capita food production peaked in 1967 and has been declining slowly ever since. The population growth rate is no less than 2.8 percent annually, and at that rate its population will double in about twenty-five years.

Africa, south of the Sahara and north of the Union of South Africa, is plagued by both individual and national poverty and by insufficient and often highly variable rainfall. The soils of central and western Africa are mostly derived from granite, which causes them to be sandy, relatively infertile, and subject to severe erosion when cleared of forest. Although the continent generally underutilizes its water resources for irrigation, there are vast areas that cannot be economically irrigated because of topography and geological formations. Development in Africa is hampered further by its division into numerous rather small countries, each with its own social and political structures. Furthermore, there are serious rivalries among tribes within countries. Above all, the educational system is entirely inadequate. In some countries such as Mali, Burkina Faso, and Senegal, the literacy rate is only 10 percent; to the best of my knowledge, no sub-Saharan country has a literacy rate above 50 percent.

Although Africa receives more foreign aid per capita than any other region, its population is growing so fast that development programs cannot keep up with needs. As a result, not only food production but per capita incomes are decreasing. The fact that there is more arable land per capita in Africa than in any other continent gives us hope, however, that it can be rescued from its current state of economic decline.

Foreign assistance organizations are learning by experience what works and what does not.[1] I believe, however, that progress will continue to be slow until substantial gains are made in controlling population growth rates, no easy task.

Education, especially for women, has been shown to reduce family size, and the higher the level of education for both men and women, the greater the opportunity for employment. Historically, as economic conditions improve, fertility rates decline. Ideally, health clinics should be within a thirty-minute walk of the houses in the more populated areas, and all clinics should be equipped to provide both advice and materials for family planning. It is essential that national governments develop policies that promote population control, and foreign assistance agencies should contribute substantially toward the necessary facilities for family planning.

The U.S. government, unfortunately, has an inadequate policy for supporting family planning in the poorer countries. I believe it is true that in all the developed countries that have attained a population growth of essentially zero, abortion has been legalized. It is my contention that the United States should not only strongly support family planning programs in all countries with a high population growth rate but should increase our research to develop improved methods of contraception—a declining area of research and development in recent years.

It was heartening to read in its 1988 Annual Report that the Rockefeller Foundation has a strong program in the population sciences. Private foundations enjoy a flexibility and independence that governmental organizations may not possess and often can work more effectively on vital problems whose solutions are hampered by controversial policies.

The advantage of private foundations applies not only to population control problems but to all areas of development. For example, Lele and Goldsmith contend that India's progress in agricultural research and development was greatly enhanced by the sound policies and competent personnel provided to that country by the Rockefeller Foundation. They suggest that many of those principles could be advantageously applied to Africa, although they recognize some of the barriers to progress in Africa that did not exist in India.[2]

Environment

This subject is so broad, so open to speculation and widely different views, that I find it daunting to do more than mention the ways in which we human beings are damaging our world. The list would include depletion of forest cover; soil erosion; desertification; the pollution of air, groundwater, lakes, and oceans; the depletion of underground water supplies; the eventual exhaustion of oil and coal reserves; the decreasing numbers—and in some cases the near extinction—of plant and animal species; the possibility of global warming due to increases in atmospheric carbon dioxide and other "greenhouse gases"; and the depletion of the ozone layer in the stratosphere. Moreover, in our relatively affluent society we are plagued by highway traffic jams around our major cities and frustrating airport delays due to overcrowded runways, and we are fast running out of suitable sites for disposing of our wastes.

Because of the limitations of time and my lack of hands-on experience with environmental issues, I shall touch on only three topics: the depletion of the world's forests, especially in the tropics and subtropics; the need for a sustained system of crop production to replace shifting cultivation; and the much publicized greenhouse effect.

Forest Depletion

According to 1985 estimates by the Food and Agriculture Organization of the United Nations (FAO), there are three billion hectares of closed-canopy forests worldwide, another 1.3 billion hectares of open woodland (wooded savannah), and to this can be added about one billion hectares of shrubland and forest regrowth, bringing our planet's total forest reserves to about 5.3 billion hectares.

Unfortunately, tropical forests are being cut much faster than they are being replanted. Estimates indicate that over twelve million hectares of tropical forests are being cleared annually, whereas only about 1.1 million hectares are being replanted. Thus ten hectares are being cleared for every hectare being planted. As population pressures require more land for food production, vast areas in Brazil are being cut—much of it burned—and settlers are moving in to engage in cattle raising or in growing crops. Brazil is destroying an area each year that is twice the size of the state of Connecticut.

One of the serious problems is supplying fuelwood for urban populations, especially in the semiarid regions of the less-developed world. Around the major cities forests have essentially disappeared, and wood gatherers must go long distances to collect firewood, still the principal source of heat for cooking in the poorer countries of the world. In many areas fuelwood is being harvested at five times its growth rate.

There seems to be no other cure for the diminishing forest resources in the Third World than extensive replanting of trees, not only in large open areas, but in cities, around village houses, and wherever there is land not suitable for agriculture.

In the semiarid regions, especially in the Sahel of Africa, extensive planting of *Acacia albida* would help relieve the firewood crisis. Unlike most other trees, this deep-rooted, drought-resistant species loses its leaves during the rainy season, thus allowing the planting of crops without undue shading, and during the dry season, when the leaves appear, provides shade for grazing animals.

In the richer, industrialized countries of Western Europe and North America, there are many more trees today than, for example, in 1850. These regions have controlled their populations and have increased the yield of crops and animals so that land once cultivated can be returned to forest. There is no reason why the developing countries could not gain in area devoted to forest if they would just limit their populations so as to be in equilibrium with their needs for wood products.

Sustained Crop Production to Replace Shifting Cultivation

It is estimated that over 250 million people eke out a living from shifting cultivation (also known as slash-and-burn agriculture). Research must be accelerated to develop sustained crop-and-tree production systems that will eliminate the deplorable destruction of forest resources now taking place under shifting cultivation.

The time-honored practice of clearing new areas of forest every few years, allowing forest regrowth to restore soil fertility, although wasteful and inefficient, was a sustainable practice for centuries. This procedure is becoming unworkable as population pressures cause farmers to shorten the forest fallow period to such an extent that there is not enough time for the land to recover its fertility. The "resting period" between clearing of the land in many areas, formerly ten years or more, has been reduced to three years and less. FAO estimates, as reported by the Worldwatch Institute, indicate that in the tropics shifting cultivation accounts for 70 percent of the closed-forest clearing in Africa, about 50 percent in Asia, and 35 percent in Latin America.

Alley cropping, also known as hedgerow intercropping, is one of the better substitutes for shifting cultivation. It consists of planting widely spaced rows of trees between which are grown food crops such as maize, upland rice, or grain legumes. The woody plants are pruned regularly, and leaves and twigs are used as mulch for the crop plants. To quote Rocheleau et al.:

> The primary purpose of alley cropping is to maintain or increase crop yields by improvement of the soil and microclimate and weed control. Farmers may also obtain tree products from the hedgerows—including firewood, building poles, food, medicine, and fodder—and on sloping land the hedgerows and prunings may help to control erosion.[3]

With proper management, as Nicholaides points out, sustained and high yields of crops can be obtained under high-input technology.[4] Yet most farmers accustomed to low-technology shifting cultivation will be hesitant to make such an abrupt change and usually adjust more readily to agroforestry techniques than to modern and costly methods.

The Greenhouse Effect

Though a nonexpert, I selected this topic because of the great prominence it is being given by scientists, the media, the U.S. Congress, and international bodies concerned with the environment. Indeed, if some scientific forecasts come true, the impact of this phenomenon could be disastrous.

As we know, the greenhouse effect is so named because certain gases, mainly carbon dioxide, methane, nitrous oxide, and water vapor, trap heat—much as the glass of a greenhouse does—and keep the earth warm. Without them our planet would be extremely cold and uninhabitable.

The concern of scientists is that the carbon dioxide content of the atmosphere has been increasing steadily since about 1850. Even since 1960 it has risen from about 316 parts per million (ppm) to a little over 345 ppm. The principal sources of the excess carbon dioxide are the combustion of fossil fuels and the burning of forests. The predicted consequences are that the earth will continue to get warmer, there will be serious and frequent droughts in the temperate zones, and the warming of the ocean and the melting of glacial ice will cause a rise in sea level of several meters, flooding low-lying coastal areas and raising havoc in such cities as New York, New Orleans, and Miami, and in low-elevation countries such as Bangladesh and Egypt.

Not long ago I had a conversation with Dr. Berrien Moore, a scientist at the University of New Hampshire's Institute for the Study of Earth, Oceans, and Space, which recently received a $14 million grant from NASA. He stated that although there is no question that the carbon dioxide content of the atmosphere is rising, the ultimate effect on the earth's atmosphere is still uncertain.

Computer models of the amounts of carbon dioxide released by mankind's activities and the quantities absorbed by plants and by the oceans leave a deficit in the atmosphere that is unaccounted for. In round numbers, scientists estimate that six billion metric tons are being released from fossil fuel combustion and an additional two billion tons from the burning of forests. Of the theoretical eight billion tons, only six billion tons can be accounted for. Thus, two billion tons annually vanish from the estimates.

I do not wish to state that the greenhouse effect is unreal but I am listing a few facts that often remain unmentioned in the literature on the subject:

1. When exposed to full sunlight, the limiting factor in photosynthesis is carbon dioxide, not solar radiation. Thus the more carbon dioxide that is in the atmosphere, the more that will be fixed by plants (up to a certain limit, of course). To take advantage of this phenomenon, producers of greenhouse plants often increase the carbon dioxide content of the air artificially to enhance yields.

2. In the past century or so, the temperature rise has been only about 1.5 degrees Celsius. The cause, rather than being a rise in the carbon dioxide content of the atmosphere, could be the increased radiation from brick, concrete and asphalt surfaces, and the heat being given off by the numerous

sources of energy produced today. Significantly, many of the temperature recording stations are in large cities where these effects are the most pronounced.

3. From the literature I find that estimates of the rise in temperature during the next half century vary from two to nine degrees Celsius. Such variations lead one to question the certainty of present-day calculations.

4. When I went to college over sixty years ago, we were told that a portion of the carbon dioxide in the air was dissolved by rain and entered the soil, combining with hydrogen to make carbonic acid or in alkaline soils to form carbonates. Although I have not seen it mentioned in recent literature, I assume the process still goes on, which may account for some of the discrepancy in calculations of the carbon dioxide balance.

5. The oceans are the largest depository of carbon dioxide, much of it eventually found in the carbonates in the shells of crustaceans, mollusks, and coral. It appears that scientists have not yet been able to determine to what extent the seas will absorb the extra carbon dioxide that is being released into the atmosphere. Considering that about 70 percent of the globe's surface is covered by water, this is no easy question to answer.

In closing this topic I must emphasize that I am completely in favor of cutting down on the emissions of carbon dioxide and other atmosphere-polluting gases. Certainly all agree that we must make every effort to develop economically profitable uses of renewable energy sources such as wind, solar radiation, tides, and eventually, we earnestly hope, fusion.

Concluding Statement

If the governments of the developing countries and the foreign assistance organizations (both governmental and private) of the industrialized nations were to provide the financial and human resources, it is conceivable that enough food can be produced to support a global population of ten to twelve billion, albeit at current inadequate nutritional levels. (Over 600 million people in the world today suffer from malnutrition and countless others are undernourished.)

We must stop deluding ourselves that world hunger and malnutrition can be eliminated in the next decade. Such a pronouncement was made by Mr. Henry Kissinger at the World Food Conference in Rome in 1974, yet there are more people suffering from malnutrition today than there were then, largely because population growth rates have continued to be high in most Third World countries. Most Asian countries are already overpopulated and in sub-Saharan Africa and many Latin American countries development programs have been unable to keep pace with population growth.

Substantial growth in food production to keep pace with expected population growth, in any case, cannot be achieved without massive expenditures, unequalled in the past except in times of war, and it cannot be done quickly.

It is still imperative that the developed and developing countries alike mount intensive family planning campaigns with the goal of attaining zero population growth. Obviously, this will be a long-term and herculean task. In Africa, for example, over 45 percent of the population is under fifteen years of age, which means that even if fertility rates were cut immediately from the current level of about seven down to two, the population would continue to expand for decades.

In 1973 a book appeared, entitled *Toward a Steady-State Economy*, edited by Professor Herman E. Daly of Louisiana State University. It contained chapters not only by him but by specialists from many fields, all of whom recognized that an equilibrium must be established in this world between its natural resources and the human population. With zero population growth, which eventually will become essential for human survival, a steady-state economy must come about as well. I agree with the postulates in this book as well as those on the predicament of mankind presented in the 1972 book, *The Limits to Growth*.

Without question we must reverse the trend of over-cutting of forests. We must likewise make every effort to produce more food more efficiently, developing systems of sustained yields, yet protecting the life-supporting resources of our planet. Such efforts, however, will be but a temporary stopgap unless we bring the human population under control.

There are uncertainties about global warming, but there can be no doubt that in a finite world the human population and the natural life-supporting resources are on a collision course. To avert such a calamity is the greatest challenge that confronts our species.

Notes

1. Jessica Tuchman Mathews, "Rescue Plan for Africa," *World Monitor* (May 1989): 28–36.

2. Uma Lele and Arthur A. Goldsmith, "The Development of National Agricultural Research Capacity: India's Experience with the Rockefeller Foundation and Its Significance for Africa," *Economic Development and Cultural Change* (January 1989).

3. Dianne Rocheleau et al., *Agroforestry in Dryland Africa 1988* (Nairobi: International Council for Research in Agroforestry).

4. J. J. Nicholaides III et al., eds., *Agronomic Research on Soils of the Tropics* (1980–81 Technical Report) (Raleigh: Soil Science Department, North Carolina State University, 1983).

Readings

Barker, Randolph, and Robert D. Herdt with Beth Rose. 1985. *The Rice Economy of Asia. Resources for the Future.* Washington, D.C.: Resources for the Future.

Daly, Herman E., ed. 1973. *Toward a Steady-State Economy.* San Francisco: W. H. Freeman.

Food and Agriculture Organization of the United Nations. 1985. World Forest Resources. Rome: FAO.

International Rice Research Institute. 1988. World Rice Statistics. Manila, The Philippines: IRRI.

Lele, Uma, and Arthur A. Goldsmith. 1986. "The Development of a National Agricultural Research Capacity: India's Experience with the Rockefeller Foundation and Its Significance for Africa." *Economic Development and Cultural Change* (January 1989). [Reprinted in MADIA Discussion Paper no. 2, The World Bank, 1989.]

Mathews, Jessica Tuchman. 1989. "Rescue Plan for Africa." *World Monitor* (May 1989): 28–36.

Meadows, Donella, Dennis L. Meadows, Jorgen Randers, and William H. Behrens III. 1972. *The Limits to Growth.* New York: Universe Books.

Nicholaides, J. J. III, et al., eds. 1983. *Agronomic Research on Soils of the Tropics.* 1980–81 Technical Report. Raleigh: Soil Science Department, North Carolina State University.

Rocheleau, Dianne, et al. 1988. *Agroforestry in Dryland Africa 1988.* Nairobi: International Council for Research in Agroforestry.

World Almanac and Book of Facts 1989. Section on Nations of the World, 649–737.

World Bank. 1988. *World Development Report.* New York: Oxford University Press.

Worldwatch Institute. 1988 and 1989. *State of the World.* New York: W. W. Norton.

CHAPTER 10

World Agricultural Development: India's Experience with Technologies, Markets, Management, and Trade

Address by the Laureate of the 1989 World Food Prize

Verghese Kurien
Chairman, National Dairy Development Board, Anand, India

Ladies and Gentlemen:

I am deeply honored to be the recipient of the third World Food Prize, an award distinguished by its inspiration, Dr. Norman Borlaug.

The honor is further enhanced by my joining the company of such accomplished scientists as Dr. M.S. Swaminathan and Dr. Robert F. Chandler, Jr. Let me, however, warn you that you cannot expect from me — a milkman from a little town — the erudition and eloquence of my predecessors. Let me also share my fear that this prize for past achievements will only serve to set even greater standards for the future. If we are to live in a world without hunger, we face a challenge of such importance and magnitude that when our meager abilities are measured against it, we must all stand humbled before such an awesome task.

As gratifying as it is personally to receive such an award, the World Food Prize recognizes not so much what I may have accomplished as an individual, but the achievements of so many who have contributed to the work with which I have been privileged to be associated.

When I first came to Anand many years ago, I was inspired and guided by several Gandhian leaders — men of great ability, integrity, and commitment to a cause. One of these men, Mr. Tribhuvandas Patel, devoted the greater part of his life to building the dairy cooperatives of Kaira District. To him, my country, our farmers, and I owe a great deal. He was my "guru."

The officers of the institutions where I have worked, and which I have been fortunate enough to serve, have been men and women of courage, of ability, and integrity. Many have sacrificed more lucrative careers to work with our farmers. Some have even sacrificed their lives for their beliefs. This award recognizes all that they have given.

Our work has received support from several international and national aid agencies. This has come in the form of commodities, financing, and a shared belief in our vision. They have helped make our achievements possible.

Over the last forty years I have also been privileged to have received total support at the highest level from my government, and particularly from our prime ministers.

I would not be standing before you today had it not been for the support and encouragement I have always received from my wife. A husband who works in a small town as an employee of farmers is considered neither fashionable nor prestigious. She has shared my commitment with unflagging courage and grace.

Above all, this award recognizes the Indian farmer, whose courage in the face of adversity, whose skill as a farmer, and whose wisdom as a human being have transformed dairying in India. Our farmers have proven that, given command over the resources they create, they can and will produce miracles. The remarks I make today are an attempt to speak to you on behalf of more than six million dairy cooperative members in India, whose elected chairman I am. It is from them and their families that I have drawn my strength.

Operation Flood, the program that has transformed India's dairy industry, is not a story of the triumph of science and technology: there have been no such miracles. How then was our dairy revolution made possible? I would submit that one very important reason is that we have created structures that give our farmers control over the resources they create.

Over the last two decades, more than six million dairy farmers have joined 60,000 milk producers' cooperatives spread throughout every part of my country. Imagine, if you will, every morning and evening, six million farmers pouring milk at their cooperative — milk that will travel from remote villages to towns and cities throughout India. Today these farmers earn more than one billion dollars annually and own some of the largest, most successful businesses in India.

These structures have, first and foremost, returned a greater share of the consumer's rupee to the farmer. They have built markets, supplied inputs, created value-added processing and products. All this has happened because our farmers' productive capacity has been linked with professional management in cooperative organizations that have staked out a place in the market. Put bluntly, these structures have forced others in the dairy business to compete fairly, and they have helped turn the terms of trade in favor of the rural producer.

When producers have such structures at their command, we know that they have the means — and the will — to ensure that the results of science and technology reach all those who will benefit. It is only when such structures exist that confidence in a remunerative price stimulates investment in productivity. It is only when such structures exist that farmers can demand the delivery of the services and inputs they need to realize returns on that investment. And, if I may hazard a prediction about the future, it is only such structures that can educate farmers around the world about the fragile nature of our environment and the need to exercise the greatest care in exploiting our limited resources and in controlling our population.

The great lesson we have learned is that we must respect and trust our farmers. They represent 74 percent of India's population. They may not be educated, or even literate, but they possess uncommon sense and even uncommon wisdom. Time and again they have shown the ability to rise above narrow self-interest and parochial concerns to act together in pursuit of longer-term goals and a greater common good. Programs and projects that are designed and managed from the top down, that treat farmers as "targets" and that ignore this untapped capacity of rural producers to manage their own affairs, such programs invariably fall short of their goals. Those which respect the right of the farmer to manage his own affairs cannot fail.

We have learned, however, that even producer-controlled structures are not enough to ensure progress. For these structures exist in a social, economic, and political environment that may extend well beyond national boundaries.

How, for example, can milk production increase in a country if other nations with well-established dairy industries are allowed to simply dump their surplus at whatever price they can get? Until two or three years ago, world supplies of dairy commodities were in great surplus. Governments — the same governments that urge us to "liberalize" our economic policies — competed to subsidize exports. And a great many countries with fledgling dairy industries succumbed to the temptation of those low-priced products. Subsequently, herd buy-outs, new policies, and unexpected events such as Chernobyl have combined to reduce surplus commodities drastically. World prices of dairy commodities have now more than doubled. Imagine the plight of those countries that relied on the productivity of other nations' dairy farmers and the generous subsidies of those governments.

We are now in the midst of a new round of GATT negotiations, a round in which agriculture has become a central subject of discussion. Those with surpluses are trying to find ways to keep the other fellow from subsidizing production while they continue subsidies themselves. The economists who serve these interests provide a great many fancy arguments about why we should do this and not do that. What it boils down to is an agreement that you should produce, and I should buy — in perpetuity.

Well, I, for one, will have none of it. We shall not hand over India's markets to the dairy farmers of New Zealand or to the soybean producers of Iowa simply because, today, they enjoy a temporary comparative advantage.

Where it makes sense to do so — and only where it makes sense — we intend to ensure that tomorrow we, too, will have a comparative advantage.

What is far more important, however, is that we must all work together to increase trade — in all directions — to mutual benefit and with mutual respect. Not by taking a short-term view and erecting direct and more subtle trade barriers, but by sitting down together to determine how — together — we can feed, clothe, and provide shelter to our fellow man.

When we look at what we have achieved in India with Operation Flood in milk — and now with oilseeds — we are not looking simply at the application of science and technology, though both have played a role; we are not looking simply at the creation of farmer-owned structures — though such structures have been necessary to success; what we are looking at is all of this, combined with the orchestration of all the policies and programs that affect production to ensure — to the extent possible — that these support and strengthen our efforts, rather than standing as obstacles, which all too often is the case.

There has been one last, and critically important, ingredient in our success: food itself.

For those of you who may not be familiar with Operation Flood and how it works, let me provide a brief background.

Twenty-five years ago we set about to replicate Anand's very successful dairy cooperatives. We believed we knew something about structures and something about the science and technology of dairying. But we had few resources. Those resources that were available were in the hands of government departments that did not feel inclined to share them with us.

Now, at the same time, mountains of butter and milk powder were growing in Europe. It was only a matter of time before those responsible for those mountains looked at India and decided that it was just the place to sell that butter and powder. And we knew if they did sell it — or worse still, if they gave it to us as a gift — our dairy industry, already weak, would be destroyed.

What we devised was a way in which to use those commodities, but to do so in a manner that strengthened, rather than undermined, our own dairy industry. With the help of the World Food Program, and then the European Economic Community, we arranged for the donation of some of that mountain. These donated commodities were then used to create a market that our own increased domestic production would later fill. The donated products were sold at prices that did not undercut our own farmers. The funds generated were used to finance our own infrastructure—dairy plants, feed factories, training, education. This financing was largely in the form of loans, so that the funds were recycled again and again.

Subsequently, we have used a similar approach with our oilseed projects. The governments of Canada and the United States, through their cooperatives, have donated edible oil, which we have used for this purpose. We are now even looking at a nonfood commodity—paper pulp—as a way to finance a project to "green India."

I must frankly say that in trying to get Operation Flood implemented, and later with the oilseed project, we did face severe practical difficulties. In the early years of Operation Flood, we received mouldy milk powder and rancid butter oil. When we complained, we were told, in effect, that beggars could not be choosers. Finally I had to intervene and reject the milk powder to make it quite clear that India would not be a dumping ground for commodities unfit for human consumption. Surely this should not have been necessary.

A little later, in fact just as our Operation Flood investment was getting into high gear, there was a temporary decline in world dairy surpluses. Our supplies of donated commodities were virtually cut off. A similar situation occurred with our oilseed project when donations were shipped to meet the donors' convenience. Again, we had to take a stand to make clear that we could not accept food aid on a stop-and-go basis.

The relationship between the person who gives and the one who receives is an uneasy one. It must be remembered that we who receive are not beggars and those who give are not doing us a favor. In undertaking such collaborations, both the donors and recipients are recognizing and acting on a mutual interest. The recipient must learn to receive with dignity, the donor to give with grace.

I have mentioned this because although we have experienced some problems with food aid, we have also benefitted greatly from it. It is a benefit that we firmly believe can and should be more widely shared.

"Food aid" has three important uses. The first is as emergency relief in the case of natural disasters. Such food aid may be vitally important to the survival of those affected. Second, and perhaps more commonly, food aid is used for the medium- and long-term alleviation of hunger. Third, food aid can be used as an investment in the production, processing, and marketing of food, thereby helping to eliminate the future need for such aid.

If I may, I would like to suggest that there has been too much use of food aid for the alleviation of hunger, and too little use of food aid as an investment. Food aid has been too often used to alleviate the symptoms, and not often enough to cure the disease.

Feeding programs have played a useful role—and can continue to do so in a limited and carefully planned way. However, all too often, such use of food creates dependency, alters food consumption patterns, and depresses demand for local production. I regret to note that such "humanitarian" use of food has also led to abuses. In some instances donated food is sold, benefitting the sellers but not the intended recipients. In other instances this food has been used to promote political or religious interests. This, I hope you will agree, is improper and immoral.

However, the arguments for food aid as an investment do not rest on problems associated with other uses of commodity assistance: they stand on their own merits.

First, food aid, used as an investment, is anti-inflationary. The food is sold, helping to mop up the consumers' money for investment in development.

Priced consistent with the local market, and imported in appropriate quantities, such food aid supplements food supplies without causing detriment to market prices or depressing domestic production.

Given a comparative advantage and selection of the appropriate commodities, a donor investment of one dollar can produce two dollars and more in local currency resources for development.

At a time when international debt is mounting, the least productive use of scarce foreign exchange is for food imports. To the extent that donations reduce that outflow, they free such funds for productive investment.

Funds generated from the sale of commodities and then loaned can finance the creation of structures to produce, process, and market commodities; as loan funds are repaid, they become available for investment in expansion and diversification. The resources can be recycled again, and again, and yet again.

In the last two years, a hungry world has witnessed some of its most productive member nations adopt policies and programs to reduce production. Commodities available for sale—and for donation—have diminished sharply. We understand that this has not only reduced world supplies, but has also caused hardship to producers and consumers in the very countries that have taken such steps.

What must be the effect on the farmer who is told not to achieve excellence, who is bribed to do less than his best? Knowing, as I do, the enormous benefits that result when food is used as an investment, I feel even more strongly that to constrain production in a world with hunger is wrong, even immoral.

Instead, let those nations that have—or that can produce—a surplus sit down together with those that are as yet unable to fully feed themselves, and let us evolve a plan in which surplus food will be used as an investment to increase the production and productivity of those presently in need.

Let our goal be the ability of each nation to feed itself. By that I don't mean that a nation need produce everything it consumes, but that it will produce enough to ensure that what is not available can be purchased. Nor do I mean that a nation is feeding itself when significant parts of its

191

population can afford only the barest minimum. A nation is feeding itself when the nutritional requirements of all its men, women, and children—especially its children—are fully met.

Let us plan, produce, and channel surplus to meet the requirements of countries in need, not haphazardly dispose of the occasional excess of surplus-producing nations.

Let us plan and commit resources over the span of a generation, sufficient time to build genuinely sustainable results.

Let us jointly examine and agree upon the types of policies and programs that serve a world in need, not the interests of the few. Let us agree that food aid investment is in the interest of both donors and recipients, and commit ourselves to the highest standards of quality, continuity of supplies, and integrity—not only in commodities, but in our efforts.

Let us pledge not to use food either as a political incentive or as a weapon, but rather to contribute to those who need such support and who are prepared to use it well.

Such a plan is one that serves all our interests. It is a cost to a nation to have people who suffer from hunger; it is equally a cost to constrain producers from pursuing the best they can achieve. If today's donation reduces tomorrow's market for one commodity, experience has shown that it will open new markets for other commodities tomorrow. By working together we can, I believe, bring some order, progress, and sustainable growth to our shrinking world.

The challenge we all face is far too important to leave to our politicians and bureaucrats. Let the leaders of genuine producers' organizations from around the world, from rich nations and poor, take the initiative to use food to our mutual and sustaining benefit. Just as cooperation has proved successful in individual countries around the world, let it prove successful on a far broader scale to solve the greatest problems of our time.

Only last week six countries of Asia at the ministerial level sat around a table at the National Dairy Development Board in Anand to discuss how the Anand pattern could be replicated, with suitable modifications, in their countries. These six countries were Vietnam, Indonesia, the Philippines, China, Pakistan, and India. The meeting concluded with a resolution to establish an international center in Anand for sharing our experiences in the field of dairy development with our neighbors.

That countries so vastly different in their social, political, and economic structures should so quickly come to a unanimous decision is a measure of what can be achieved if there is a will.

As this year's World Food Prize laureate, my colleagues and I are committing ourselves to set up such an international center, which we hope will serve not only Asian countries but those of Africa and Latin America as well. Let me express the hope that the advanced countries will join in the support of this effort, particularly with food aid as an investment in dairy development.

We have enjoyed a decade of "almost enough," enough to cause complacency. If there is a touch of hunger in the Sahel, then we have tried to patch it up with a few concerts and shipments of food. However, we are now looking toward a much more difficult decade, one in which many will face a rude awakening. The world faces a grave agenda: poverty, hunger, a deteriorating environment, growing populations, new and dreadful diseases. These problems respect no artificial boundaries. Nor are these simply the problems of governments and international organizations. I firmly believe that it is only when people and their structures become directly involved, when responsibility is with those whose interests are genuinely at stake, that solutions are possible. We can no longer afford the luxury of leaving problems entirely to governments to solve. We must seize the initiative and involve ourselves and the people of the world in attacking hunger, disease, and poverty. The future of our world depends on it. Thank you.

CHAPTER 11

Excerpts of the Discussions at the Morning and Afternoon Sessions

[Editor's Note: The colloquium speakers presented their papers in a morning and an afternoon session. Following the papers in each of the sessions, a panel discussion was convened to examine further the issues and ideas presented in the papers and to provide for an exchange of ideas between the speakers, the discussants, and the audience. The following are excerpts from the transcripts of the panel discussions, slightly edited to improve clarity. Barbara Huddleston chaired the morning panel, and Robert D. Havener, the afternoon panel.]

Morning Discussion

Barbara Huddleston (moderator): We will begin the panel discussion. I am going to ask each discussant to speak to the issues for about ten minutes and then, if time permits, we will have questions from the floor and, perhaps, some responses from the speakers.

Our first panelist is Michael Lipton, who is program director of the Food Consumption and Nutrition Policy Research Program at the International Food Policy Research Institute in Washington, D.C.

Michael Lipton: I shall concentrate almost entirely on Dr. Aboyade's fascinating and very useful paper, but first, a comment on water resources. I think that the issue of water management and water control is absolutely critical to getting acceptable rates of growth of cereal production, in particular in sub-Saharan Africa. We are dealing with a continent where at most 3 percent of the land area is irrigated or water controlled, even in the most extended sense. We have heard that China is 45 percent irrigated, and India is moving toward 35 to 36 percent water control. Even the areas in these countries that are not irrigated are much more water controlled than most areas in sub-Saharan Africa. If you go to Sri Lanka and ask them to show you unirrigated areas, you will find all sorts of water-management systems in place in the field. There are reasons for this disparity: most of sub-Saharan Africa, until rather recently, has had a labor shortage and quite a lot of land, and people often have moved around from land area to land area. Even where they were settled on a piece of land, it did not really pay to put water-management systems in place.

But with the enormous growth in populations, which are dependent on land, and with more and more areas coming to the point of land scarcity, it is absolutely critical to develop the water-management capacities in sub-Saharan Africa, much more so than has been done up to now. I think that transcends issues of the balance between irrigation and rainfed emphases in agriculture. Much more efficient use of water is needed in both irrigated and unirrigated areas. I don't see how population growth at 3 to 4 percent, and in Kenya at 4 percent per year now, is going to be handled without a very substantial increase in irrigated areas in sub-Saharan Africa. I don't mean big dam schemes. I certainly don't mean the sorts of things that have been such a disaster in many parts of northern Nigeria. I mean small, farmer-controlled impoundment, use of underground rivers, use of groundwater, but much more control of the water systems without which farmers simply will not be persuaded to adopt large amounts of nitrogenous fertilizer and without which they are not going to be able to get very much benefit out of high-yielding varieties of crops, either. End of commercial.

I fully agree with Dr. Aboyade that micro- and field-perspectives, such as he has provided, are vital to assess what works and what doesn't work in achieving the goals of agricultural development. And, it is a marvelous thing, he started his paper with an extended microperspective. But we do need indications of the benefit-to-cost ratios and the poverty impact of particular schemes. No doubt this is all there, but he hasn't, for example, told us about what the development costs of the Awe program are, how many people were benefitted, whether they were poor, and what the benefit-to-cost ratio was. We also need to know whether schemes like this are typical. And that means we need to put together a lot of experiences of the Awe-type and then draw conclusions.

Now as far as the ratio of benefit to costs from different sorts of schemes is concerned, quite a lot of work on that has been attempted by the World Bank. They've looked at their agricultural and rural development projects by region. On the whole, it really isn't clear that agricultural credit has a crucial role in sub-Saharan Africa. It apparently did in the Awe community, but it looks as though Awe might be exceptional. It appears that the great majority of sub-Saharan African development schemes, where they have failed, have failed because the technology has not been properly specified or because the local rural institutions have not been put in place, or because people have not been trained to cope with the problems. Incidentally, in most of the World Bank's evaluations of their agricultural and rural development projects, it does not turn out to be the case that it was price mismanagement or a bad macroeconomic policy that primarily caused the failures. But, overwhelmingly, the main cause of project failure in rural development in sub-Saharan Africa has been a failure to specify correctly the technology that would work locally and to test it and institutionalize it in the context of local farming systems.

As far as the typicality of the Awe experiment is concerned, I don't think there are many African farming systems left where it is possible to do what has been done in Awe, which, according to Dr. Aboyade, is "to bring more land and labor into the production process." Now there are areas where you can do that. You can do that in the eastern province in Zambia. When the price of maize rises, the farmers of the eastern province manage to produce a lot more maize and to bring new land into cultivation. Labor comes back from the towns, comes back from the mines, and you get more output, and there is also hybrid maize technology around the corner once it pays to introduce it. But less and less of sub-Saharan Africa is like that. More and more of it faces a land shortage. Quite a number of places that don't face a land shortage, as in Sierra Leone, face a labor shortage.

There really is a problem of generating new technologies that will enable people to make better use of both their land and their labor. And I think it is very important that we get an idea of how typical or atypical these particular microexperiences are. And I am pretty sure that when we do look at these experiences together, we are going to come to the conclusion that fairly rapid technical change is needed. And the question is, to what extent is it feasible? It is going to be increasingly vital to lift technical constraints on African agriculture as more and more of it moves into conditions of land shortage.

Now Dr. Aboyade says that there is a long lead time for agricultural research, and that is quite true in many cases. I think that makes a quick start particularly important. There is an enormous amount of money going into national agricultural research in sub-Saharan Africa, but unfortunately many countries in sub-Saharan Africa fail to give adequate governmental priority to that support. I think that to put foreign money into international agricultural research systems without the national support is like pushing on a piece of string. It is no good if the government is not prepared to pay its own scientists adequately, to turn on the electricity, to turn on the water, and I am not speaking of imagined research stations. I am talking about research stations I have seen in Zaire and Sierra Leone and elsewhere. Under those circumstances, it is no good pouring in international support. One has to concentrate on those cases. I am convinced by Dr. Aboyade's presentation that Nigeria is likely to be one of those cases where there really is substantial national support from the government for the agricultural research systems. And in those cases, certainly major international support is justified.

Dr. Aboyade is quite right that it is usually a myth that there are scientific and technological institutions readily available on tap. That isn't so. But there are local varieties and there are local farming systems. And these local varieties and local farming systems can interact reasonably quickly with introduced germ plasm that is crossbred with local varieties. It can't be done instantly, but we may be talking about a three- to five-year time horizon in some cases, rather than a ten- to fifteen-year time horizon.

Finger millets. We have heard a lot about finger millet today, called "ragi" in India. Now ragi, which is an entirely rainfed crop and a crop grown in drought-prone areas and almost always a poor person's crop, has been a dramatic success for high-yielding variety breeding in the Indian state of Karnataka. Hybrid sorghum has more problems, because you have got to be able to distribute the hybrids to the farmers each year on time; it is not like a variety that can pollinate itself year after year. Yet hybrid sorghum has also been a roaring success in large parts of drought-prone areas in India's Maharashtra State. Now you can't, of course, take these varieties and simply transplant them into environments in sub-Saharan Africa — in semiarid areas. Of course, Awe, Nigeria, is a semihumid area. I am not talking about that particular area, but about the general problem here of technological transfer. You can't just transfer these varieties, you have got to test them. A lot of the time you are going to have to do a certain amount of crossbreeding to take in the best of local germ plasm as well. But I am convinced that there is a lot that can be done by breeding approaches combined with improved water management, even in unirrigated areas, in sub-Saharan Africa.

I've mentioned that technology change will certainly have to focus on better knowledge with regard to water supply. In very little of sub-Saharan Africa do we know how far down the water table is, let alone how much it will cost to get it up. Regarding major irrigation projects, I was interested to hear Dr. R. P. Singh tell us that $1,700 per hectare was the cost of irrigation development in India and how that cost was worrying irrigation planners. Yet in West Africa and in East Africa, too, we take for granted land development costs in bringing in an irrigation scheme, not of $1,700 per hectare, but of $17,000 per hectare. And I think we need to ask ourselves why these costs are so appallingly high. Why isn't it possible to get the costs of irrigation and of water control down to reasonable levels? I think we have to consider much smaller scale, much more farmer-managed systems, fewer bureaucracy-managed systems, and certainly a shift from surface water to ground water development.

I think that we are going to be talking in more and more of sub-Saharan Africa about seed-, fertilizer-, and water-based technologies. You've heard the expression "the only game in town." As far as I can see, that is in most of the African countryside the only game that there is. Yes, one needs to respect the farmer's own farming system, priorities, values, crop mixes, and farm practices, certainly. And it is possible for seed-, fertilizer-, and water-based research to grow out of all these things and not to be an extraneous imposition. But we're talking about dealing with a major requirement for extra food and for extra jobs that in many nations of Africa is rising at a rate of 3 to 4 percent a year.

With all the good will in the world toward traditional African systems and the attempt to minimize the rate of technical change, I don't think we're going to make a great deal of progress without seed-, fertilizer-, and water-based technological change of a fairly dramatic kind. I would agree with Dr. Aboyade about not wanting to raise expectations too much. But this sort of thing is going to need to be done. Of course, there are major constraints and problems in sub-Saharan Africa — water control, for one thing. But crops are not relatively easy, either. Rice and wheat were not easy crops with which to make the progress that has been made. We have some distinguished contributors to that progress in this room, and they wouldn't let me get away with saying that these were easy crops. Certainly sorghum, millet, and maize are harder; cassava and yams, much harder. But I'm not convinced that this can't be done and, indeed, I know that major progress has already been made in some of these crops and in some of these places. Resources are simply going to have to be put into national research systems to help make that progress in sub-Saharan Africa and to transmit it in a way consistent with the ecosystems and with the farming systems which farmers are already using.

I don't think that it makes sense to talk about so-called low-input, low-output agriculture. And it certainly doesn't make sense to talk about low-input, high-output agriculture. Low-input, high-output agriculture is a polite way of mining the soil of the nutrients which are in it. There may or may not be such a thing as a free lunch, but certainly there is no such thing as a free crop. Biological nitrogen fixation can help and it is very nice if you can get it, and let's hope that more progress will be made. But on the whole, low-input, high-output agriculture means crop mining, and there are going to have to be transitions to higher inputs to meet the needs of Africa's growing population.

Dr. Aboyade places great faith in shifting the structure of Nigerian agriculture, at least subhumid Nigerian agriculture, by raising the value of output per hectare by changing the crop mix. Now, I think we need to ask what exactly that means. If he's talking about export crops, which have a higher value per hectare, fine, let it be tried. I don't think it is going to be consistent with what he calls "selective closure" of the agricultural food economy, because that tends to encourage import replacement and production of nontradeables. It doesn't tend to encourage production of exports. If you're going for an export-oriented policy, then you can't go for a selective closure policy.

What about a domestic crop-oriented policy? Well, he mentions two sorts of crops to go for. One, increased production of coarse grain staples, and, the other, of roots and tubers. I very much agree that far more can be done here and should be done. There's been too much emphasis relatively, not perhaps absolutely, on research into exotic or locally unknown crops such as soybeans. In Nigeria, more money is spent by national agricultural research on soybeans than on cassava, which accounts for ten to twenty times the growing area. Much more can be done in research on locally grown main staples. But that's not going to increase the value per hectare, probably not the value per worker, either, of agricultural output. It will increase the calories generated, but it won't increase the value added per hectare, which is what Dr. Aboyade rightly is after.

So then if we look at fruits and vegetables and nuts for local consumption, small ruminants, dairy production, yes, a lot can be done. It will raise value added per hectare and value added per worker. And it's promising. But it's got a problem. These crops are not eaten or, in the case of milk, drunk by poor people. There are better crops and if we want to make a major impact on the diet, then that particular path has its problems. I think there's a limit to how far one can move by changes in the crop mix alone. Some things can be done in this area, but it is not an alternative to raising the productivity of staples by means of improved water, soil, varietal development, research, and management. So I think Dr. Aboyade is shifting too far into the future and into the long run the urgent task of beginning now with the process of major staple-specific crop research in sub-Saharan Africa.

Barbara Huddleston: Thank you very much. I think this comment will be very useful both in discussing Dr. Aboyade's paper and also the point that was raised by Bruce Stone with respect to China on the role of technology, the relative importance of technology versus other avenues. We will turn next to Dr. Thomas Odhiambo, who is director of the International Centre of Insect Physiology and Ecology in Nairobi, Kenya, and who has taught at the University of Nairobi since 1965.

Thomas R. Odhiambo: First of all, let me say that I enjoyed very much Professor Aboyade's presentation. It is a starting point for discussion of what the shape of Africa's agriculture and food production could be in the future. And the first challenge I see from his presentation is the issue of diversification that he emphasized in the paper. Perhaps over the last forty years, we have been overemphasizing the wrong things in this regard. First of all, Africa, in this century and before, was a continent of very diversified staples. It is really in the last forty years that we have been deemphasizing diversification and have tried to make Africa dependent on a few cereal grains: maize, particularly; recently sorghum; maybe in some ways, cassava. But Africa has been known for diversified staples. And I think that is part of the strength of Africa, and we should go back to the situation in which Africa relies on a large number of staples.

In saying this, I feel that there are some strengths we have been underemphasizing, both in research as well as in program implementation. Why has Uganda survived all the civil disturbance over the last twenty-five years? Why is a poor country like Rwanda still in many ways food secure? Why are Sudan and Ethiopia not food secure? When you look at this, you find that in Uganda and Rwanda their immediate staples are not grains. Their immediate staples are something else—sweet potato, banana, to some extent, cassava. The northern parts of drier areas depend on millet and sorghum, which in the colonial period were regarded as a poor man's food. They were never regarded by Africans as poor man's food. This is something that came up only in this century. And it seems to me that there is work to be done to change the status of these food staples back to what it was before, as the major food staples of Africa.

What that means is that we may have been investing in the wrong things. In much of Africa even now, maize is only grown really in high potential areas. And we spend a lot of funds to get maize more widespread in Africa, perhaps more funds than we ought to. That misplacement of funding is something that the policy people should be looking at again. As I said earlier, and given what has been shown this morning, irrigation is not a very important part of agriculture in Africa, traditionally speaking. Other than in Sudan and Egypt, irrigation is a fairly minor component of agriculture. There has been a notion that putting too much investment in irrigation, whether at the local level or national level, is not going to advance Africa from the problems that it has been facing in the last twenty-five to thirty years.

Rather, the technology focus should be shifting to dryland agriculture. An important issue is to examine what new technologies can be brought about to ensure that those crops that already are well suited to dependable rainfall, in some cases almost semiarid conditions, can be made productive in other areas, despite all the constraints that Africa has been familiar with prior to the twentieth century. Therefore, this means that we need to devote more attention to sweet potato, to sorghum and millet, to cassava, to tree crops, which have been a major feature of traditional African agriculture but very much neglected. So that's one challenge I can see stemming from Professor Aboyade's presentation.

Another challenge involves the issue of the domestic market. Africa in the last twenty years has been concentrating not simply on food security, but also on the export element of it. Yet, the domestic market is very strong. If you look at the many vegetables that are grown in Africa and at specific staples like sorghum, sweet potato, and banana, it is the domestic market that is paramount in those areas. We have not done enough to understand that domestic market. And it seems to me that agricultural economists in Africa should really begin to understand better what goes on in the rural markets, much more than what is happening at the national market or in the export-import business.

The third challenge that I can see here is the issue of water management. This obviously is a major problem. But I would not characterize it as a problem of irrigation. I think it's a problem of managing our watersheds in a better way than we have done by bringing in tree crops, but ensuring that traditional methods of water harvesting are upgraded to modern requirements, and ensuring that we can still intensify our agricultural production given the diminishing areas that are available for agriculture. And, of course, a serious constraint in Africa is soil erosion. Indeed, this is one area where we need new research and new technologies, because soil instability in Africa is rather different from what takes place in other areas of the tropics. We need to understand how soil erosion can be diminished from the levels that exist now in Africa, so that this doesn't become a dominant problem in the future.

In this particular case, there is no question that the advances we are making at the moment in terms of high-yielding varieties will be negated if we are not certain that we can manage the diseases and pests that affect those new varieties. A good example is the case of cassava. If we are not able to control these pests using new methods for controlling them, cassava as a major crop in Africa could be in a very dire position. The intensification of research in this area is very important indeed.

Lastly, one area that has not received enough discussion in Africa is the question of leadership. If we are going to have sustainable agriculture, we have to also sustain our institutions with leadership at the policy level, the technology development level, the research level, the marketing level, and the institutional management level. This ingredient is paramount in Africa. We need more of it at the present time. It will not do any good for Africa to continue to have its policies decided on the basis of other models in the rest of the world. Today we heard Dr. Singh discuss a very good model for integrated watershed management in India. I would like to see a situation where we look at our own problems the way the Indians and the Chinese have looked at their problems.

This will depend on knowing the situation in Africa and understanding what roadblocks you need to remove to ensure sustainable agricultural production. Without sustained scientific, managerial, technological, and policy leadership in Africa, I do not think that Africa's agriculture is going to change. That is a question that many people are not really prepared to look at. Our own governments have not realized that technology transfer is not going to work in the way that it has worked elsewhere where technology has been implanted over a long period of time. We will have to build that leadership to ensure that over the long run, Africa will develop its technology, while recognizing what the policy constraints are, knowing the constraints in adopting other models, and in recognizing the critical importance of working closely with farmers and understanding what farmers actually need. Thank you.

Barbara Huddleston: Thank you very much. Our last discussant is Robert Herdt, director of Agricultural Sciences at the Rockefeller Foundation.

Robert W. Herdt: Thank you very much. Well, we've had a wide range of papers this morning. We've heard about two countries in Asia, about Nigeria, about other countries in Africa. I want to step back a little bit and put some of this in a broader perspective.

Virtually all developing countries, including those discussed this morning, face four great challenges over the next decades, indeed over the next century. The first is to provide employment and food entitlements to the people, many of whom are already here, many of whom inevitably will be born.

The second is to provide a steady increase in food output, food production, at between, perhaps, 2 percent a year, in the case of Indonesia — maybe a 2 percent increase in grain production in China would be adequate, up to 6 percent a year in the case of very rapidly growing countries where both population and income are increasing significantly.

The third is to do this by using agricultural systems that can be sustained over the long run, without degrading the resource base on which agriculture must depend. And, lastly, to stabilize and eventually bring down the population growth rate and, ultimately, total populations. Because if population continues to grow forever, there is little that agriculture can do to keep up with it.

Our focus today is on food and agriculture, not only because this is the occasion of the World Food Prize, but because economies that are heavily dependent on agriculture for their economic base must meet these challenges through agricultural growth and agricultural development. In Africa today, agriculture makes up more than 50 percent of the economic base in most countries and that was true in India, China, Indonesia, and in many other places twenty-five to thirty years ago.

The speakers and the discussants have talked about the contributions of technology, on the one hand, and institutions, on the other, to the agricultural growth process. Dr. Singh and Mr. Stone concentrated on technologies. Dr. Aboyade and Dr. Lin concentrated on institutions. And so we have these two broad categories.

I want to focus on the conditions for agricultural production growth. What is it that makes agricultural production growth possible? To put it simplistically, farmers have to be able to produce more food and to have the incentive to be willing to produce more food. At the same time, we don't want to lose sight of the fact that consumers have to be able to consume increasing amounts. That is, they have to have the economic capacity or have the food entitlements to consume the increased production.

If we look at the essentials for production growth, the ability to produce increasing amounts of agricultural output requires the knowledge of how to do so, an area in which China has excelled, and of getting the technology out there, as mentioned by one of our speakers. This includes the knowledge of how to increase production, the inputs and natural resources on which production is based; increasing the amounts of inputs; achieving soil fertility from whatever source, biological or chemical; using water and soil resources wisely; and, in all cases, being able to acquire those inputs, which in some cases requires credit. Dr. Aboyade discussed the case in which credit was very critical to getting the increased inputs.

Once there is the ability to generate increasing amounts of agricultural production, then the issue arises, how do we get that ability translated into reality? Functioning markets are crucial to linking up the output that these farmers can produce with the consumers who want to buy it. So, functioning markets are crucial to generating the incentives necessary. And the role of prices adequate to compensate farmers for their efforts and transmitted through those functioning markets is equally important. At the same time we recognize that technology and prices are two sides of the same coin. If farmers have a more productive technology available to them, the price can be somewhat lower and the incentives are still there to produce. So it's not a question of either prices or technology. It's a question of the complementary role of prices and technology in generating the appropriate incentives.

Since much of my own career has been spent in the area of technology, let me discuss a little bit more about technology. Often this is interpreted as being synonymous with machinery or, in the United States, electronics. Technology has bells and whistles and it moves. In reality, as a number of our speakers and discussants have pointed out, technology in agriculture is how things are produced. That is, it is a combination of crop varieties, plant nutrients, the physical operations, the sunlight, the water, and the biological balance of pests and nonpests. All of these things in combination make up the technology that farmers use. The role of these components of technology has been mentioned here, so I'm not going to go into that. All of these things are crucial. And the particular emphasis that any given country or location requires at a given point in time depends on the local situation. Dr. Odhiambo has stressed the need for diversity and looking at the crops that grow well under the conditions existing in some locations; in other locations, other crops. Where there is water, irrigation is a possibility. The fact is that much of Africa is a semiarid climate.

In each case, for the proper technology, one has to depend on knowing the local situation and bringing in adequate knowledge to deal with that situation. And one has to remember always that appropriate technology is only part of the solution. Other parts include adequate prices, functioning markets to link those prices to farmers, the knowledge acquired by farmers, inputs and their availability, and credit, where it is required. Agricultural growth is a complex process, and with that I'll close. Thank you very much.

Barbara Huddleston: We are approaching our closing time but I want to give the speakers a chance to comment briefly. And I would like to ask each of the speakers to concentrate particularly on what, I think, have been the key issues that have been raised. Namely, in thinking about food policy for the next decade, what should be the relative balance between technological development and institutional development? We've heard different views expressed on this point. Within technology, what kinds of technology should be emphasized and what mechanisms should be used to encourage the development of new technology? And what kinds of institutions are most appropriate and how can they be encouraged in policy terms? Dr. Aboyade, would you take the floor first.

Ojetunji Aboyade: I would like to thank the discussants for their keen interest in my paper and for the criticisms and comments that will help me revise the paper. I'll concentrate on just three or four points from the discussion.

In terms of the so-called debate between technologies and institutions, frankly, I don't see it this way at all. Really, technologies are institutions — different sides of the same coin. I think that sums up what I tried to do. I tried to demonstrate that, given the long historical decline in African agriculture, the first thing to do is to ensure that the decline is stopped. And you do that through economic policies and adjustments. Once you reverse it, halt it, then what's the next question? The next question is to utilize the economic base and the best technological packages available at the time. From my experience there are three major determinants. One is the institutional factor. Second, access to credit. And third, product mix.

The idea behind this is not to extend into the future decisions that can be made in the shorter term. It's just to buy time. While you are waiting for the resource systems to take off to address the key issues, including mobilizing science, research and technology, you utilize these stopgap measures to keep the momentum moving. And, indeed, from my experience in the African context there are two major factors. One is in terms of trade, and the other one, the import capacity. And with these two, you do the best you can at the policy level. Of course, you don't wait until all these issues exhaust themselves before you start addressing the question of technological innovations. I do agree with Michael Lipton that perhaps the lead time is not as long as people tend to imagine.

The second thing I'd like to comment on is Thomas Odhiambo's emphasis on the importance of diversification in agricultural products in Africa. And one of my contributions, when I was at the International Food Policy Research Institute, was to oppose the way they tried to convert everything to grain-based statistics. Everything was converted to grain. I think the focus was too much on grains. Now, I'm happy for Dr. Odhiambo's emphasis on diversity. Bringing more land and labor into production was the essence of the Awe experiment, and it may not be typical. You cannot really avoid the importance of product mix, at least in the short term. Vegetables are important. Fruits are important. Horticultural products are important. Not to say, as I think Michael Lipton asserted, that perhaps these other crops are not as important in the consumption pattern of small-income households. Well, I will not say he is wrong. That is an empirical question. Because in some parts, these other crops are important. But how important, I cannot say. This may be something which the policy research institutes would like to tackle. What are staples, and what is the importance of the staples vis-a-vis other products within the milieu of the African production-consumption pattern? My own suspicion is that these things are more important than scientists and policy analysts are acknowledging.

My third comment concerns the typicality of the Awe experiment. Clearly, and I think I said so in my presentation, one cannot say that the Awe experiment is typical. I would like to just say that our first objective in this experiment was on our part to learn about what makes African farmers tick. It really was addressed to ourselves as professionals, as scholars, as economists, to try to determine a standard—what is it that makes them tick? What is their reaction? How do they see their own production? What are those things that they think they really require to make a difference? It was not really to gather data in a formal way. It was to learn. We had monthly meetings, myself, my wife, and others over the years, meeting with these farmers, and I must say that although I'm not an agricultural economist, what I've learned from those farmers over five years probably was far more than what I've read in recent research papers and publications.

We didn't want to get involved in monitoring the experiment because it might have biased the results. We are quite happy trying to collect information. To do that, you must first get baseline data about where you are starting from, and then see what differences, if any, have occurred. So that's where we are now. And the intention of that experiment is not to document fully the results, the failures and successes, but just to show that there's an alternative way, probably a more productive way. The point I raise about the major studies done in connection with the ADPs that the World Bank sponsors is to show clearly that credit availability is a key factor. The ADPs are not generally organized that way at all. So we have tried to show this alternative way, and the importance of credit, at least in the particular case in Awe.

And finally, I did suggest that more case studies are needed. Contrasting case studies are needed. So the impression was not to show that Awe is so typical and that nothing else can be different. We are just at the beginning of trying to understand the paradigms being developed in connection with African agriculture. Are we going to have just one paradigm that is suitable for all time in all countries and for all periods? I think we have to put it in stages. Step one, step two, step three. And then recognize the turning points, the transitions, in that process. This I hope will become the subject of more policy research. Thank you very much.

Barbara Huddleston: Mr. Chen, would you like to comment?

Zhigang Chen: I would like to make one brief point that I quite agree with the comments from Mr. Bruce Stone that agricultural performance in China has been very remarkable during the years 1952 to 1987. That raised for me the question that Professor Herdt emphasized, of the importance of the combination of choice of technology and of price. I would like to add that institutions, to me, are the basis for these two factors. The problem is what should we emphasize? In the case of China, rural farming institution reform in place since 1979 has dramatically improved the incentive structure of agricultural production and the performance of the rural economy.

Grain production in China has been constrained by several factors. One, certainly, is the price problem as Dr. Lin argued. The second one is the technological constraint. And the third one is the environmental issue, which has been largely overlooked in China. The question was raised, which factor should the government put more emphasis on? Is it price reform or is it technology reform, or should more emphasis be placed on the environment issue? On the technology side, long-range investment in agriculture involving irrigation and fertilizer production has been lagging behind farming institution change. In the case of fertilizer, even though demand for fertilizer in China has increased rapidly over time, the availability of fertilizer domestically has decreased. And imports of fertilizer from other countries also have decreased. So that raises the issue that the price side of technology has lagged behind the demand side.

So my thought is that to ensure the further success of institutional change, China should be emphasizing price reform, to provide the right incentives to farmers to produce grain, and long-range investment issues will be solved in that way. Thank you.

Barbara Huddleston: Mr. Stone.

Bruce Stone: Let me respond to the questions about technological versus institutional development, what kinds of technology, what kinds of institutions. I agree with Dr. Aboyade that technological development and institutional development are very closely linked. In the case of China, I've been arguing, in particular in the case of food grains after the 1950s, following upon the land reform, it was the technological development of the seed-soil-nutrient balance and of water control that was the major source of change and growth. The appropriate institutions to focus on are those institutions that serve that development. And what I'm arguing is that the kinds of institutions that China developed at that time were very suitable to that focus. However, they're not very suitable and even can become a liability in the second stage of technological development.

Let me give you an example. There's been some reference to China's food procurement system. The government established a grain monopoly. And it was through the grain monopoly that the government was able to artificially depress the price that farmers could receive for their grain. A lot has been made of that. At the same time, it was a mechanism for solving some problems.

There's technological change going on all the time. China presents a great story of both nondirective technological change as well as of directive change. If fertilizer is made available to farmers, gradually they'll sort out the problems of what to buy and how much to buy. But, if we want to collapse or accelerate that process — that's what we're really talking about here — and make much more rapid gains than societies might make on their own, then we're talking about what kinds of institutions are most suitable at that particular stage and in that particular environment for rapidly increasing the acceptance of technology, the efficiency of technology, and the distribution of the benefits.

Specifically, what do you need for rapid fertilizer growth? You need essentially four processes operating fairly well. You need an agronomic potential for fertilizer use. It helps if there are high-yielding, fertilizer-responsive seed varieties available, if there is good water control, and if there is good farming technique among farmers. Then, the agronomic potential is high, and as those inputs increase, then the use of fertilizers will increase. Then you need on the demand side an ability to convert that potential for fertilizer use into effective demand for fertilizer. In any system of prices, fertilizer use might be profitable, but there might be many reasons why farmers would not choose to purchase fertilizer. They might not have the cash. They might feel that it was a bad investment because of risk. They might not know about fertilizer. They might be using it improperly. So the question is, well, you might need to develop institutions to serve those particular needs. One of the interesting things about the system China developed is that it took a neat end run around those kinds of demand problems. They had a very high agronomic potential for fertilizer use, because of the relatively high degree of water control, of seed varieties, and of farmer skill. The demand problems were essentially solved by providing fertilizer directly to farmers and giving the state a claim over the crop. The pricing issue was sorted out after the fact. It got around the problem of fertilizer credit and risk and a variety of problems on the demand side. And I think it did so quite effectively. It was a system in which the government could distribute fertilizer in areas where they got a lot of bang for the buck and they could be sure that they were putting all the units in place early on and using fertilizer in places where they would get large increases in food production.

Well, you can imagine that when China reaches a stage in which their increase in fertilizer availability is at the rate of an additional 1.2 million tons of nutrient a year, what it was in the 1980s, then the institutions that were developed for targeting fertilizer to high-application, market-oriented areas simply aren't able to adjust rapidly enough. The point is reached where more and more fertilizer is dumped onto the same areas. A situation arose in which there were very different rates of fertilizer use in different areas and very different marginal response rates to fertilizer use. Some places showed almost no response and in some places the response was very great, but they simply couldn't get the fertilizer. Adding a market system at this stage is a helpful way of getting around this problem, without suddenly eliminating the huge public system upon which the whole thing is based. That's the kind of transition that China's going to have to be making. It's unfortunate that with the current leadership, there's been a retreat from some of these kinds of experiments in adding supplementary markets, which can solve some of these second-stage problems.

Barbara Huddleston: I would like to give Dr. Singh the opportunity for one last word.

R. P. Singh: It appears to me that for a country like India, rainwater management is priority number one. And whether it is irrigation or rainwater management, it cannot be done unless there is sound land management. Land management and water management go together.

The technology for rainfed lands has to be location-specific technology. The requirements vary from one area to another as does, of course, the level of rainfall. In other words, the technology to absorb the amounts of water and the runoff collection has to be different, depending on the area involved.

My second point is that the components of the rainfed technology should be such that they can be easily adapted by the farmers. Therefore, the first thing we observed in our experience was that seeds are the first to be taken out—the seeds, again, of varieties, not of hybrids. Now, the question is, should we be advocating technology that is rather costly and that cannot be adopted readily by poor farmers? Or, should we have a sustainable technology? My view is that, first, we should try to understand the farmer's wisdom, what his traditional practices are, and then to try to build on those practices and systems and try to find out how best we can improve the farmer's resource base. Much of the efforts that have been made in the developing countries so far, including India, have been to improve the productivity, not so much to conserve the resource base. The example of soil erosion was given by my colleague from Africa. It is a serious problem. Things like that which are long standing have to be looked into.

Another point concerns the transfer of technology. Technology, however dependable it may be, is very difficult to transfer, particularly with respect to dryland areas. You have to have infrastructure. You have to have the skills, the training part, which is often missing. Then, the other questions automatically arise—input supply, credit supply, recovery of loans, and so on. Therefore, the presence of skills and training is critical to the transfer of the technology. After all, technology is like a wagon that has to be taken from one place to another, but it needs the farmer's participation.

Barbara Huddleston: Thank you very much.

Afternoon Discussion

Robert Havener (moderator): We are going to proceed with comments from the discussants who have been asked to prepare responses to the essays that have been presented. I urge you to make those within five to seven minutes, or thereabouts. Summarize the best you can.

I would like to start with Alberto Valdés. He is the director of the International Trade and Food Security Program at the International Food Policy Research Institute (IFPRI) and is a native of Chile.

Alberto Valdés: Thank you. I think I should concentrate more on the experience of the Chilean case rather than try to cover all the other countries of Latin America. I think it presents an interesting case of institutional innovation, economic development, and incentives, and I will link this with Anthony Wylie's presentation. These are reflections on one experience in South America, and I think there are others. The other case that comes to mind to analyze is soybean and citrus development in Brazil.

So what aspects of Chilean fruit and vegetable development present lessons in terms of the entire region? I think that the growth of Chile's agriculture is quite spectacular. Fruits and vegetables are only one of several sectors whose exports have expanded significantly. Most of them are natural resources-based: fisheries, forestry, minerals, but now also industrial products are beginning to grow. It's interesting that in the early-to-late-1970s, Argentina exported about three times as much in total as Chile. Today both countries export the same in terms of total value of exports, although Argentina's population is more than twice that of Chile's. It's obviously not a question of natural resources. Argentina has plenty.

I think it points out the differences in what is essentially economic environment and economic policies. It is an important point that Wylie made that the growth in Chile is not primarily the result of the government's agricultural policy. There was really very little one can identify as the promotion of the fruit sector by the government in Chile. One of the aims of economic policy in Chile in the mid-1970s was not to have subsidies for any particular sector, except perhaps some subsidies for forest planting, for example. This is an important point, because the growth was essentially driven by farmers, by the growers' association, by the private sector, with the government playing a very selective role in only certain activities like health, sanitary regulations, and basic infrastructure improvements such as roads.

There has been no expansion in government expenditures on agriculture. In fact, there has been a decline. During all these years of expansion in agriculture, there was a decline in government expenditures. So it's not a question of money. It's the productivity of money that counts. It was an effort in the public sector to identify what it did well, quite unlike the tradition in Chile, which was to have a highly socialized economy, in which the government was spending money on practically everything from food subsidies, to fertilizer subsidies, to marketing, to whatever. In the period we are examining these types of public activity contracted a lot.

This very important point was made by Wylie: growth was spurred by deregulation in the nonagriculture sector, in the service industry, in a variety of export activities. This applies to many other sectors, such as transport, communications, and banking. So, you cannot develop this kind of growth without these changes in the other sectors, which reinforces the idea that growth was not the result of sectoral policy changes, but rather the result of an overall attitude toward the economy.

Very important also is the point that there has not been in Chile a real trade-off between export production in agriculture and domestic food production. This concern was raised in terms of Africa, funding one or the other. I don't think this has been the case in South America. I think that the Chilean experience shows that it is possible to get simultaneously the expansion Wylie was describing in food production, essentially through higher yields on wheat and rice. The level of self-sufficiency of food has increased considerably. So I think the export pessimism that I find in so much literature on agricultural development is not warranted, certainly at least for some regions, certainly not for Chile and other parts of South America.

The social implications of these policies are very important. As was mentioned, the employment effect of these policies is of critical importance, the contribution in generating employment in rural areas. There has been a reverse migration to the rural areas, with an expansion, initially, in employment, now in real wages. I think that's going to be one of the challenges, how long you can continue without a very significant increase in real wages and labor costs. I think there has been a very important multiplier effect in the rural areas, because of the high labor intensity of these activities. In my opinion, over the long run, that's the main contribution of these developments for the Chilean economy.

In terms of policy reform, I think the thrust has been in the form of a commitment to export-oriented policies using uniform rules rather than discretionary behavior of particular officials. That is a very fundamental principle of economic policy: the sense that there are no quantitative restrictions on exports, no great problems with export licenses so that exporters, producers, and importers, for that matter, know that if they need something, they have to apply for a license, and the procedure is consistent and uniform.

From what I have learned in East Africa, for example, it's so difficult to develop a dynamic export sector if you cannot get spare parts, or be able to produce cheap parts. This type of product cannot wait. And so, everything has to move very fast. This has implications for the type of economic policies that exist, for the credibility of policies, so investors will be willing to wait the number of years it takes, but also have confidence in the possibility of moving around the products, getting imports, getting the foreign exchange quickly without having to go through months of negotiations, which had been the case in Chile prior to the early 1970s. I think that's the main difference, if one looks at Argentina or Peru, and Brazil today, though it wasn't the case four or five years ago. The regulatory framework of an economy, the lack of credibility in the policies, the discretionary character of policies have been tremendous handicaps for the development of nontraditional exports. Brazil did very well before. Unfortunately in these last years it has not done well.

In terms of the challenges ahead, there are real questions about the backlog of technology, and how to mobilize more resources from the producers, the nonagricultural sector, and from the government to generate all the new technology that will be needed. In terms of labor supply, Chile is beginning to face the prospect of increases in real wages, and with projections in five or eight years at this rate, one could see a significant increase in labor cost that could very much affect competitiveness. I think there could be problems for fruit exporting.

Finally, an important factor is the continuing need to look for new markets overseas. It takes so long. It's so difficult. It's something that at least in the case of Chile the government was never able to do effectively. I think that the private sector really has to receive all the credit for trying to open up markets while at the same time being supported by a very consistent policy of the government.

I think these are the lessons for South America. There have been several other successful cases, as I mentioned particularly Brazil, but the region in the past overall has grossly undervalued the potential of agricultural exports. Thank you.

Robert Havener: Thank you very much, Alberto. Next we will hear from Per Pinstrup-Andersen, professor of food economics and director of the Cornell University Food and Nutrition Policy Program. Per is a native of Denmark.

Per Pinstrup-Andersen: Thank you very much. As the saying goes, don't argue with success. And I'm not going to. I'm convinced that what we heard this afternoon represents three solid successes. What I'd like to do is to talk about some of the factors that seem to have contributed to the success in all three cases.

First of all, all of the three cases have recognized that households are the key actors. Whatever action is external to the households will succeed or fail depending on the initiative or response to new opportunities by the households. This may appear obvious to some of you, but think about all the many attempts to circumvent or to tell households what they ought to do and what they ought to be, and almost all of them have failed.

The second factor is that all of the efforts have been based on a thorough understanding of the constraints faced by households, and the proper balance between efforts to remove these constraints and efforts to change household behavior. And that balance has been obtained by understanding what the households were facing. In the case of the Tanzania project, the proper balance has also been obtained between food and health-related constraints, a balance that we frequently miss in many predesigned projects and programs. The need to understand the constraints is illustrated by the approach used in Tanzania, and similar approaches characterize the successful agriculture research in Indonesia.

Third, all of the cases reflect the transfer of appropriate technology, what we might call soft technology, transfer of knowledge, and so on. Fourth, all of the cases recognized the importance of facilitating macroeconomic and sectoral policies. And, fifth, all of the cases recognized the importance of leadership at various levels of design and implementation, a point that should not be missed in a colloquium associated with the recognition of leadership in agriculture and food development. One final factor that is more obvious in the case of the Tanzania project is the importance of community organization, of community action.

Based on these factors, what are some of the issues that we need to consider in the design and implementation of programs in the future? I'm going to limit myself to one set of such issues, because of time constraints, and I'm going to focus on the Tanzania project. The set of factors I'd like to focus on is represented by the question: what is the proper role of the public sector and of the foreign assistance community in facilitating success in the area of food, agriculture, and nutrition?

First of all, we must have macroeconomic and sectoral policies that facilitate household behavior and community action and that do not attempt to replace them. Again, it may seem obvious, but let's think about some of the past failures where in many cases we were trying to use policy not to facilitate local action, but in some cases to circumvent or replace it. We must build on what is there. And this leads into the next issue that is very important. We must identify, specify clearly, the role of what I'm calling "the magic bullet": what can be done at a more general level. What is it we can do that is applicable to a large number of cases, a large number of local situations, and what are the policy options that will not lend themselves to those kinds of magic bullets?

Agricultural research has shown that there is a great deal of technology that can be used widely. So, if you like the term magic bullet, maybe that is one example. Some of the components of the child survival efforts one could argue are magic bullets: vaccination, as one instance, has wide applicability. The issue is to focus on the problem and identify those elements of a magic bullet sort that are appropriate in each case. We must design the solutions based on the problems and the environments within which we find the problems. We should avoid the situation we have run into in the past of finding solutions that are in search of a problem.

It seems rather important that we start by understanding what problem we're trying to solve, its nature, and its courses. And related to that, we should not despair if all of the problems cannot be solved by magic bullets shot from Washington, Rome, or Geneva, because they cannot. We cannot solve the nutrition problem in such a way. It is too complex. It is too much part of a complex world out there. We cannot solve it simply by shooting out bullets from the capital city of the country we are talking about, and much less so from capital cities of other countries.

Related to that, we frequently run into the problem of the scaling up of pilot projects, the attempt to increase their size and their reach. We frequently find successful pilot projects, but when we try to scale them up, they fail. Clearly we should look for opportunities to scale up successful local projects. But we should not discard those local successful projects that cannot be scaled up. In fact, in many cases, the main reason for success is that those projects were smaller and well-designed; they were based on a thorough understanding, and very good local leadership. When we try to scale these projects up, they very often fail. It gets very messy if you have to deal with a thousand points of light out there, but maybe that is part of the game. Maybe we cannot have a generalized solution to the nutrition problem.

It seems to me that even more important than the scaling up question is the question of sustainability and continuity. Are these projects, at whatever level—local or national—sustainable over the long run? I'm not arguing that these projects should be self-financing. It would be very nice if they were. But, in a time when even in this country and in mine governments are providing a fair amount of public-sector resources to health care and other activities, it is not reasonable to argue that health and nutrition projects should be self-financing in developing countries. But they must be sustainable. We must identify what it is that needs to be provided from outside the community or the household, and what it is that the household and the community can provide themselves. The question then is, is the project sustainable or was it something we played around with for a couple of years and now we're tired of it, so we try something else?

The question in this particular context is whether the Iringa nutrition program, in fact, can be scaled up, which I think is probably an irrelevant question. Much more important is the question, is the Iringa project sustainable? What is the cost of a project of this nature, not relative to doing nothing, but relative to some other approach? I'm not arguing we should put a cost on good nutrition or put a cost on the life of a child. I'm saying, what is the opportunity cost? Is there some other way we can do this that is less costly? My hypothesis is that there probably is not a better alternative in the Tanzanian context, but I would like to hear the answer from the experts. I am concerned, because the Iringa project, as well as many other similar projects that are successful, are targets of scaling up by international organizations. I'm worried that in some cases a scaling up will prove to be unsuccessful, and it will also kill the projects that otherwise would have continued successfully. Thank you very much.

Robert Havener: Michael Lipton already has been introduced in the morning panel. I will call on him next.

Michael Lipton: These are, indeed, all good case studies that we've heard this afternoon. I'm a bit concerned that the Tanzanian case, while excellent in itself, is entirely distribution-based; the production side, the necessary creation of resources to finance that distribution, hasn't been so successful in Tanzania. And it makes me think of other examples in India and in Sri Lanka, where substantial resources were devoted to distribution, but the distribution programs proved very difficult to sustain, because the production base was not being looked after.

But one also needs to ask the question the other way. One needs to ask whether programs such as in Chile are, in fact, delivering a very large part of their benefits to a small number of people and whether that is either politically sustainable or humanly desirable. The good side of the Chile experience is that these are very labor-intensive, employment-generating crops. As was briefly mentioned in the Chile paper, there is a splendid record in Chile going back fifty years at least of attention to child nutrition and child health care, which has served to mitigate the adverse consequences of undesirable income distribution elements of some programs.

We've had substantially encouraging stories this afternoon. And I want to concentrate on the Indonesian story, because a comparison of Indonesia with the Nigerian case that we heard about this morning is of particular interest. These are both economies which discovered oil and discovered trouble both when oil prices went up, and, later, when oil prices went down. You might think it is wonderful when the price of your new discovery goes up in the world. But if the result is that your exchange rate is overvalued, which places a whole range of exports at a disadvantage, and resources are pooled heavily into that single product without making room for other products which are going to form your base for diversification in the future, then that becomes a serious problem. We've seen it in Britain; we've seen it in Holland, where it's known as the Dutch disease; and we've certainly seen it in Nigeria and in Iran. Indonesia managed to avoid the problem because those resources were to some extent secured by the government and to some extent reinvested in other sectors, particularly in agriculture.

If we look back to the mid-1960s, Nigeria was actually slightly richer in income per capita than Indonesia. They were both in the $270-290 per capita mark. If we look at 1987, however, Indonesia is much better off, on average, than Nigeria: $450 per capita in Indonesia as against $370 in Nigeria. And that is mainly because of the much greater success in agricultural production in Indonesia. Between 1965 and 1987, agricultural production in Indonesia was increased in real terms by about 30 percent per capita. It rose faster than the population, whereas in Nigeria, there was a sharp fall. We do know agricultural output per capita fell in Nigeria and this dragged income per capita down with it, as well as damaging the conditions of life of the poor. Agriculture is very important to the poor through food production and important to national growth through its income contribution. Of course, there are huge differences in climates and in other agroecological factors between Nigeria and Indonesia, but I think there's reason to accept the central implication of Sadikin's paper, that policy in Indonesia did substantially help advance agricultural development, at least after 1985, and did so in a way that was conscious of the need to alleviate the poverty problem.

I want to say three things about Dr. Sadikin's paper — about technology, about institutions, and about outcomes. On technology, we've seen through Dr. Sadikin's paper that a key role was played by the International Rice Research Institute (IRRI) in the fight against the brown planthopper, in introducing new germ plasm both in itself and as crossbred with Indonesian germ plasm, and so on. But we've also seen that there was a dramatic need for local research backup both to generate relevant local, indigenously-based, high-yielding varieties and, in particular, to respond to the evolution of that serious pest. It's quite clear, and there's a lot of independent evidence for this, that if countries are to use the benefits of international agricultural research such as that of IRRI, they also will need their own developed off-take system of agricultural research. They need a system of their own. And it was really quite remarkable to learn of the terrible conditions in which the educational and research establishments in Indonesia found themselves after independence—far worse than the conditions in which most African agricultural research systems find themselves today. And we learned how very rapid and effective the build-up of that research system was by means of diverting resources to it. In other words, a national agricultural research system was in place that was able to cooperate with the International Rice Research Institute not only to develop appropriate varieties, but, in addition, respond rapidly to farmers' needs and farmers' signals with respect to plant diseases and pests.

We also heard on the technology side about the response to environmental sustainability considerations—for example, the use of pesticide subsidies to move away from chlorides and, now, increasingly, the switch toward integrated pest management. One is, however, still concerned with the heavy emphasis in countries such as Indonesia and in the rice research work of the international institutes on vertical resistance, including the brown planthopper pest, and the danger of a lack of diversity in countries in which modern varieties are becoming more important. One is particularly worried about what this might do in the countries of sub-Saharan Africa, particularly in the areas of rice and wheat. We may see countries developing very homogeneous populations of one or a small number of modern varieties that will be particularly prone to a new biotype of a pest, and lacking an adequate range of organizations to take care of these developments. That seems to me extremely risky. Species diversity is very important, as well as what has been emphasized here about soil and water.

One final point about technology. I was very interested in learning from Dr. Sadikin about the growth of reliance on urea for fertilizer. Urea in Indonesia is economical because there is a nearby feedstock, there's natural gas, which makes it very sensible to produce that locally. There is a warning, however, against transferring a search for self-sufficiency in fertilizer to countries that do not have nearby availability of feedstock; and the prospect of protecting or creating local industries that are never going to be efficient.

I also want to comment on institutions. I think that it has been very important in the case of Indonesia that they have had an outstanding agricultural and economic survey capability, which has led to skilled people who work on the survey, and natural scientists, economists, sociologists who use the survey material. They have a very good bulletin of Indonesian agricultural economic studies going on month after month. This has provided all the elements of a high-powered critique of government policy within a research framework that is not being used, however, to undermine or to denigrate policy. But there is an understanding that government agricultural policy needs criticism. That every government in the world is going to do silly things or going to fail to do sensible things sometimes, and that you need to have a critique of that government's agricultural policy develop on the basis of broad research. The presence of intellectuals and journals is often emphasized. But, in addition, farmers' institutions are necessary. One of the great strengths of Zimbabwe is its use of small farm institutions, smallholder institutions, that essentially create from below the sort of civil society that makes it possible for agricultural policies to be developed and to be criticized. I think that's very important in the Indonesian context too, and particularly important for African countries.

Finally, regarding results, it's important that Dr. Sadikin and even the Government of Indonesia have emphasized poverty reduction through employment generation as an outcome of the policies that they are seeking. I'm not entirely satisfied that the policy sequences that Dr. Sadikin has described are going to maintain the outcomes that he and the Government of Indonesia want. Credit to small farmers is very important. But an increasing proportion of the poor in Indonesia are not small farmers, but mainly landless laborers, farm employees. Much of international agricultural research, as far as it is poverty oriented, has been concerned with small farmers, and to a large extent with the food supply. But it has been inadequately concerned with the generation of labor-intensive techniques that can help poor people to find productive employment as the population grows and as development proceeds. As it happens, more and more of those poor people depend on employment and not on farm ownership and operation for a livelihood. We need to look at ways of substituting labor for scarce fertilizers, substituting labor for scarce water — such as the placement techniques of fertilizer, improved irrigation management techniques, that the International Institute for the Management of Irrigation is emphasizing. All these things need to be looked at with a view to asking how the poor can use their employment, as well as how society can save some of these scarce nutrient and water resources.

Robert Havener: Our time has drawn to a close. I want to thank the discussants on the panel for being with us, and for stimulating us to examine the range of issues presented at the colloquium. This discussion has been extremely productive. Thank you.

CHAPTER 12

Research Directions on Sharing Innovation: Proceedings of a Discussion at the International Food Policy Research Institute

[Editor's Note: In cooperation with the Smithsonian Institution, the International Food Policy Research Institute (IFPRI) in Washington, D.C., hosted a two-hour roundtable discussion on the morning following the colloquium (October 18, 1989) to examine the research implications of the colloquium proceedings. The discussion, titled "Research Directions on Sharing Innovation," was chaired by John W. Mellor, director of IFPRI. The discussion was taped, transcribed, and edited for publication. Participants included Dr. Verghese Kurien, the 1989 World Food Prize laureate, Dr. Robert F. Chandler, Jr., the 1988 World Food Prize laureate, the colloquium speakers, discussants, and moderators. Other participants included Alan Berg, senior nutrition advisor, the World Bank; Raymond E. Meyer, of the Office of Agriculture at U.S. AID; and Nurul Islam, of IFPRI. Dr. Mellor contributed a brief introductory essay to orient the reader to the discussion.]

Introduction

John W. Mellor
Director, International Food Policy Research Institute

Increasing the productivity of people producing the basic food staples—in particular rice, which is so important in Asia—is the first key to lifting people out of poverty. Bob Chandler and his colleagues at the International

Rice Research Institute (IRRI), in pioneering in short stiff-stemmed rice varieties, which could produce much higher yields of rice at much lower cost per unit of output, paved the way for much that has followed. Once there is enough food to feed poor people, one can think about how they may be employed so that the food can be purchased. It was the first step of the Green Revolution, which was so critical in that respect.

We tend to think of milk and dairy products generally as food, but they have another important role. They are employment, particularly in poor countries. What Dr. Kurien and the dairy-based "White Revolution" have done is to provide markets for milk produced by over six million low-income people, including women and particularly including women with no land resources. With those markets, they were able to move into labor-intensive dairy production and make themselves jobs that would enable them to buy more of the basic food staples that the Green Revolution was providing. With those rising incomes they could begin to acquire other types of food to improve the quality of their diet, something that can only follow upon improving the quantity of the diet, and gradually to obtain other things to make a better life.

As people begin to meet their basic caloric needs and achieve general improvement in the quality of their diet, we come to much more complex elements of nutrition in which scientific knowledge and education become important.

Thus, we have in this room the individuals who helped to bring about the Green Revolution of inexpensive basic food staples and the White Revolution, which provides employment and improved quality to the diet, as well as nutritionists who can help us spend our money more effectively in improving our nutritional status, our health, and our well-being.

But, beyond the economics of these relationships, we have something else represented in this room and again particularly by Dr. Kurien. If people are to avail themselves of the scientific opportunities open to them, they must bond themselves together to create the institutions that are needed to take advantage of those opportunities. It is in this regard that Dr. Kurien has excelled. He has bonded together over six million people as producers, not into one large organization, but into many small organizations, dairy cooperatives, which they control and operate for their own benefit. And the result of this is a set of institutions that reaches a market estimated at 170 million people as consumers. Those small organizations, of course, pyramid into a larger one, but it is the small ones in which they participate and make decisions, and run things for themselves, that form the base of the entire system. It is such a decentralized system that distinguishes Dr. Kurien's contribution. And as people organize themselves for various economic activities, such as milk cooperatives, they begin to acquire the knowledge, the experience, and the power for organizing local governments more generally to achieve a wide variety of their ends.

Today we are gathered to discuss the interrelation of food production, employment creation, nutrition, and the ending of poverty, on the one hand, and the way people can organize themselves and bond together in order to achieve those ends, on the other.

We are particularly concerned with knowledge generation in this context, the kinds of knowledge that have to be generated on the scientific side and on the social side in order to create the opportunities of which we speak. Thus, it is our purpose today to raise questions, to see their interactions, and to proceed from there back to our own organizations for finding answers to those questions. We will make assertions on many occasions today, but those assertions are intended to get ideas out to be questioned and to raise further questions so that we can push back the frontiers of knowledge and move more effectively and efficiently to alleviating poverty, removing hunger, and making this a better world.

Research Directions on Sharing Innovation

John Mellor: Good morning. I feel a considerable sense of humility chairing this meeting, in large part because of the extraordinarily distinguished company. The other thing that subdues me is the very broad agenda. We want to try to focus on the issue of how can we find more knowledge about the very important things that we are dealing with.

I want to now turn to the most pleasurable part of the whole occasion for me, and that is in welcoming our many distinguished guests, but particularly Dr. Kurien and Mrs. Kurien. Many of us here at IFPRI have been for a very long time impressed with the tremendous potential for creating income and employment among poor people in the world, and particularly in Asia, by helping them to get into very labor-intensive activities, particularly dairying. We have been inspired by what Dr. Kurien has done in Anand, India. And the total output of the work Dr. Kurien is involved in is staggering, although it actually isn't all done by Dr. Kurien, as he made clear last night. There are six million other people out there doing the things for which we honored him.

But it really is an extraordinary pleasure for those of us at IFPRI to honor Dr. Kurien and to have him honor us by his presence here, and we look forward to some remarks and help from him.

I would also like to note that the father of IRRI, Dr. Robert Chandler, Jr., is here also, and a former recipient of the World Food Prize. And I can't help but remark that we have in this same room the person who inaugurated the Green Revolution by pulling together the team of people and creating the environment in which those people at IRRI generated IR8, and ushered in the Green Revolution in Asia. And we have in the same room the person who brought us, if you will pardon the term, the "White Revolution," which is clearly spreading way beyond India at the present time. I think in all fairness, it requires the Green Revolution to make it succeed, since there has to be more crop production and more incomes to help make that market for milk successful. This is quite extraordinary and drives home to us that we are living in extraordinary times when really incredible things are happening in the developing world. Things are happening there in five, or ten, or fifteen years that took a century for others of us to see and participate in.

I would like to turn in starting this meeting to Barbara Huddleston to kick us off with what I think will be a summary of her colloquium remarks yesterday and to help us zero in on the issues. And then I would like to turn to Dr. Kurien and ask him to make some remarks. And, just in case he misunderstands the kind of people we are, particularly at IFPRI, we are a bunch of academic researchers in a sense, but we think academic research begins by talking to very ordinary people. And we do a tremendous amount of survey work in which we interview farmers and consumers and try and find out what is happening.

And we consider it particularly helpful to hear comments about what is needed in the way of knowledge, and how, therefore, our kind of research might be helpful, from someone who is in daily contact with six million people and who has his feelers out to a very large number of people.

And then after that I will ask Bob Chandler to make some comments, if you would, and then we will sweep around the room, in a helter-skelter way.

Barbara, may I turn to you?

Barbara Huddleston: I think some people may not have heard the discussions yesterday, so I will just very briefly summarize the main points and conclusions that were presented, drawn from the day's debate.

Basically, the theme that emerged from the discussions of the different papers yesterday is that the development process — the agricultural and rural development process — is a synergistic process, and we cannot focus in on just one element of the process and suggest that there is only one line of action that is an overriding priority.

Three main elements emerged as interlinked and interactive, and they were the institutions, the policy environment, and the technological basis required to advance the agricultural development process.

The entire theme relates to how the development process should not only promote growth in the agriculture sector, but how that growth would ultimately contribute to food security. So the questions about the institutions, the policies, and the technologies have to be addressed not only from the standpoint of whether they are going to promote agricultural growth but also whether the kind of growth generated will promote food security.

Many of the speakers focused particularly on the question of institutions. Remarkably, during the entire day the focus was almost entirely on relatively small-scale institutions at the local and household level; there was virtually no discussion of institutional questions relating to the role of the public sector or government, other than with respect to the economic policy framework. All of the speakers, on the other hand, alluded to different kinds of institutions at the community level that could be innovative in terms of moving forward the development process.

We had a presentation from Dr. Aboyade on community development processes under way in Nigeria. We had a reference by Dr. Sadikin to the need for group farming, which emerged in Indonesia as a way to achieve an adequate farm size. We had a very interesting paper by Dr. Lin on China, in which the experiences with different sizes of communal organization were discussed and the difficulties with very large-size organizations were highlighted, and some of the relative successes of the smaller-size communal organizations were pointed out.

We heard from Mrs. Mtalo about the role of the community with respect to people's participation in the integrated nutrition project in Tanzania. Probably I am forgetting one or two. But the point here was that various types of communal organization were seen to be the vehicle or the instrument for carrying forward the development process.

At that level, one needs to see a package of activities that can be carried out, including taking advantage of existing traditional farming practices or traditional modes of production and traditional consumer patterns and building initially on what is present, while at the same time trying to develop new technological packages that could be gradually introduced that would improve productivity and improve the quality of nutrition.

With regard to the policy framework, there was a general sense that there was some role for the public sector in ensuring that policies were coherent for outputs, inputs, and consumption goods, and that macroeconomic policies were not undermining the goals for the agriculture sector. But there was little discussion of the need for a specific public intervention to provide price incentives.

With regard to technology, there was a very considerable discussion on the importance of water resource management and different possible approaches to this important topic. There was considerable allusion to the need for technologies that would be sustainable and that would sustain the environment, and for combining improved production practices with soil conservation techniques. And there was considerable discussion, particularly for Africa, about the role of mixed cropping, the kinds of crop mixes that need emphasis in research, and the ways in which cropping systems may be combined with animal husbandry or with tree cropping or forestry practices.

In terms of a research agenda to carry forward the ideas that were brought up yesterday, one very important area has to do with the question of the appropriate size for a farming community. And perhaps Dr. Kurien may have some thoughts on this, since I think that the cooperative movement is one that has had much experience in how communities organize and what size organizations work.

It was suggested yesterday that we should not think that there is just one size, or that we should always go for that one size no matter what the group or the ecological conditions. But nevertheless, the question of the appropriate size and organizational structure for rural farming communities, which can serve as the basis for development at a local level, is one that needs more attention. And Dr. Aboyade had suggested also that it would be useful to have more case studies of a community development process. That is a bottom-up type development process: how people enter into the task of defining their own needs and stimulating the external services to be provided so that they can move forward.

A second area requiring further research is the area of water resource management, and here I think there are two elements to consider. It seems to me that the debate was not definitive on the respective merits of irrigation versus dryland agriculture, relying on natural rainfall or natural methods of collecting rainwater.

And a second topic beyond this question of the relative advantages of the two approaches to water resource management is the question of the role of the public sector in financing water resource management activities for dryland agriculture, where many of the techniques that are suggested are ones that are appropriate to a community-based development process. They are smaller in scale, and they don't require the large capital investments that a major irrigation project would require. But, nevertheless, they probably do require an external resource input — and what is the size of it, what is the nature of it, and what is the bureaucratic process by which one can inject external resources? This is true both for water resource management and for other activities. What is the process by which one can move external resources to community-level development activities, as opposed to activities where the bureaucracy itself manages them?

Finally, I think that drawing on Dr. Kurien's remarks last evening one may ask, in particular, what is the role of food aid? And whether we can think that as part of the process of a community-based development we can imagine a community-generated demand for food aid, rather than a demand for food aid that is determined primarily by the donors.

In general, is there a technique or mechanism by which we can turn to the communities and ascertain from them what it is they need? I think in the Nigerian example, in the community that was studied, it was observed that demand for credit was very important, and the provision of credit made an important difference. However, Dr. Aboyade noted that not every community would think that credit was the most important element.

So we have here the need for finding ways in which the communities themselves can generate the demands for the external services and the resource transfers that they require. To discover how to do this, I think, is a central point on the research agenda that came out of yesterday's discussion.

John Mellor: Thank you, Barbara. I would like to turn to Dr. Kurien, and he has a tough act to follow after Barbara, but he has a much tougher act to follow after his own presentation last night. Nevertheless, could we turn to you, sir, for some comments to lead us off. We are particularly concerned today about pushing the frontiers of research forward, and your experiences in Anand are most appropriate to that end.

Verghese Kurien: Well, ladies and gentlemen, I am greatly honored being here. But I am also a very worried man in having to speak to such a distinguished gathering of—

Robert Chandler: Can you speak a bit louder? The old man can't quite hear.

Verghese Kurien: I'm speaking Hindi.
    (Laughter.)
    I am a bit worried at being here before such a distinguished audience. Because, as you know, I am not a scholar by any manner of means. I am just a manager. I would like, however, since you have asked me, to speak about some simple, elementary matters and elementary truths regarding Operation Flood (John Mellor referred to it as a "White Revolution") and, if we have the time, about vegetable oil.
    I would like to explain to you the basic principles underlying Operation Flood. They are so simple that nobody has bothered to understand them. I am talking about my country, not of course of the International Food Policy Research Institute.

John Mellor: Thank you.

Verghese Kurien: The first principle is, there can be no Anand if there is no Bombay. There can be no production if there is no market. Therefore, to create an Anand, to create the production center, to create the cooperative structure, we need a concentrated market. And Anand was capable of being created because we had Bombay 270 miles away.
    The second principle is that you cannot create an Anand next door to Bombay, because you do not need an Anand next door to Bombay to take the milk from next door to consumers of Bombay. All you need is a bicycle. You do not need a processing plant; you do not need this manager to run it; you do not need any pasteurization plants.
    In fact, if you try to create an Anand next door to Bombay, you are bound to fail because it is unnecessary. Economically, it will be a monstrosity to try to create a processing plant to collect milk when it is not necessary to create that processing plant.

You know I discovered that my wife, as soon as I got married, had no respect for the dairy technology I had studied in this country. The first thing she did with bottled milk was to unbottle it. The next thing she did with pasteurized milk was to put it in a pot and boil it. She felt that these processes were unnecessary for India. Anyway, we won't go into that now.

So the second point is, you cannot create an Anand next door to Bombay. The next principle underlying Operation Flood is, you cannot start a milk scheme by simply collecting milk from the farmers through cooperatives, or through any other way, and by simply marketing it in the city. Because if you do that, you have to market only what milk you collect.

You cannot market more, of course, because you haven't got it, and you have to sell what you collect. And, as your collection increases, your market must increase just to that extent, no more. And you have linked procurement and marketing so rigidly that it cannot work. As your markets expand, your production and your procurement must expand just to that extent. And when summer comes and production declines, your market is not going to shrink. And so by collecting and marketing in a rigid system you have doomed your efforts to failure.

I am saying these are simple things. I am sure that this Policy Research Institute finds this all too simple. But you know we built a hundred plants in India. We spent millions of rupees doing exactly this. So you should not be simply collecting milk and selling it and have to depend on the uncertainties of the market, because that will not work.

The next principle presents a solution to this problem. For example, when Anand grew and became successful, we discovered that we could not sell all the milk that we were collecting. The Bombay people said we don't need all of this milk at one time. And the Bombay milk commissioner or the milk scheme people said, "Stop sending all this milk."

I said "I studied at Michigan State University, an excellent university, but nobody taught me how to plug the udders. So what shall I do with this milk?"

They said "That is not our business. We have not learned how to make our people here drink two bottles of milk in winter and one bottle in summer. So that is your problem."

I said, "No, it's not my problem. I will send you the milk." So we got into conflict because there was no system to meet this variation in procurement and in market.

And, therefore, we found it necessary to have a balancing station, which would convert seasonal surpluses into milk products, milk powder, butter, etc. And of course then everybody told us this cannot be done because buffalo milk had never been made into milk powder before. Buffalo milk is unstable to heat and when you try to make powder, it will coagulate. We encountered a great deal of opposition.

Many great experts in dairying, from advanced dairying countries, told us that milk powder cannot be manufactured from buffalo milk. It is technically impossible, they advised us.

It is then that we began to understand that very often the technical expertise we get from advanced countries is colored by the commercial interests of those countries. And we then learned to be more judicious in accepting technical advice from advanced countries.

But the other approach was what we did in our neighboring district, that was the district of Baroda. Now, those people were stimulated by the experience of the Kaira district, by the example of Anand. They followed our lead, they started a cooperative dairy. They started collecting milk from cooperatives set up in the villages around Baroda, and marketing it in Baroda. And then they found that every summer, collection became a serious problem because milk merchants offered a higher price, and they can add water and sell it. A cooperative cannot.

So the chairman of that cooperative came to me and said, "You know I've been telling them, 'All for one and one for all', the cooperative principle. We should be loyal to our cooperative. But loyalty to a cooperative in the face of the higher price offered by milk merchants is becoming very difficult. I have managed so far. Our collection is 25,000 liters; we are selling 25,000 liters. But I am afraid come summer I am going to be in serious trouble. This coop is going to fail. Can you give us some advice?"

And the advice was very simple. "I'll tell you what, Mr. Chairman, I will give you this coming summer 25,000 liters of milk from Anand to Baroda."

And you know we Gujaratis are supposed to have a business instinct. So he immediately asked, "At what price? At what price will you give it?"

I said, "You know you are my brother. We are doing this to help you."

He said, "Yes, but at what price?"

I said, "My dear brother, you decide the price. I suggest you take my milk. You meet all the cost involved in marketing it, and what is left after meeting all the cost is the price you pay me."

He said, "Really? That's good. The quality of your milk is better. You are going to give it to me in summer, then I will enlarge my market."

I said, "Exactly. Go ahead and do it this summer. I give you 25,000 liters."

He said, "Can I take the first 12,000 liters next day?"

I said, "Take it as it suits you." So he took more and more milk from Anand and started marketing in Baroda, more and more milk that summer over his 25,000. And what did he discover? He discovered the other principle underlying Operation Flood: as you capture a market, the milk falls in your lap. In other words, his competition could not collect milk because they lost the market.

What is the role of food aid? This I alluded to in my remarks last evening in accepting the World Food Prize. The milk came as donated

226

commodities from Europe. It had no value to the Europeans. It, therefore, was a secret tank of milk for India. So we set up dairies in Bombay, Delhi, Calcutta, Madras. We began to pump in milk and capture the market.

As we captured the market, we pushed the cattle back out of these cities into where they should be, into the hinterland. And we set up coops there in the hinterland. That required five years. That is Operation Flood.

Now, one more piece of philosophy. In the city of Bombay in the early 1970s there were 100,000 buffaloes. They produced something like 600,000 liters a day. The Bombay milk scheme was marketing 400,000 liters of milk. So the total market of Bombay was a million liters.

Now, assume for a moment we are magicians and by dumping milk, by capturing the market, we push these 100,000 buffaloes back to where they belong, in the hinterland. I suppose you realize that these buffaloes do not give milk always, that they become dry in Bombay after eight months.

As soon as they become mothers in rural areas, up to a thousand miles away, they and their calves are brought into the city because the buffaloes produce milk not for us but for their calves. No calf, no milk. Then the calf drinks milk. It takes the cattlekeeper fifteen days to teach the buffalo to let down the milk without the calf. After which, he doesn't want the calf to live.

But we are holy people, we Indians; we don't kill cows and calves. We just starve them to death. We dip their mouth in a bucket of water; we kick them until they die. But within fifteen days of taking them to Bombay they all die. The mortality rate is 100 percent.

Now, these buffaloes that are taken to Bombay are the finest buffaloes of India. And what we have killed, the 100,000 calves that we kill in Bombay alone, are the progeny of the finest buffaloes of India.

So this is a very serious, genetic drain. Then what happens when the buffalo becomes dry after eight months? It doesn't bed "Mr. Bull" in Bombay.

Bombay is not a good place for dating for cows. So what happens then?

So when the buffalo becomes dry, it is not pregnant. So it is sent to the slaughter house half the time, if it is beyond the fourth lactation; or sent back a thousand kilometers or 500 kilometers, to be salvaged. That is, it is sent back to meet "Mr. Bull," to become pregnant, to calve ten months thereafter. And then we will make the second trip with the calf, only to have the calf killed.

This is how these hundred thousand buffaloes produce 600,000 liters. Now, assume for a moment that these 100,000 buffaloes are, by waving my magic wand, wished away to the rural areas. How much milk will they produce in the rural areas?

In Bombay there is no fodder and feed; so, not only do you have to keep the 100,000 buffaloes, you have to take the fodder and feed into

Bombay to feed them, too. So, if you keep them where the fodder and feed are, in the rural areas, and take the buffaloes from the city to the rural areas, they will produce 600,000 liters. There is no reason to assume they will produce any less.

What will they produce in the second year if half of them are not killed or sent to the slaughterhouse when they are dry? Because in the rural areas, they wouldn't be. Then, their production would be 900,000 liters, assuming you have increased the feed production to support this increased production of milk.

What would they produce in the third year? It is 1.2 million liters, assuming, again, that you have produced more fodder and feed. The fourth year, 1.5 million. Now, the new female calves — 50,000 of them — have come into production.

Now, plot the graph. Assume mortality rates for the buffaloes. Assume similar mortality rates for the calves, and you draw your graph. You will find the milk production in rural areas will shoot up and reach eight million liters in about the fifteenth year. That is Operation Flood.

Merely by not taking milk on four legs to Bombay and leaving the buffaloes where they ought to be, you can create a flood of milk — provided you increase the fodder and feed available in the rural hinterland.

"Oh," said one of our economists, and we too have some economists, very few, though. "Oh," he said, "but if you continue to send 50,000 buffaloes from the rural areas to feed the meat market of Bombay, you don't even have to increase the fodder and feed production." These, ladies and gentlemen, are the principles underlying Operation Flood. I have nothing more to say at this stage. Thank you.

John Mellor: We hope we will stimulate you to say something more very shortly, but thank you very much. I think we are benefitting greatly from this.

I would like to turn to Bob Chandler and ask you to make some comments. We will get a few more things on the table, then we will see where we go.

Robert Chandler: Thank you, John. You people have heard me before and I don't have many new ideas, although I think I have some strong prejudices about matters of concern.

As you know, the Green Revolution took place in Asia with rice. And in the twenty-five-year period from 1960 to 1985, there was an average increase of 114 percent in rice production. Seventeen countries in Asia now produce more than one million metric tons of rice per year.

Only four countries have had a lagging rate of increase. They are Taiwan, and that is because it has a limited area and got its yields up where it can't get them much higher; Japan, which actually has had a 13 percent decrease; and Kampuchea and Nepal, which have had some real problems.

The rest of the countries have had increases of 50 to 200 percent in rice production.

But the thing that disturbed me as I was looking at these figures was that, in Asia, as a whole, there has been no increase in land allotted to rice production since 1977 for India, and even longer for China. The only country that I can find that had any continuing increase since ten years ago is North Korea, which is still increasing the land devoted to rice.

I was in Bangladesh with some of the people around this table and I was amazed to find in that country—which I first visited in 1954—113 million people living in an area the size of Wisconsin or Georgia. And the World Bank predicts that when that population becomes stabilized they will have 300 million—not 113 million people. It seemed to me an impossible situation in Bangladesh, with so many of the people still in the rural areas, landless and poor. You walk around the streets of Dhaka, and most of the people are quite thin. There are a few merchants and businessmen that are stout. It seems to me that here is a country that is already overpopulated.

We tried to estimate among ourselves what the potential would be for increasing rice production as a result of increased fertilizer use, and increased irrigation. And the best that we could come up with, considering the cyclones, floods, and poverty that Bangladesh is subject to, is that the country might get an 84 percent increase in rice production in the next twenty years. That is not a very optimistic prediction. After all, Bangladesh is a major rice-producing country, and it has not been able to double its rice production in the course of the Green Revolution—with only a 56 percent increase in the twenty-five-year period.

Well, what I want to say is this, that of all the problems of the world, and there are many, I think the biggest problem we have on this planet, and I have said this before, is overpopulation.

India is slated to be the largest country in the world in terms of population. The World Bank estimates that the population will double before it stabilizes. And there will be 1.56 billion people in India. I wonder what is going to happen to the cows. Can they get enough to eat to produce enough milk to feed the people of India? I don't know how they are going to do it.

In Nigeria, as another example, the World Bank estimates that there will be 500 million people, not 120 million people, when it stabilizes its population. I don't believe it is going to reach that. What I think is going to happen is that you are going to have a significant reduction in the well-being of people. You are going to have an increase in the death rate, and you are going to have a destruction of the country's natural resources.

The thing that we need to do as a world is to influence the leaders of countries and the donors of foreign aid to redouble their family planning efforts. I wish the United States had a better population control program. It has a very weak one. But I believe that this is a thing that we have to realize, that the world is a finite thing. No land area is being added, other than a little increase in the delta here and there. And that we have just got to stop population growth, and that we have got to put more effort into this.

The thing that amazes me is that I go to these various meetings, even that one in Bangladesh, and find so little emphasis placed on the urgent need for action and investment and ideas on policies with respect to population control. I think that natural resources and population are on a collision course, without any question.

Now there are some hopeful things. I made the suggestion yesterday at the end of the session that perhaps next year when we have this collo- quium that we might have as a theme the balance between population, food production, and the environment. We can make predictions. Experts know more or less what the maximum yields of crops will be. By and large we know what we can expect and we know what the land area is. We know what its carrying capacity is. We know what the water resources are. A lot of information can be brought together. It would be very nice if we could have a discussion in which population control is a central focus of concern. Thank you very much.

John Mellor: Thank you, Bob. Michael Lipton, I wonder if I couldn't turn to you for some comment with respect to Bob Chandler's statements on population. Or do you have some response on other issues that have been raised?

Michael Lipton: At the moment there are many more questions than an- swers. It is a small piece of the pilot work that is being done here by Steve Vosti and myself, with the support of Bob Herdt of the Rockefeller Foun- dation. What we are doing is trying to get at the questions that Bob Chandler has been raising from a slightly different perspective.

The thing that I think we have learned about population decisions and household behavior in the last fifteen or twenty years — and we have learned a lot of things — is that, on the whole, when parents decide to have a lot of kids it is because they need to — not because they are behaving irrationally, or stupidly, or antisocially, or anything of that sort.

Now, on that assumption, we can ask what are the choices of agri- culture policy, of labor intensity, of crop mix, of agriculture incentives and their effect on population growth? We don't know the answers to that. We have a lot of hunches, and we have for India some pretty good data sets. Pakistan has some relevant data sets that we are also beginning to take a look at.

But the question is: Are the fast-growing agriculture areas bringing down their rate of population growth? Are the areas that are growing, in more labor-intensive ways, doing better or worse in terms of the impact on household decisions? Why? We suspect that these may be very important long-run factors.

One very interesting fact in India is that the state of Kerala, which has had an appalling agricultural growth performance, as you know, but a very good performance as far as health, education, and human physical infrastructure are concerned, brought the infant mortality rate right down. That state has brought the total fertility rate of women down to 2.2, and the net reproduction rate is hardly more than necessary to maintain population. I mean, population growth in Kerala is very low, below 1 percent, while in India it is still just over 2 percent.

Now, that is very suggestive, but we want to see what has happened to the rate of natural increase in those parts of the Indian Punjab, for example, which have had a very fast growth in rural agriculture-related incomes. We want to try and close this circle and see what the effect of different agricultural growth patterns on population change is.

I wonder if I might take this particular argument into other directions. One regards the knowledge base; the other, the role of governments.

In the extremely interesting set of presentations we had yesterday I was struck by what a huge difference there was with regard to the knowledge bases. We can think of India or, indeed, of Indonesia, or perhaps of Kenya in doing this sort of work. Of saying, why are the population patterns different? How does this relate to agricultural production, agricultural policy options, as they influence what we know? Are rational couples deciding at the household level, rational couples who need their incentive patterns oriented to less population growth?

Now, we can ask those questions in those countries. But in most countries in the developing world we can't answer those questions because the basic information is just not there. There are not more, at best, than half a dozen, probably four countries, in sub-Saharan Africa where I can tell you what the total agriculture production was in any of the last three or four years, within 40 percent to 90 percent confidence. The data are just so bad.

There are lacking in most of these countries reliable farmer surveys, which, when done properly, can give you pictures of what the total level of agriculture production was. So a huge gap exists in the knowledge base both in agriculture and, indeed, in population policy.

And we can't say this part of a country is doing better than that part, this crop is doing better than that crop. We can't make statements like Bob Chandler was just making about Asian rice production. Because the areas under major crops in most of these countries are guesswork. We talk in a very would-be learned fashion about which agricultural policy works, and which doesn't work. But in most of sub-Saharan Africa the data base is just not good enough to make those sorts of statements.

And I think it is scandalous that the international community has not encouraged more of those sub-Saharan African countries that are interested in reporting reliable data. There are some countries that are not so interested, but with those that are, I think that much more could be done.

The last thing I want to mention is this whole question of the role of government. Barbara Huddleston, I think, correctly presented a picture that came out of yesterday's discussions and that rather worried me. I thought it was a bit old hat, a bit of yesterday's conventional wisdom. This idea of cutting governments down to size, and that community or production unit size be kept at a minimum, and that everything can be left to the community itself. I think that is nonsense.

There are certain things that governments do well and other things that they do badly. What they do very badly is to seek to establish marketing monopolies in major food crops, indeed, agricultural crops, and interfering with and seeking to control and monopolize agricultural markets. However, there are an awful lot of things in and with regard to the agricultural sector, and certainly population policy, that nobody except government is going to effect. Even with excellent population policies adopted now, we are talking about the doubling of population in most of the countries of sub-Saharan Africa within the next twenty to twenty-five years.

We are not going to deal with those situations without massive changes in production techniques and methods in most of sub-Saharan Africa. And that doesn't mean pushing ploughs around, but building on their farming systems with improved water control, improved supplies of plant nutrients, mainly through inorganic fertilizers, and improved, greatly improved, agriculture research yielding the stream of improved varieties and, yes, with mixed cropping systems. This means not trying to pretend that these are rice and wheat areas, which the great majority of them are not.

As far as I can see, there is no other way to meet that sort of population increase and extra demand for food. And there is no way, particularly in the area of water control and water management, environmental issues, and even if we are talking about minor irrigation, small-scale, farm-level irrigation, there is no way of doing this without a large expansion of government/public sector activity.

And the question is, how is that public sector activity to be kept honest, efficient, publicly controlled, nonbureaucratized? The question isn't, how to cut it back to a small scale. That in my view is a nonstarter.

John Mellor: I would like to pick up on something that Michael said and, earlier, that Barbara stated. Let me make a brief comment myself, and I hope this will stimulate Dr. Kurien to respond. Of the three areas Barbara put forth, one was the institutional issue. Michael referred to the role of government, and I would like to raise a specific question in that context. I would preface that with an historical statement about the present-day industrialized countries, and what I see as a major contrast between the present-day industrialized countries and the present-day developing countries with respect to their early stages of development.

That difference I will put in two contexts and then raise my institutional question. I am convinced that in the rural areas of present-day industrialized countries, when they were in the early stage of development, there existed vastly more investment in physical infrastructure and roads than is the case in present-day developing countries—and a vastly more developed system of rural education than is the case in present-day developing countries.

I believe the reason for that is that in Japan, Western Europe, and North America, you had rather highly developed systems of local government. In effect, these governments developed from little feudal principalities or some other kind of local system and pyramided up. So that there were structures which allowed people to get together and say, we want a school, we want a road, we want a clinic, if that were feasible at the time, and to say, we will tax ourselves or somehow come up with a system to get the resources to accomplish these goals. And they did it.

In most present-day developing countries, you have, first of all, a colonial heritage in which it was quite against the interest of the colonial powers to get rural people organized to do things for themselves, because they might do something adverse to the colonialists as well, which would not have been a very good idea from the colonialists' point of view. And then it seems to me that the independence movements tended, with some striking exceptions such as Kenya and one or two others, to be basically urban-based movements.

Hence, we find present-day governments in many developing countries to be very centralized, and they find building local structures, whether it is a local government, to use the Indian terminology, "panchayats," or locally people-based cooperatives, or whatever, very threatening, and, therefore, something not to be encouraged. So we are left with a situation now of a need for massive physical investment in infrastructure, education, and so on—a need for a lot of organization at the local level.

The reason I want to turn to Dr. Kurien on this is that in his work he has helped to develop local structures. We are seeing him as the head of six million people, but I think he made it quite clear that his organization is quite a decentralized structure, which does work from the bottom up. This is something which has, in general, been quite lacking in modern developing countries, and the lack of it represents a very major barrier to growth. Could I stimulate you, Dr. Kurien, to respond to these concerns? This even gets into population issues. I don't see how you can solve the population problem without people being able to get at their problems in this way.

Verghese Kurien: I would like to ask Dr. Chandler whether he would totally rule out the possibility of migration in large volumes from a heavily populated country like India to less populated areas, as a means of population control.

Robert Chandler: I hope I did.

Verghese Kurien: Well, can you visualize migrations to less populated areas of the world?

Robert Chandler: One of the problems of moving people is that the best parts of the world have been already inhabited by people and they are growing crops and so forth. So people would have to go to poorer lands.

You also have great difficulty moving people away from where their environment is, where their relatives and friends are. Indonesia has had real problems moving people to the outer islands. I saw this happening as far back as forty years ago. We can't go to the moon, and it seems to me that this is not going to be a solution. I think the solution is right in the countries themselves.

India has had population control, a family planning program, for over thirty years. But still it leaves a 1.8 percent increase annually. And you are less apt to cut down still further without incentives of various kinds. China, of course, has had some strong regulations. Thailand is doing a fair job now. And so those things could be analyzed and we can see what can be done. I know it is a difficult thing, a very difficult thing.

Verghese Kurien: Well, after all, most of the population of Europe was kept under control by migration to other continents, including America.

Robert Chandler: This is a finite world, however.

Verghese Kurien: What would have been the population of Europe if that migration had not taken place?

Robert Chandler: But Europe has gotten down to essentially zero population growth.

Verghese Kurien: This European migration enabled you to have a higher standard of living, which, in turn, enabled you to control your population. One can keep on arguing, but I suppose this is not a practical thing.

Robert Chandler: But I don't think this is the solution.

Verghese Kurien: Yes, but you hold what you have.

John Mellor: Dr. Kurien, I was trying to stimulate you a little bit on this issue of decentralization.

Verghese Kurien: Well, it is fairly well known that one of the principal obstacles to development in developing countries is the growing part of our bureaucracies and their unwillingness to allow popular institutions to emerge. After all, we got our freedom rather cheaply.

The British did us dirty. They didn't make us fight for freedom as much as they should have. The result was that we got freedom rather unexpectedly. Along with freedom, we inherited a machinery of government designed by the British to rule, not to serve. And we Indians have maintained it intact and probably made it worse.

So our government still, in my judgment and I am sure many Indians will not agree with me, particularly those in Delhi, I maintain that our government is still one that is designed to rule, not to serve. And I pass the blame all to the British, as we always do for all our ills.

Now, it is also true, as you are implying, that the answer to these problems is the creation of a plurality of democratic institutions, and to cease our almost total dependence on the political structure, the parliamentary structure, for the emergence of our future leaders; and to increasingly look to structures that are constructive in their approaches, structures that are developmental in their tasks, to create the future leaders of our country.

With this plurality of democratic institutional structures we create in the country, we will be erecting meaningful democratic structures throughout and not confining democracy only to Delhi, but spreading it right down to our village levels and giving democracy more meaning. It means people's participation. I think that is what we are driving at.

John Mellor: Thank you very much. I turn to Nurul Islam for comment, and then to my friend Ojetunji Aboyade.

Nurul Islam: The example is given of developed, industrialized countries having well-functioning local governments throughout history. Is this not related to the development of the national government in the first place? Are they independent of one another? What I am saying, Dr. Kurien just said: unless you have democratic institutions at the local level and a plurality of democratic institutions, you do not have an effective government at all. The suggestion is that local government is a function of a democratic government, of a national government. Yet Japan did not have a democratic national government while they have had effective government. They had feudal institutions at the local level, which did developmental functions. So there is a critical question here, of the processes and factors that lead to effectively functioning local government in various types of societies.

The United States is a special case, in which the local institutions came along with independence and, therefore, local governments and national governments were both democratic and both developed simultaneously. The European cases are different. So, in order to understand the reasons why effectively functioning local governments have failed to emerge in developing societies, I think we have to be very careful in drawing parallels and analyzing factors relating to this.

Democracy does not necessarily imply effective local government. We know of cases where the central government and local governments conflict. The politicians of the local government have interests different from those of politicians of the central government, and conflicts, and sometimes insoluble conflicts of opposing parties, arise.

So a local setting itself does not necessarily imply an effective local government. Of course, a dictatorial, authoritarian government would make it impossible for an effective local government to operate. So we really do not know the forces which can shape an effective local government.

John Mellor: I was very careful not to use the word democracy anywhere. I do believe, however, that when you decentralize, it is very difficult to avoid all the wisdom that resides with the mass of people.

I want to call on Ojetunji Aboyade, who has been talking, particularly yesterday, about the grassroots level, but who also operates at rather high levels as well.

Ojetunji Aboyade: I was not thinking of speaking at this stage. However, since you have called on me I will make only two observations at this point. Maybe I'll come back later. I agree with you, John, that the evolution of developing countries is not as successful for a variety of reasons, partly because of this need for building infrastructures locally. There is no doubt in my mind that this is absolutely important.

I was reflecting also on what some may call the doomsday approach of Dr. Chandler and the observation by Michael Lipton. Whatever you do now to the population size for the next ten to fifteen years, you are basically stuck with what you have in the pipeline. And that must be addressed from a food and policy standpoint. That does not mean that you cannot or should not think ahead about doing something more serious, more rigorous in reducing the population growth rate. But, as of the moment, you just cannot send off people like you send the cows or buffaloes to Bombay, kill them off or whatever. You just have to address the issue. Partly through technology, improved varieties, or mixed varieties, or water management, or whatever. Those are the issues that we ought to address. And I am happy that IFPRI is taking an interest in institutional matters.

I know institutional study is not as analytical, as coherent, and as statistical, and manipulative, as is technology-based or quantitatively-based research, but it is important, I think, to show that there are things that you can do in terms of institutions. There are creative ways you can use institutions or create new ones. That is not a subject for a technology-based approach that Michael Lipton has been talking about and that is discussed in his recent book.

But as I was advocating yesterday, policy research institutions like IFPRI should be interested in undertaking these studies at the community level. Now, what is the community? How do we define that community? The problem I am talking about is one of the optimum size. Of course, it will vary from country to country; it will vary from one social structure to another. But whatever it is, however it is defined, however it is measured, there is no doubt in my mind that we now need different inputs of knowledge, more studies at the community level. More studies of the constraints to the expansion of food and crops, how to utilize what is on the ground, and by using these local institutions how to get better results from them.

These were all the three items or four items that I suggested yesterday for a research agenda. But I hope most humbly that we will recognize the need to look more seriously and in more scholarly ways at how societies are going to function at the local level. I would like to look at community-based structures, rather than look at governments, because that is a common structure, the local level. And the more differences we find, the better. Certainly in my part of the world, that would be very, very helpful.

John Mellor: Thank you very much. I might respond just before I turn to Alan Berg, who is particularly able to cut across a lot of these issues. I think we do want to focus today on the issue of where analysis, where research knowledge, should be going. It is true that on the surface at IFPRI, we do not appear as though we emphasize institutions very much. I would like to make just two comments on that.

One, we do emphasize institutions in one sense. From the sort of numerical research we do, particularly down at the grassroots level, we are contributing to defining what kinds of institutions are needed and what kinds of decisions need to be made to make them better institutions.

What scale of operation? That is an institutional question—little institutions or big institutions? The extent to which they diversify? The details of what they work on, and so on? That is my first point, that we are doing a lot, and I think it is very important and perhaps has been underemphasized.

The second point is that there are an awful lot of things that we just aren't touching. I think one reason for that is because of the disciplinary bias that we have at IFPRI. We are very proud of the fact that there are a good number of noneconomists here, but they are still scarce and we do somewhat co-opt them, at least at the fringes of economics. However, some of us are concerned whether the other academic disciplines are really very good at dealing with those institutional issues that we don't deal with, but maybe that is just a disciplinary bias.

We are searching at IFPRI for the best ways to move into that vast set of institutional issues that we aren't presently touching. And I think we are getting closer and we very much look forward to comments and help on this. And I might say, Michael Lipton being at IFPRI has been very helpful because he is pushing us rather vigorously in that direction. But we are listening.

Michael Lipton: Very briefly. I would very much agree with everything you have said and warn against the view that economics is rigorous and all these other things are vague. It is possible to tackle the question of, for example, the size or scale of a cooperative credit society that makes it likeliest that the credit will be used productively and paid back.

That is a question that can be analyzed as empirically and as rigorously as any of the questions that economists tend to uncover. Anyone who doubts it should look at David Leonard's marvelous book on agricultural extension in Kenya: where it works, where it doesn't, and how that links to the social organization and to the attitudes of the staff. Rigorous and thoroughly useful research.

John Mellor: Thank you. Alan Berg.

Alan Berg: I was going to shift slightly. May I do that? I want to take advantage of Dr. Kurien's offer at the outset to tell us a little bit about his oilseed project. Where it stands. What has been learned. What the implications are. What applicability it has for elsewhere.

Also, in the process, if you could add a sentence or two about an item that was introduced almost parenthetically last night as part of the introductory remarks, if I understood correctly, which indicated that you were being asked to get involved in salt distribution.

I ask this, given the fact that India has now come up with this new technology to fortify salt with iron. I think a lot of us are aware that the major nutritional deficiency in India is iron deficiency anemia, and it is just crying out for a Dr. Kurien to make advances in this area.

Verghese Kurien: First, a word about oilseed. Perhaps you are all aware that India is perhaps the largest importer of vegetable oil. It imported in the year 1987–88 over $1 billion worth of vegetable oil per annum.

But what is disturbing is that some years ago it used to export oil. And India started importing oil, and the curve of imports was rising steeply. Two years ago, the drought was responsible for larger imports. The trend is a disturbing one. And it was quite clear, at that rate, that we would soon be asking for $2 billion of imported oil, and that would upset the economics of the vegetable oil economy of the whole world. Because I don't think the world production would support it if India were to import $2 billion worth. The price would go up to such an extent that it would cost us $3 billion to import the same quantity of oil.

Now, therefore, the Government of India raised these serious questions as to whether an Anand pattern was possible for oil. Can we create Anands around vegetable oil? Now, quite clearly there are certain special reasons why dairy coops or milk is extremely suitable for a cooperative endeavor. And there are some wide differences between milk and vegetable oil.

But my reply was that I did not know anything about vegetable oil but we would study the problem. I assumed that if what the government meant—namely, should the farmer be placed in the middle of things; should he own the procurement, processing, and marketing of vegetable oil?—was, in fact, the case, then we would be prepared to study the matter.

We found that vegetable oil was being handled in several ministries of the Indian government. Of course, the Ministry of Commerce was concerned with the imports. It was a canalized item. There was a state trading corporation to import the oil. They were importing so much oil that it became their main business. They were making so much profit that they developed a vested interest in these imports. In fact, if these imports had not come, state trading corporations would be in serious trouble. These imports of vegetable oil were, in fact, subsidizing the losses incurred in the export of certain other commodities. So this was very necessary for the good health of the state trading corporations. They had a vested interest in the imports of oil, and preferably larger and larger quantities of oil.

There was another ministry involved, called the Department of Food, which is concerned with the distribution of food. This department likes to be popular: its projects are based on the distribution of food, preferably, as cheaply as possible to what they call the "vulnerable sections" of the population, who are always discovered to be living in Delhi, and in Bombay, and in Calcutta, and never in the villages of India. So they set up distribution schemes, which they call "public distribution schemes," most of which are city oriented. And this distribution of vegetable oil is based on the imported price of oil.

Now, the advanced countries producing this oil, from whom we buy this oil, I think are also heavily subsidizing the oil export. In fact, it is my feeling that the European Economic Community countries are exporting oil at half the full cost of production, and I don't think the United States is far behind in the subsidies they pay on the export of vegetable oil.

Now, we bring in these subsidized imports. You know, at all these locations, a fellow called GATT [i.e., an international trade agreement] is asleep. He goes to sleep whenever advanced countries' interests are involved. He only wakes up when developing countries do something to protect their farmers. Until then, he is asleep. So these imports at low prices were brought in by the Ministry of Commerce, given to the Department of Food, distributed at prices lower than that at which Indian farmers can produce the oil.

Now, it is in the interest of these ministries that India does not become self-sufficient in vegetable oils. If India were to become self-sufficient, the sale price of vegetable oil to the public distribution schemes would have to go up, which would make them unpopular. And, after all, we are a democracy and we must all be popular. So there is that department.

The Department of Agriculture, on the other hand, has of course the task of making the country self-sufficient and it must do the research, it must do everything necessary to increase production, to see that the imports are diminished.

The prime minister [Rajiv Gandhi] is a modern man. Our prime minister has a keenness for technology. The prime minister said, "We shall have a mission to do certain worthwhile things in India." And worthwhile things were identified as immunization of all children, literacy, drinking water in all of our villages, vegetable oil self-sufficiency, and so on, and the last one was dairy technology. And these missions were given targets, specified periods in which these targets are to be met, and so on.

Now, I happen to be a member of this technology mission and in a technology mission all ministries concerned sit down for the first time. And no longer do you pass a note from one ministry to another, but you argue and come to conclusions. So then I raised some issues. All the departments are represented, incidentally, at the level of the permanent secretary. So I said: "I am a magician. I have been put on this mission to ask this question. Supposing tomorrow or midnight tonight India becomes self-sufficient in vegetable oil, at what price, Mr. Secretary of the Food Department, would you distribute oil tomorrow? At what price? Would it be at the world market price or would it be at the Indian price? Would you be importing anything, Mr. Secretary of Commerce?"

He said, "No, we won't import, of course."

"Then, if you don't import it, at what price will you distribute it? At an Indian price? And if we have a lower consumer price, who will subsidize the distribution?"

The Finance Secretary said: "We won't subsidize." "So then," I said, "if that is so, why aren't you increasing the distribution price now?"

We have another product called "vanaspathi." I don't know if you are familiar with this product. There is a company called Unilever, you may have heard of it, which came to India a long time ago, and to their disgust they found that Indians don't use butter. And so they are specialists in oils and soaps, fats and soaps, and they were very upset that we were not using butter.

But they found that we were using a product called "ghee." They used their technology to make vegetable oil not into margarine but to hydrogenate it just enough to imitate ghee, and they call it vanaspathi. And we were importing 5,000 million rupees worth of vegetable oil at a low price to feed the vanaspathi industry in order to make this product to harden our arteries.

It is a totally unnecessary product because most of the countries of the world do without it except for India and Pakistan, which were the only two countries that used ghee.

Now came a problem. What will be the pricing policy for the vanaspathi industry? So came the whole problem of arriving at policies that are consistent, policies that would help India to become self-sufficient, policies that will help Indian farmers to produce the vegetable oil within the country, policies that will militate against the imports. And, therefore, it is that within one year of this mission being created India's imports went down from $1 billion to roughly $300 million.

Now, what are some of the reactions of the government ministries? Finance Ministry says, "Good Lord, what have you done? We have calculated the import duty of 7,000 million rupees as revenues to the government. Now, that has disappeared. Our budget deficit will go up by 7,000 million rupees. You don't have to put up foreign exchange to import. Dr. Kurien, for god's sake, you never will understand economics. Foreign exchange is met by borrowing, which is repaid after twenty years. I will not be here. The problem tomorrow is rupees."

So what I am trying to say is to have a vegetable oil policy, to create conditions where India can produce the vegetable oil, a consolidated, comprehensive policy has to be evolved. It is not enough to say: let us use fertilizer; let us have research to get the best seeds. That alone will not do. A framework has to be erected within which you can have a coherent policy and, once you can do so, all problems are solvable.

That is more or less what the oil mission is doing. Our vegetable oil project, therefore, aims to create the cooperatives, and we are very fortunate that we got the donation of oil from the cooperatives of Canada and the United States to the value of some $400 million, which we sell in India, generate funds, which we use to create cooperatives. At the moment we have about 500,000 farmers organized into cooperatives, and we have about twelve large oil mills already working.

But then, of course, there are many powerful interests who are opposed to this project. I think so far five of our officers are dead. An oil mill, a cooperative oil mill, has been burned seven or eight times. But this is all normal in trying to bring about change. It is not a very easy thing to change existing structures and to erect new structures.

Coming to salt. The salt project became of interest to us only because the state of Gujarat, where Anand is located, has one-third of the coastline of India. You know, if you take that coastline and straighten it out, it becomes one-third, and this state produces 60 percent of the salt of India.

One day, the chairman of one of our district cooperatives for milk came and met me. After we finished with milk, he began to talk about the plight of those who are producing the salt, the "salt farmers," as they are called.

Each salt farmer had two hectares of land, and he and his family work on that two hectares farming salt for ten months of the year. They make a hole in the ground. The salt water comes in and, during the other two months, it is dry but the water is down below. You make a hole, pump it out, and fill up the salt pans and allow the sun to evaporate them, and move the water with diesel pumps from one pan to another, as it gets concentrated. He explained the plight of these people and their children.

There is not a single tree there because it is a desert. The children have no education. There is no electricity. They work ten months of the year and at the end of it they produce the salt, and they are paid the equivalent of 2 cents of a rupee per kilo for the salt; out of which one cent they have to pay back to the salt merchant for the water he has supplied them for drinking, for the diesel he has supplied them, and for the credit he has supplied them. So all they are left with is one cent of a rupee per kilo of salt, and the price of a kilo of salt in the marketplace is the equivalent of 75 cents of a rupee.

He started weeping as he explained the plight of these farmers and he said, "When they die, and they die young, and when you burn their bodies, the feet cannot be burned because they are impregnated with salt and they don't burn." And then he went on to say, "This is the free India after forty years. And Mahatma Gandhi's symbolic gesture of picking up salt in defiance of British exploitation, and today what is happening? This is what is happening in salt," and he wept.

I said, "Get up from here! Why must you come here and weep? Am I here to solve all the problems of the world? I have enough problems of my own. Please, out! You go somewhere else and weep!"

But I heard two days later that he died in an accident and so that made it necessary for us to look at salt. And so now we are creating salt farmers' cooperatives to purchase the salt, to provide them the diesel. And then we say, why diesel? Why not solar pump, energy-based pumps? Why not voltaic cells to provide them light? Why not better marketing of the salt? Can't we make pumps that will run on the electricity which we can generate with voltaic cells, and so on?

So the whole of this movement is begun and the big salt merchants are very upset, and god knows what will happen. So we are working on it. In the first year we handled 15,000 tons of salt; this year, 100,000 tons of salt. Already we have pushed up the earnings of salt for the farmer from 2 cents to 6 cents, and already there are things happening. That is our salt project.

We have put a plan into effect to iodize salt because it is considered to be desirable to do so and some laws are being passed that only iodized salt can be sold, and we want to sell.

Alan Berg: Iron and iodine at the same time?

Verghese Kurien: Yes, probably.

Alan Berg: That's the new technology?

Verghese Kurien: Yes, probably you're right. Yes. But we are still at the fringes of this project and breaking our teeth on it. There are too many problems. But what is interesting is that such exploitation of man, such gross exploitation of man, takes place in India even today. That is what is shown.

John Mellor: It was quite clear in Dr. Kurien's presentation last night, I think this is fair to say, that you take the importance of technology as a given but you march on from there.

I wonder if we could turn to Dr. Sadikin to push us more in the technology direction, since that was very essential in your paper. We probably should come back to the technology issue.

S. W. Sadikin: I don't feel very comfortable to talk in this room among so many economists.

John Mellor: You shouldn't feel so discomforted.

S. W. Sadikin: From the discussion yesterday about the threat to increased food production, there are some disturbing trends. It is not only in the technology but also in the institutional field and in the economic field.

I will give you one example, coming back to my topic of rice production in Indonesia. There are some complaints lately among farmers that there is a declining trend of profitability in rice farming. Even while we now apply modern technologies and advanced technologies, the profitability of rice farming seems to be declining, especially when it is compared with the profit from, say, soybean growing, or corn growing, or vegetable growing. Is it true that rice is the most expensive grain to produce? I wonder whether there are plans or programs at IFPRI to study the ways to lower the cost of production of rice. Maybe you can have a cooperative project with IRRI to lower the cost of production of rice so that you can improve the profitability of rice farming in many places in the world. In the last year, it has gotten to be a serious problem in Indonesia. I don't know what all the implications are and the impact of this on the sustainability or self-sufficiency of rice production in Indonesia.

John Mellor: I would like to make a brief response to that and then open this up for other comments.

I think that, on the one hand, we can see tremendous increases in farm incomes arising from these other kinds of agriculture, other than the basic staples, such as the cereals, rice, and so on. This is shown in the tremendous strides in marketing that Dr. Kurien and his colleagues are making in the livestock area, dairy in particular. We see the same thing in the extremely interesting paper on Chile dealing with the horticultural area. I think that particularly for the relatively lower-income countries of Asia and certainly in Africa a number of us at IFPRI are very concerned with what we see as a slackening in the rate of progress of cost-decreasing technology.

I would say that the really exciting thing about the IR8 rice variety was not just that it allowed a lot more rice to be produced but it allowed rice to be produced at a much lower cost than previously. And that brought, in some ways, the complaint that it wasn't the highest quality rice. IR8 is not quite Basmati rice, I think it is fair to say. It was criticized somewhat for that, but that was one of the beauties of it, that it was very cheap rice and that it was a great boon to lower-income people.

I would like to make just two or three quick responses to what you said. One, I think that we are putting out far too complex instructions to the biological scientists for what they have to do. Bob Chandler, you may think this is putting it too simply. But my impression is that you set a relatively simple task for the people you brought to IRRI when you were the founding director, and that was to double or triple the yield of rice. And you didn't complicate it with environmental issues, and you didn't say to do it in the worst rice-growing areas and not in the good rice-growing areas. You didn't worry a great deal about the quality in that first round. It is a simple, straightforward job, and the biological scientists went out there, and they did it. Well, obviously as time goes on, the task has to become somewhat more complicated.

But perhaps we have been complicating it too rapidly relative to the needs of poorer people in the world, and so we are not making as much progress now in pushing down that cost of producing rice.

Bob, I think I'm correct in saying that IRRI has really not succeeded in pushing rice yields up, their maximum yields up, significantly from the old IR8. Now, I want to add to that. The work that Mark Rosegrant is doing on Indonesia and the Philippines, and that Gunvant Desai is doing on India — both of IFPRI, I should add — is very much keyed to this issue of the cost of production and the institutional and technological factors that are involved in that. In both cases we are very much concerned, perhaps particularly on the Indian side, that the cost of production is not declining.

I would just like to close that comment by saying that we must not forget that what the farmer is concerned with is the profitability of what he produces. And, yes, pushing up the price for their rice increases profitability; but pushing down the cost of production through improved technology also boosts profitability and increases incentives. And the latter is very good for poor people, and the former is decidedly not.

Robert Chandler: There is no question that the yield potential of IR8 is as high as IRRI has obtained or anybody else has obtained, as far as I know.

John Mellor: And that's bad, right?

Robert Chandler: That is the yield potential, forgetting quality. But we have improved quality, we have improved disease and insect resistance. We've got more stable yields than we had in the early days.

Looking at Indonesia's problem, yesterday Mr. Sadikin in his talk mentioned that at the beginning of the Green Revolution they had 85,000 tons of urea in use and this went up to 4 million tons of urea used. I would think the Indonesians might be concerned with the cost of production, and might want to look at whether or not they are using too much fertilizer. They may have on that curve diminishing returns.

In the early days of IRRI, Randy Barker showed that during the wet season, as far as nitrogen is concerned, you shouldn't go over 60 kg per hectare in the wet season, and never more than 120 in the dry. Even though you might get yield responses higher than that, it was not economical. When it comes to using insecticides, they found that they got a good yield increase by using insecticides but it was not a benefit because insecticides cost too much. They have got to get the price down before they can do it.

Well, that is the type of thing I think you have to look at: What is the cost of growing? I think saving nitrogen, achieving nitrogen efficiency, is going to be a very important thing because you are losing a lot by volatilization and poor application. Those are some of the things that you have to look at and I think you are absolutely right, reduce the cost of production but maintain stable high yields.

John Mellor: One thing that we are working on at IFPRI that I think is very relevant is looking at the returns to training and education, including secondary education of rural people, as it relates to these kinds of issues.

I was on a panel in the last few days, that involved heads of major farm organizations in this country. There were two farmers on the panel talking about exactly this issue, how much less nitrogen they were using now than four or five years ago.

When I look at the problems in developing countries, I am appalled at the complexity of the technologies being used to get those nitrogen levels down. It takes a very sophisticated extension service and soil testing service and so on. These farmers emphasized they were not raising their costs; rather, they are reducing their costs but this involves very complex systems, and obviously this has to be the wave of the future in developing countries. But someone has got to get cracking on education and training to push ahead on that.

Robert Chandler: One more comment and then I'll stop. In the seven different studies that IRRI made a few years ago of unit costs in several areas of Asia, in which they were studying the factors associated with increased yields, they found that two things were common to all. One was irrigation and the other was the degree of education of the farmer.

Robert Herdt: One big source of productivity increase has been the reduction in the duration of the crop, of the rice crop. So that while traditional varieties were of long duration, IR8 was only moderately long. The newer varieties were not higher yielding, but they stay in the ground a shorter time, they use less water, they are less exposed to pests, and so the cost of producing a kilogram is lower.

Another factor is the reduction in pesticide application to get that maximum yield. Farmers no longer have to apply a pesticide for most pests because there is a built-in resistance to those pests. And so there have been significant gains in reducing these costs, even though, as Bob Chandler has said, the maximum yield you could get has not gone higher than IR8.

Raymond Meyer: Let me raise a few other issues that merit attention. I think the depth of knowledge we have regarding the natural resource systems in these countries is tremendously less than what we have with respect to the crop systems. And I think this is extremely important from the standpoint of carrying capacity. What we know about carrying capacity I think is very minimal. A lot of it is erroneous because we don't know enough about the natural resource system. By natural resource system I mean the soil, water, and climatic resources.

I am reminded of something I heard a year ago that John Mellor said, that one of the major needs is stability of production. Well, how do you deal with a case like Sudan where you go from a million tons shortfall to a million tons excess in one year? And that is the norm in rainfed agriculture, that is what you can expect. I think Dr. Singh hinted at this yesterday. I recall something Uma Lele of the World Bank said about a year ago, that a major cause of failure in Africa is due to the fact that we are making policy recommendations without understanding the natural resource constraints. And, if you are looking for a need for information, I think this is where it is. It is understanding the natural resource constraints, the natural resource system.

This is very relevant to the institutions issue, too, because data needed for natural resource management is much more site specific. You can't deal easily with crop commodities across disparate areas. And we aren't making the effort in this.

I only have to look at the international agriresearch centers to see how little emphasis they are putting on soil and water resources as compared to commodities. My estimation in U.S. AID, for instance, is that we are putting less than $1 million a year into really understanding the basic soil and water systems in Africa. And I think that is appalling because I think that is where the need is. If we are really interested in looking at this, I think we have to get back to some of the basic understanding of soil and water and climatic resource systems.

Barbara Huddleston: I just would like to say that FAO does have a substantial amount of knowledge on this issue in its Land and Water Division, and has done work on the population-supporting capacity of different soils and different ecological environments. But I think that the point is very well taken in that we see, even within the discussions that we have at FAO on these issues, that available knowledge does not feed into the policymaking process adequately, especially with regard to production strategy or decisions about crop mix.

In other words, when we are doing analysis of domestic resource costs of different crops and evaluating crop mix, the question of the soil and the water base, of the natural resource capacity for those different crops, is not adequately fed into the process of thinking through the strategies. I think this is where the lack is. And as you say, it is location specific and it forces the policymaker to go to a level of disaggregation that policymakers don't normally like to go to.

John Mellor: I would like to ask Dr. Kurien to comment on the education issue.

Verghese Kurien: Considering the magnitude of Operation Flood, as well as the other related projects we are now launching, like oil seeds, like fruits and vegetables, like the greening of India, like rural rationing distribution systems, one of the principal constraints in implementing projects of this magnitude is the shortage of managerial personnel.

As you are aware, agriculture has never been considered to be a prestigious occupation in our country. And those who work in the field of agriculture are not considered to be doing something that is as glamorous as working in other fields. And agriculture did not, until recently, attract the very brightest of our youth to work in that field. The result has been that we were not able to command, or obtain, or tempt the finest of our youths to work in the agricultural field.

And all this surfaced very quickly when we found we had to run large commercially-oriented schemes, like large dairy plants, large procurement systems, large vegetable oil mills.

One of the deficiencies was in the field of management of these plants. To emphasize this still further, it is somehow prestigious to work for a multinational company manufacturing shampoo in Bombay, though manufacturing shampoo is a triviality in the context of India. It is not prestigious, however, to work in a dairy cooperative. So these were some of the problems that we had.

And, therefore, one of the solutions we came up with is to set up an Institute of Rural Management in Anand, an institute specially created in order to provide us with 100 new managers every year.

We offer a management course of two-year duration in which we take in graduates of all disciplines, including engineering, agriculture, veterinary science, dairy technology, and including chartered accountants, arts, science, and marketing people — a whole blend of graduates who have been admitted. The role of this management institute was new. We also agreed that we would pay for the student's education, that education at the Institute would be free, provided the students agree to work as employees of farmers for three years after graduation.

Therefore, we got as many as 10,000 applications for 100 places. So we were able to attract to this the finest of the youth of India. And, then, having attracted them, we had to set up a faculty, mostly basing their courses on management courses, but insisting that these students spend 40 percent of their time in the villages trying to understand rural society, and trying to understand the problems of rural India, and at the same time training them to become good managers of industrial enterprises.

And so the gap in top managerial cadres, hopefully, will be solved through this management institute. At the same time, we have had a whole series of short-duration courses for middle-level management to orient them towards their tasks and teach them how to handle certain specific tasks better.

We have had a farmer induction program and farmer training hostels set up in order to bring farmers from all over India to Anand, put them through a four-day orientation course so that they would begin to understand what a cooperative is, what are the rights as a member of a cooperative, what are the things they should insist upon as a member of the cooperative.

From farmers to supervisors, from middle management to top management, a whole series of management training courses has to be set up not only in this institute but all over India.

And India has a fortunate situation, a large education base, a large number of institutions of technical and scientific agriculture, and so on. So we have a large base to draw from. So the Institute has served to invite and draw people into this field and get them trained to shoulder these massive enterprises.

Without this educational program, and most importantly the program of educating the farmers, for which we have to use all sorts of technologies, including audio-visual programs and all the rest that goes into it, our cooperative enterprises could not have met with the success they have.

I am very glad somebody mentioned the importance of training and education, and it has to be with farmers all the way through to top management.

John Mellor: Dr. Sadikin, for a last comment.

S. W. Sadikin: We have some experience with the training of farmers. As I said yesterday, the participation of children in the schools of Indonesia has more or less doubled. I remember the difficulties we had in 1967–68 when we tried to introduce modern ideas and also to introduce the use of pesticides to illiterates. The pesticides had to be diluted with water, and the ratio of dilution was very, very hard to explain to the farmers. Now twenty years or so later, we have to talk with farmers about the ability to control the brown planthopper using modern plant varieties. In fact, every year we come with a new variety to the farmer, and this requires an explanation of the possibilities of the emergence of new biotypes. You can talk to the farmers more easily today because they are better educated, they are better trained now. I think the increased participation in the primary schools— now 90 percent—has helped a great deal.

That's the big difference as compared with twenty years ago. Farmers now even talk about the recycling of old varieties. I was amazed to hear this from a farmer. "Why not recycle the old variety?" This idea comes from an ordinary farmer, but he is better trained than his father or grandfather of twenty years ago. There is tremendous progress made in education and training in the rural areas. That's our experience in Asia.

John Mellor: Thank you very much. I think we have to end this roundtable discussion. It has proven to be very productive. I want to thank Dr. Kurien in particular for taking the time to be with us when I know there are many other heavy demands on his time, particularly during this week. And I would like to thank Dr. Chandler and all the other participants for joining with us. We are especially grateful to our overseas participants who travelled so far to join us here today. Their participation in the colloquium yesterday and in this morning's discussion has been invaluable. So thank you all very much.

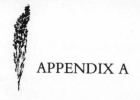

APPENDIX A

Colloquium Program, October 17, 1989

9:00 AM   Welcoming Remarks

Robert McC. Adams, Secretary, Smithsonian Institution
A. S. Clausi, Chairman, Council of Advisors, The World Food Prize

9:30 AM–12:30 PM   Morning Panel: *Perspectives on Agriculture, Food Policy, and Rural Economic Development*

Ojetunji Aboyade, Chairman, Presidential Advisory Committee, Lagos, Nigeria
"Perspectives on African Food Policy and Agricultural Development in the 1990s: A Nigerian Perspective"
Justin Yifu Lin, Deputy Director, The Development Institute, Research Center for Rural Development, Beijing, China
"Farming Institutions, Food Policy, and Agricultural Development in China"
[Paper presented by Zhigang Chen, Group of Rural Economic Research, Économie Rurale, Université Laval, Quebec, Canada]
Bruce Stone, Project Director for Chinese Research, International Food Policy Research Institute, Washington, D.C.
"Evolution and Diffusion of Agricultural Technology in China"
R. P. Singh, Director, Central Research Institute for Dryland Agriculture, Hyderabad, India
"Dryland/Rainfed Agriculture and Water Resources Management Research and Development in India"
Discussants:
Robert W. Herdt, Director, Agricultural Sciences, The Rockefeller Foundation, New York, New York

Thomas R. Odhiambo, Director, International Centre of Insect Physiology and Ecology, Nairobi, Kenya

Michael Lipton, Program Director, Food Consumption and Nutrition Policy Research Program, International Food Policy Research Institute, Washington, D.C.

Moderator: Barbara Huddleston, Chief, Food Security Service, Food and Agriculture Organization of the United Nations, Rome, Italy

12:30 PM   Luncheon

2:00 PM–4:30 PM   Afternoon Panel: *Innovations in Agricultural Research, Technology, Trade, and Food Policy*

S. W. Sadikin, Director General Emeritus, Indonesian Agency for Agricultural Research and Development, Bogor, Indonesia
"The Diffusion of Agricultural Research Knowledge and Advances in Rice Production in Indonesia"

Calister N. Mtalo, National Program Coordinator, Joint WHO/UNICEF Nutrition Support Program, Iringa, Tanzania
"The Iringa Integrated Nutrition Program in Tanzania: Research and Development"

Anthony Wylie, Director General, Fundación Chile, Santiago, Chile
"Agricultural Development and Technology: The Growth of Chile's Fruit and Vegetable Export Industry"

Discussants:

Per Pinstrup-Andersen, Director, Cornell Food and Nutrition Policy Program, Cornell University, Ithaca, New York

Michael Lipton, Program Director, Food Consumption and Nutrition Policy Research Program, International Food Policy Research Institute, Washington, D.C.

Alberto Valdés, Director, International Trade and Food Security Program, International Food Policy Research Institute, Washington, D.C.

Moderator: Robert D. Havener, President, Winrock International Institute for Agricultural Development, Morrilton, Arkansas

4:45 PM–5:15 PM   Summation

Barbara Huddleston, Food and Agriculture Organization of the United Nations, Rome, Italy

6:30 PM   The World Food Prize Award Ceremony, Baird Auditorium, National Museum of Natural History

Verghese Kurien
World Food Prize Laureate, 1989
Acceptance Address

7:30 PM   Buffet Reception

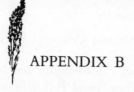

APPENDIX B

Biographical Notes on Contributors

Ojetunji Aboyade

Ojetunji Aboyade, chairman, Presidential Advisory Committee, Federal Republic of Nigeria. Educated at Hull University (A.B., economic science) and Pembroke College, Cambridge University (Ph.D., economics). Professor of economics at the University of Ibadan (1966–81) and vice-chancellor of the University of Ife (1975–79). Head of National Economic Planning, Federal Ministry of Economic Development and Reconstruction (1969–70). Publications include: "Growth Strategy and the Agricultural Sector," in *Accelerating Food Production Growth in Sub-Saharan Africa*, ed. by John W. Mellor, Christopher Delgado, and Malcolm J. Blackie (1987); "Administering Food Producer Prices in Africa: Lessons from International Experiences," *IFPRI Report* (1985); *Integrated Economics: A Study of Developing Economies* (1983); *Issues in the Development of Tropical Africa* (1976); "Income Distribution and Economic Power," *Nigerian Journal of Economic and Social Studies* (1975); *Foundations of an African Economy: Study of Investment and Growth in Nigeria* (1966); *Capital Formation in Nigeria* (1960). Member, Council of African Advisors, World Bank (1987–). Founding member of the board of trustees, International Food Policy Research Institute. Honored as a Groves Prizeman, Commander of the Order of Niger, and as a fellow of the Nigerian Economic Society. Born in Awe, Oyo State, 1931. Address: PAI Associates International, 25 Osuntokun Avenue, P.O. Box 2681, Bodija Estate, Ibadan, Nigeria.

Robert F. Chandler, Jr.

Robert F. Chandler, Jr., founding director, International Rice Research Institute, the Philippines. Educated at the University of Maine and the University of Maryland (Ph.D., 1934). Held several posts at the Rockefeller Foundation: as associate director for agricultural sciences; assistant director, natural science and agriculture; soil scientist with the Mexican Agricultural Program. Directed the Asian Vegetable Research and Development Center in Taiwan. Served as dean of the College of Agriculture and as president of the University of New Hampshire. Professor of forest soils at Cornell University; state horticulturist at the Maine State Department of Agriculture. Author of *An Adventure in Applied Research: A History of the International Rice Research Institute* (1982); *Rice in the Tropics: A Guide to Development of National Programs* (1979); and *Forest Soils*, with Harold J. Lutz (1946), along with some sixty articles in professional and trade journals. Recipient, World Food Prize (1988), U.S. Presidential End Hunger Award (1986), Special Award of the Republic of China (1975), International Agronomy Award (1972), Golden Heart of the Republic of the Philippines (1972), Star of Merit of the Republic of Indonesia (1972), Star of Distinction Award of the Government of Pakistan (1968), and Gold Medal of the Government of India (1966). Awarded eight honorary degrees from universities throughout the world. Born in Columbus, Ohio, 1907. Address: P.O. Box 852, Raymond, ME 04071.

Zhigang Chen

Zhigang Chen, agricultural economist, Group of Rural Economic Research, Économie Rurale, Université Laval. Educated at Zhejiang Agricultural University, Hangzhou, China (B.A., economics, 1982), University of Maryland (M.S., agricultural and resource economics, 1987), and the Université Laval. Recipient of a Ford Foundation Fellowship (1988); research assistant, International Food Policy Research Institute (1988); and teaching and research assistant, Department of Economics and Management, Zhejiang Agricultural University (1982–85). Coauthor, with Peter Calkins, of "Rural Credit System in China: Lessons for Rural Development," research report to Société de Développement International Desjardins (1989), and coauthor, with Peter Calkins, "Applied Econometric Analysis of Dahe Data Set," research report to the Ford Foundation (1988). Born in Zhejiang, China, 1963. Address: Group of Rural Economic Research, Économie Rurale, Université Laval, #4320 Pavillion Comtoir, Quebec GIK 7P4, Canada.

Robert D. Havener

Robert D. Havener, president and chief executive officer, Winrock International Institute for Agricultural Development. Educated at Ohio State University (B.S. and M.Sc., agriculture, animal science, and agricultural economics) and the Kennedy School of Government, Harvard University (M.P.A., 1972). Former director general, Centro Internacional de Mejoramiento de Maiz y Trigo (CIMMYT), Mexico. Served at the Ford Foundation as director of the Arid Lands Agricultural Development Program (ALAD) in Lebanon (1972–76); project development officer at the International Center for Agricultural Research in Dry Areas (ICARDA) in Syria (1975–76); and program advisor on agriculture, Asia and Pacific region (1976–78). Held positions as county agricultural agent, state extension specialist, county manager with the Ohio Farm Bureau Cooperatives, merchandising manager with two meat packing firms, and served on the staff of Michigan State University. Served on the boards of trustees of ICARDA, IRRI, CIMMYT, the International Agricultural Development Service (IADS), Honduran Agricultural Research Foundation, and International Development Conference. Served as an agricultural advisor in Bangladesh and Pakistan. Numerous papers presented at international conferences include: "Analysis of a Successful Livestock Project" (1988), "Emerging Domestic and International Issues in Agriculture" (1987), "Food Production in the Third World: Implications for U.S. Agriculture" (1986), and "Strengthening National Agricultural Research Organizations: Some Lessons Learned by CIMMYT" (1984). Born in London, Ohio, 1930. Address: Winrock International, Route 3, Morrilton, AR 72110.

Robert W. Herdt

Robert W. Herdt, director of agricultural sciences, the Rockefeller Foundation. Educated at Cornell University (B.S. and M.S., agriculture and agricultural economics) and the University of Minnesota (Ph.D., agricultural economics, 1969). Visiting fellow and adjunct professor at Cornell University (1981–). Served as senior economist, Agricultural Sciences Division, the Rockefeller Foundation (1986–87); scientific advisor, Consultative Group on International Agricultural Research (1983–86); agricultural economist and head, Economics Department, International Rice Research Institute (1973–83); professor, Agricultural Economics Department, University of Illinois (1969–75); agricultural economist with the Rockefeller Foundation serving at the Indian Agricultural Research Institute (1967–68); training associate in India with the Ford Foundation's Intensive Agricultural District Program (1962–64). Consultant to governments and international institutions. Coauthor, with Jock Anderson and Grant Scobie, of *Science and Food: The CGIAR and Its Partners* (1988); with Randolph Barker, *The Rice Economy of Asia* (1985); with L.L. Castillo and S.K. Jayasuriya, "The Economics of Insect Control on Rice in the Philippines," in *Judicious and Efficient Use of Insecticides on Rice* (1984); with Celia Capule, *Adoption, Spread and Production Impact of Modern Rice Varieties in Asia* (1983); with S.K. Ray and R.W. Cummings, Jr., *Policy Planning for Agricultural Development* (1979); and with W.W. Wilcox and W.W. Cochran, *The Economics of American Agriculture* (1974). Associate editor, *American Journal of Agricultural Economics*. Born in Glen Cove, New York, 1939. Address: Agricultural Sciences, the Rockefeller Foundation, 1133 Avenue of the Americas, New York, NY 10036.

Barbara Huddleston

Barbara Huddleston, chief, Food Security Service, Commodities and Trade Division, Food and Agriculture Organization of the United Nations (FAO). Educated at the College of Wooster (B.A., 1961), the Johns Hopkins School of Advanced International Studies (M.A., 1963), and George Washington University (M.Phil., 1975). Supervises FAO's Food Security Assistance Scheme and the Committee on World Food Security. Involved in food aid, food insurance, and food security programs in developing nations: as a research fellow, the International Food Policy Research Institute; as an economist with the Africa Division, U.S. Department of Commerce; and as an economist and director of Trade Negotiations Division, U.S. Department of Agriculture. Coeditor, with Charles P. Mann, of *Food Policy—Frameworks for Analysis and Action* (1985). Author, *Closing the Cereals Gap with Trade and Food Aid* (1984); and coauthor, with D. Gale Johnson, Shlomo Reutlinger, and Alberto Valdés, *International Finance for Food Security* (1984). Member, international editorial board, *Food Policy*. Has served on the editorial council, *American Journal of Agricultural Economics*. A consultant to the U.S. Presidential Commission on World Hunger, the Rockefeller Foundation, the Agriculture Development Council, the American Universities Field Service, and the World Food Council of the United Nations. Born in Malone, New York, 1939. Address: Food and Agriculture Organization, ESCF, Via delle Terme di Caracalla, Rome 00100, Italy.

Verghese Kurien

Verghese Kurien, chairman of the National Dairy Development Board, Anand, India. Educated at Madras University (B.S., 1940; B.E., 1943); Tata Iron and Steel Company Technical Institute in Jamshedpur (1946); and Michigan State University (M.S., mechanical engineering, 1948). Has held numerous positions in dairy, agricultural, and industrial management and development, the cooperative sector, agricultural and rural education, regional planning, and in government. Chairman of the board of governors, Institute of Rural Management, Anand, India; chairman, Gujarat Cooperative Milk Marketing Federation; executive chairman, Animal Husbandry and Dairy Development Council of Gujarat; chairman, National Cooperative Dairy Federation of India; member of the Central Advisory Council on Trade, Ministry of Commerce, of the National Wastelands Development Board of the Ministry of Environment and Forests, and of the Advisory Council for 20-Point Program Implementation. Chaired the Gujarat Electricity Board, the Protein Foods and Nutrition Development Association of India, the Development Council for Food Processing Industries, the Gujarat State Cooperative Cotton Marketing Federation, and the India Dairy Science Association. Served as a director of the Reserve Bank of India and of the Industrial Development Bank of India. Recipient of numerous awards, including the Padmashree and Padmabhushan Awards by the President of India; the Ramon Magsaysay Award for Community Leadership; the Carnegie Foundation Wateler Peace Prize; the Krishi Ratna Award for service to the farming community; the Silver Jubilee Award of the India Society of Agricultural Engineers; and the National Integration Award of the Indian Chamber of Commerce. Holder of honorary degrees from Michigan State University, University of Glasgow, Acadia University and Ottawa University in Canada, Anna University in Madras, and the University of New England in Australia. Born in Calicut, Kerala, India, 1921. Address: National Dairy Development Board, Anand 388 001, India.

Justin Yifu Lin

Justin Yifu Lin, deputy director, The Development Institute, the State Council of the People's Republic of China. Educated at Peking (Beijing) University (M.A., Marxist economics, 1982) and at The University of Chicago (Ph.D., economics, 1986). Associate professor of economics, Beijing University (1987–), and visiting associate professor of economics, UCLA (1989–90). Head of the Department of Economic Growth Studies at

RCRD (1987); special assistant to the Chinese University Development Project II (1987); consultant to the World Bank (1987-). Thirty published articles include: "Agricultural Credit and Farm Performance in China," *Journal of Comparative Economics* (forthcoming); "The Major Economic Issues and the Way Out in China's Economy," *Zhongguo: Gaige Yu Fazhan* (1989); "On the Rational Sequences and Breakthrough Point of Economic Reform in China," *Jingji Shehui Tizhi Bijiao* (1989); "Small Peasant and Economic Rationality," *Nongcun Jingji yu Shehui* (1988); "Technology Innovation in China: A Study of Public Research Fund Allocation in a Socialist Economy," Development Institute working paper (1989); and "The Household Responsibility System Reform in China: A Peasant's Institutional Choice," *American Journal of Agricultural Economics* (1987). Recipient of a postdoctoral fellowship, the Rockefeller Foundation (1986–87); and a postdoctoral fellowship, Economic Growth Center, Yale University (1986–87). Has lectured in many nations, including Bangladesh, Thailand, India, and the Philippines. Born in 1952. Address: The Development Institute, State Council of the PRC, 5 Liuliqiao Beili, Beijing 100055, China.

Michael Lipton

Michael Lipton, program director, Food Consumption and Nutrition Policy Research Program, International Food Policy Research Institute. Educated at Balliol College and at All Souls College, Oxford University (B.A., 1960; M.A., 1979); Massachusetts Institute of Technology; and Sussex University (D.Litt., 1982). Professorial fellow, Institute of Developmental Studies, Sussex University (on leave); fellow, All Souls College; director, Village Studies Programme and Grain Storage Project. Lecturer and reader in economics, Sussex University. Publications include: *Effectiveness of Aid to India* (in press); *New Seeds and Poor People* (1989); "The Place of Agricultural Research in the Development of Sub-Saharan Africa," *World Development*, 16, 10 (1988); *Migration from Rural Areas: The Evidence from Village Studies* (1977); *Why Poor People Stay Poor: Urban Bias and World Development* (1977; 1989); *The Crisis of Indian Planning* (1968); *Assessing Economic Performance* (1968). Served as senior policy adviser, the World Bank, and as employment development adviser to the Government of Botswana. Has conducted research in several nations of Asia and Africa, and has served as a consultant to international organizations. Former managing editor, *Journal of Development Studies*. Recipient of the Jenkyns Prize and George Webb Medley Prize, Oxford University, and a Rockefeller Foundation fellowship. Born in England, 1937. Address: International Food Policy Research Institute, 1776 Massachusetts Avenue, N.W., Washington, D.C. 20036.

John W. Mellor

John W. Mellor, director, International Food Policy Research Institute, Washington, D.C. Educated at Cornell University (B.Sc., 1950; M.Sc., 1951; Ph.D., 1954) and Oxford University. Previously chief economist, U.S. Agency for International Development; professor of economics, agricultural economics, and Asian studies, Cornell. Author, *The Economics of Agricultural Development* (1966); *The New Economics of Growth: A Strategy for India and the Developing World* (1976), a detailed statement of his concept of an agriculture- and employment-led strategy of growth; and numerous other publications. Edited and contributed chapters to: with G.M. Desai, *Agricultural Change and Rural Poverty: Variations on a Theme by Dharm Narain* (1985); with C. Delgado and M. Blackie, *Accelerating Food Production Growth in Sub-Saharan Africa* (1987); and with R. Ahmed, *Agricultural Price Policy for Developing Countries* (1988). Contributing editor, *Environment*. Fellow, American Academy of Arts and Sciences, American Agricultural Economics Association. Member, board of directors, Overseas Development Council. Recipient of U.S. Presidential End Hunger Award (1987), Wihuri Foundation International Prize (1985)—the first social scientist so honored—and American Agricultural Economics Association awards (1967, 1978, and 1986) for publications and research. Address: International Food Policy Research Institute, 1776 Massachusetts Avenue, N.W., Washington, D.C. 20036.

Calister N. Mtalo

Calister N. Mtalo, national coordinator, Joint WHO/UNICEF Nutrition Support Programme (JNSP), Iringa Region, United Republic of Tanzania. JNSP is a program of community-based health, nutrition, education, and economic development services reaching an estimated 50,000 young children in 62 villages. Regarded as an international standard for programs of its kind, JNSP has been credited with significant reductions in malnutrition and child mortality, and in successfully mobilizing the participation of villagers. Educated at the University of Dar es Salaam (B.A., management and administration, 1975; post-graduate diploma, regional development planning, 1980) and at ISS, The Hague, the Netherlands (master's degree, regional development planning, 1982). Served as regional planning officer in Iringa region (1983–84) and as an economist with the Regional Planning Office, Morogoro Region (1975–81). Secretary, National Coordinating Committee for Child Survival and Development. Has lectured widely in Rome, Italy; Wageningen, the Netherlands; Geneva, Switzerland; Awassa,

Ethiopia; Nairobi, Kenya; and in Bulgaria. Publications and papers include: "Community-Based Health Care Project: Case Study of Iringa JNSP" (1989); "The Iringa Nutrition Programme and the Social Mobilisation Process" (1987); "The Implementation of the Iringa Nutrition Programme" (1986); "An Evaluation of the Five-Year Development Plan for Morogoro District" (1980). Born in Moshi, Tanzania, 1951. Address: Joint Nutrition Support Programme, P.O. Box 413, Iringa, Tanzania.

Thomas R. Odhiambo

Thomas R. Odhiambo, director, International Centre of Insect Physiology and Ecology; president, African Academy of Sciences. Educated at Makerere College, Kampala, Uganda, and Cambridge University (B.A., M.A., Ph.D.). Research has focused on natural history and insect endocrinology, particularly in relation to insect reproductive biology, on which more than 100 papers have been written. Has taught at the University of Nairobi since 1965; was first professor of entomology, head of the newly established Department of Entomology, and first dean of the Faculty of Agriculture. Was a visiting professor at universities in Africa and India. Founder and editor-in-chief of book series, "Current Themes in Tropical Science"; publisher and editor-in-chief, Scientific Editorial Services, of journal *Insect Science and Its Application*. Appointed in 1967 by UNESCO as consultant on entomology and applied biology. Cofounder and member of the board of trustees, International Federation of Institutes for Advanced Study. Founder of East African Academy of Sciences; fellow, Kenya National Academy of Sciences, Third World Academy of Sciences, Indian National Academy of Sciences, Italian National Academy of the 40s, Pontifical Academy of Sciences, and Royal Norwegian Academy of Science and Letters. Member of international jury, UNESCO Science Prize; member of Club of Rome. Recipient, African Hunger Prize (1987) and Albert Einstein Medal (1979). Born in Mombasa, Kenya, 1931. Address: International Centre of Insect Physiology and Ecology, P.O. Box 30772, Nairobi, Kenya.

Per Pinstrup-Andersen

Per Pinstrup-Andersen, professor of food economics in the Division of Nutritional Sciences and director of the Cornell Food and Nutrition Policy Program, Cornell University. Educated at the Royal Veterinary and Agricultural University, Copenhagen, Denmark (B.S., agricultural economics,

1965) and Oklahoma State University (M.S., 1967; Ph.D., agricultural economics, 1969). Research fellow and director of the Food Consumption and Nutrition Policy Research Program, International Food Policy Research Institute (1980–87); senior research fellow and associate professor, Economic Institute, Royal Veterinary and Agricultural University (1977–80); and agricultural economist at the Centro Internacional de Agricultura Tropical in Cali, Colombia (1969–76). Publications include: coauthor, with Marito Garcia, of "The Pilot Food Price Subsidy Scheme in the Philippines: Its Impact on Income, Food Consumption, and Nutritional Status," *IFPRI Report* (1987); coeditor, with Margaret Biswas, *Nutrition and Development* (1985); coeditor, with Alan Berg and Martin Forman, *International Agricultural Research and Human Nutrition* (1984); *Agricultural Research and Technology in Economic Development* (1982); and coeditor, with Francis C. Byrnes, *Methods for Allocating Resources in Applied Agricultural Research in Latin America* (1975). Consultant to national programs, international institutions, and governments, including: the World Bank, the United Nations, and the Rockefeller Foundation. Chairs the food policy committee of the International Union of Nutrition Sciences (1983–). Born in Bislev, Denmark, 1939. Address: Division of Nutritional Sciences, Savage Hall, Cornell University, Ithaca, NY 14853.

Suminta Wikarta Sadikin

Suminta Wikarta Sadikin, director general emeritus, Indonesian Agency for Agricultural Research and Development. Educated at the Agricultural School in Bogor and in the Faculty of Agriculture, University of Indonesia. Served as director of Bogor's Agricultural School; agronomist at the Soil Research Institute; director of the Academy of Agriculture; director of the Botanical Gardens of Indonesia; director of research institutes of the Ministry of Agriculture, spanning research from forestry to animal production to marine fisheries; special assistant to the Minister of Agriculture; director general of agriculture, overseeing the introduction of high-yielding rice varieties; chairman of the National Seed Board; and president commissioner of the government plantations of coffee, tea, cocoa, clove, cinchona, coconut, and rubber. Former president of the International Federation of Agricultural Research Systems for Development (IFARD). Member of the board of trustees, International Service for National Agricultural Research (ISNAR). Senior associate, Winrock International Institute for Agricultural Development. Indonesia's chief delegate to the Food and Agriculture Organization of the United Nations (1968–72); and chaired the ASEAN Permanent Committee on Food and Agriculture (1969–71). Served on the board of trustees of the International Rice Research Institute and as a member of the Technical Advisory Council, Consultative Group on International Agricultural Research. Honors include: Satyalencana Karya Satya for distinguished service to Indonesia; Bintang Jasa Utama for outstanding contributions to development. Born in Garut, West Java, 1924. Address: Kompleks BPPB M-12, Ciomas, Bogor 16610, Indonesia.

R. P. Singh

R. P. Singh, director of the Central Research Institute for Dryland Agriculture (CRIDA). Educated in crop husbandry at R.B.S. College (M.Sc., 1949) and in agronomy at the Indian Agricultural Research Institute (Associate IARI, 1952; Ph.D., 1972). Served as program leader in farming systems research, International Crops Research Institute for the Semiarid Tropics (ICRISAT); assistant director general and project director of the All India Coordinated Research Project for Dryland Agriculture; chief scientist for dryland agricultural research, and head of Division of Solar Energy and Wind Power, Central Arid Zone Research Institute (CAZRI); and assistant professor of agronomy, Indian Agricultural Research Institute. Author of books, book chapters, and research papers, including: coeditor with James F. Parr and B.A. Stewart, *Dryland Agriculture: Strategies for Sustainability*, (forthcoming); with K.P.R. Vittal, "Managing Rainfed Sandy Soils for Higher Productivity," *Proceedings of 1989 CRIDA Conference* (forthcoming); with B.V. Ramana Rao, "Agricultural Drought Management in India: Principles and Practices," *ICAR/CRIDA Research Bulletin no. 1* (1988); with R. van den Beldt, "Alley Cropping in the Indian Semiarid Tropics," *Proceedings of IITA Conference* (1986). Editor of the *Indian Journal of Agronomy, Annals of Arid Zone*, and *Forage Research*. President, Indian Society of Agronomy and the Indian Society of Dryland Agricultural Research and Development. Consultant to the Food and Agriculture Organization. Born in Bulandshahr, Uttar Pradesh, 1930. Address: Central Research Institute for Dryland Agriculture, Santoshnagar, Saidabad P.O., Hyderabad 500 659, India.

Bruce Stone

Bruce Stone, project director and coordinator for Chinese research, and research fellow, International Food Policy Research Institute. Educated at the Woodrow Wilson School for Public and International Affairs, Princeton University; Nanyang University in Singapore; Hitotsubashi University in Tokyo; and at Cornell University. Recipient of a McConnell Foundation Fellowship; a Princeton-in-Asia Fellowship; and a Fulbright-Hays Fellowship. Oversees several research projects in the People's Republic of China, focusing on technological change in agriculture and on staple foodcrop production and its effects on rural and urban communities. Publications include: "Changing Patterns of Chinese Cereal Production Variability during the People's Republic Period," in Anderson and Hazell (eds.), *Variability in Cereal Yields and Implications for Agricultural Research and Policy* (1989); "Relative Foodgrain Prices in the People's Republic of China: Rural Taxation through Public Monopsony," in Mellor and Ahmed (eds.), *Food and Agricultural Price Policy in Developing Countries* (1988); "Developments in Technology," *The China Quarterly* (1988); editor, *Fertilizer Pricing Policy in Bangladesh* (1987); and coauthor, with Anthony Tang, of *Food Production in the People's Republic of China* (1980). Consultant to the World Bank and several United Nations Organizations. Born in Salt Lake City, Utah, 1948. Address: International Food Policy Research Institute, 1776 Massachusetts Avenue, N.W., Washington, D.C. 20036.

Alberto Valdés

Alberto Valdés, director, International Trade and Food Security Program, International Food Policy Research Institute (IFPRI). Educated at the Universidad Catolica de Chile, The University of Chicago (M.A., economics), and The London School of Economics (Ph.D., economics). Former dean and professor, Faculty of Agriculture, professor in the Institute of Economics, and head of Agricultural Economics Department, the Universidad Catolica de Chile. Served as an economist at the Centro Internacional de Agricultura Tropical, Cali, Colombia; and as visiting researcher at the Economic Commission for Latin America. Codirector of World Bank project, "Comparative Study of the Political Economy of Agricultural Pricing Policies in Developing Countries." Publications include: coeditor, with A.O. Krueger and M. Schiff, of *The Political Economy of Agricultural Pricing Policies: The Case of Latin America* (forthcoming); with Romeo M. Bautista, *Trade and Macroeconomic Policies' Impact on Agricultural Growth* (forthcoming); with P. Hazell and C. Pomareda, *Agricultural Risks and Insurance: Issues and Policies* (1985); coauthor, with Barbara Huddleston, D. Gale Johnson, and Shlomo Reutlinger, *International Finance for Food Security* (1984); editor, *Food Security for Developing Countries* (1981); and coeditor, with G.M. Scobie and J.L. Dillon, *Economics and the Design of Small Farmer Technology* (1978). Served as vice president for programs, International Association of Agricultural Economists. Consultant to international organizations and governments. Born in Santiago, Chile, 1935. Address: International Food Policy Research Institute, 1776 Massachusetts Avenue, N.W., Washington, D.C. 20036.

Anthony Wylie

Anthony Wylie, director general, Fundación Chile, Santiago, Chile. Fundación Chile is a private, nonprofit institution established in 1976 with the objective of diffusing proven technologies that utilize Chile's natural resources, improve and diversify productive capacity, and stimulate new business enterprises. The foundation operates in the areas of agribusiness, forestry, and marine resources, and has invested in projects both in Chile and in Latin American nations. Educated at the Universidad Catolica de Chile (Ingeniero Agronomo degree) and at the University of California at Davis (M.Sc., horticulture, and Ph.D., plant physiology, 1969). Former research director of the School of Agriculture and professor at the Universidad Catolica de Chile; and professor of postharvest physiology at the Universidad de Chile. Technical manager and general manager, the Cooperativa Agricola de Fruticultores de la Zona Central, Coofrucen Ltda, overseeing fruit growing, handling, and marketing. Former director, Food Technology Department, and deputy director general, Fundación Chile. Author of several articles and monographs, including: "Status of the Chilean Agroindustry," *Food Technology*, vol. 41, no. 9 (1987), and "Improving International Transfer of Technology," in *Malnutrition: Determinants and Consequences* (1984). Born in Valparaiso, Chile, 1941. Address: Fundación Chile, Av. Parque Antonio Rabat Sur 6165, Casilla 773, Santiago, Chile.

About the Editor

Neil G. Kotler is special assistant to the director, Office of Interdisciplinary Studies, Smithsonian Institution. He studied at Brandeis University, the University of Wisconsin, and The University of Chicago, where he received his Ph.D. in political science. For ten years he was a legislative assistant in the U.S. House of Representatives and was a staff member of the Subcommittee on the City, the House Banking Committee. He has written and edited articles and books, including *The History of Eritrea*, which was an outgrowth of his service as a Peace Corps volunteer in Asmara, Ethiopia. He is co-editor of *Completing the Food Chain: Strategies for Combating Hunger and Malnutrition* (Smithsonian Institution Press, 1989) and editor of *Social Marketing: Strategies for Changing Public Behavior*, authored by Philip Kotler and Eduardo L. Roberto (Free Press/Macmillan, 1989).

The International Rice Research Institute

One out of every three persons on earth depends on rice for more than half of his or her daily food. The International Rice Research Institute (IRRI) in Los Baños, the Philippines, is an autonomous, nonprofit agricultural research and training center whose goals are to alleviate hunger and malnourishment by applying science to agriculture and enabling resource-poor farmers to produce more rice from limited land. IRRI conducts research to increase total food production in rice-based farming systems. In the 1960s IRRI became the laboratory for developing high-yielding rice varieties that generated the Green Revolution in Asia.

Most of IRRI's research is undertaken in cooperation with national agricultural development programs and universities. Today, about 6,000 IRRI-trained scientists and rice specialists work as members of national rice research and development teams in Asia, Africa, and Latin America.

IRRI is one of 13 nonprofit international research and training centers supported by the Consultative Group on International Agricultural Research (CGIAR), a consortium of 50 donor nations, international and regional organizations, and private foundations, sponsored by the Food and Agriculture Organization of the United Nations, the World Bank, and the United Nations Development Programme.